W9-DDA-926

Intracoronary Ultrasound

This book is dedicated to my parents:
Ethel and Julius Mintz

Intracoronary Ultrasound

Gary S Mintz MD

Cardiovascular Research Foundation
New York, NY, USA

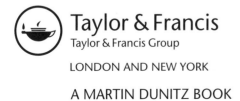

Taylor & Francis
Taylor & Francis Group

LONDON AND NEW YORK

A MARTIN DUNITZ BOOK

© 2005 Taylor & Francis, an imprint of the Taylor & Francis Group

First published in the United Kingdom in 2005
by Taylor & Francis,
an imprint of the Taylor & Francis Group,
2 Park Square, Milton Park
Abingdon, Oxon OX14 4RN, UK

Tel: +44 (0) 1235 828600
Fax: +44 (0) 1235 829000
Website: www.tandf.co.uk

All rights reserved. No part of this publication may be reproduced, stored in a retrieval system, or transmitted, in any form or by any means, electronic, mechanical, photocopying, recording, or otherwise, without the prior permission of the publisher or in accordance with the provisions of the Copyright, Designs and Patents Act 1988 or under the terms of any licence permitting limited copying issued by the Copyright Licensing Agency, 90 Tottenham Court Road, London W1P 0LP.

Although every effort has been made to ensure that all owners of copyright material have been acknowledged in this publication, we would be glad to acknowledge in subsequent reprints or editions any omissions brought to our attention.

British Library Cataloguing in Publication Data

Data available on application

Library of Congress Cataloging-in-Publication Data

Data available on application

ISBN 1-84184-047-5

Distributed in North and South America by

Taylor & Francis
2000 NW Corporate Blvd
Boca Raton, FL 33431, USA

Within Continental USA
Tel: 800 272 7737; Fax: 800 374 3401
Outside Continental USA
Tel: 561 994 0555; Fax: 561 361 6018
E-mail: orders@crcpress.com

Distributed in the rest of the world by
Thomson Publishing Services
Cheriton House
North Way
Andover, Hampshire SP10 5BE, UK
Tel: +44 (0) 1264 332424
E-mail: salesorder.tandf@thomsonpublishingservices.co.uk

Composition by Parthenon Publishing
Printed and bound by T.G. Hostench S.A., Spain

Contents

Preface

This text is the result of more than 10 years of experience with intravascular ultrasound (IVUS). It is intended to summarize both my own experiences as well as published and unpublished observations of others in the field.

This book should be read, not just used as a reference. While it is divided into chapters, there is a certain amount of overlap so that each chapter, more or less, presents a complete concept.

When appropriate, this text incorporates angiographic and pathologic data. In particular, pathologic observations are useful in filling in the gaps in our knowledge of coronary artery disease as assessed by IVUS alone. While IVUS is not equivalent to *in vivo* pathology, the two have more in common than, say, IVUS and angiography. The cases were collected during the evolution of coronary revascularization; the procedures performed and the decisions made are presented for the sake of completeness, not as a textbook of decision making.

Interventional cardiology is at a crossroads with the advent of drug-eluting stents (DES). DES has the potential to revolutionize and dominate interventional cardiology, but there is currently little information on the clinical utility of IVUS with DES. Most of the information regarding IVUS was accumulated in the pre-DES era. Therefore, this is an opportunity to summarize the field as it exists today.

One major limitation of any IVUS text is that published images are static while the actual IVUS studies are dynamic and moving. This is unavoidable. Nevertheless, a major effort went into selecting and presenting figures for their illustrative value. In most cases, each IVUS figure includes a linear sequence of equidistantly spaced image slices that illustrates the full-length morphology of the lesion and/or the pullback of the transducer through the lesion. This is clearly indicated at the bottom (or occasionally, top) of the figure. Unless otherwise stated, proximal is on the left and distal is on the right. When labeling is complicated or when it would obscure the details of the IVUS image, I have occasionally included both unlabeled and labeled versions of each figure. I have also occasionally included enlarged, labeled versions of angiograms of complex lesions to show the axial location of each IVUS image slice. I have tried to include an example of every situation, but clearly some have been missed.

Almost all of the images came from s-VHS video tape. The resolution of video is 72 lines/inch. Nevertheless, an attempt has been made to maximize the quality of the images. The tapes were played on a Sony SVO-9500MD video playback device that has a built-in digital memory so that both interlacing fields were "grabbed". The frozen signal (representing both interlacing fields) was then imported into Photoshop using a Targa 2000 card and a Macintosh computer. The individual frames were then cropped, and the composites were created. The IVUS images were not otherwise enhanced, so they are as close to the real image as possible – artifacts and all. Unless otherwise stated, the images are all presented using the same scale; big arteries look big, and small arteries look small.

I am often asked how to learn image interpretation. The answer is a lot like the old joke: "How do you get to Carnegie Hall? Practice!" The British philosopher Michael Oakeshott distinguished between technical and practical knowledge. Technical knowledge can be put into words and written down in books – like this one. Practical knowledge comes from experience. It is acquired by doing and by entering into the intrinsic pattern of an activity. To this end, there is no substitute for doing cases and looking at images. However, it is difficult to learn image interpretation while also performing an intervention. One good idea is to spend time with someone who does a lot of IVUS imaging and who can explain the images and their clinical utility during the procedures. A second idea is to look at each study again and again, in a quiet room with subdued lighting, sometimes even days or weeks apart. As you gain experience, you will see new details in the image and wonder how you missed these findings in the past. A third idea is to compare pre- versus post-intervention IVUS studies and look to see how the vessel has changed. Fourth, look at the image in pieces rather than as a whole. Identify the lumen, trace the adventitia, look at the plaque, follow the course of branches, and so on. Then put the image back together. In effect, you train your own eye. Finally, make an effort to understand the biology of coronary artery disease and intervention, relate the IVUS images to the angiogram, and recognize that there are only a finite number of possibilities when interpreting an image.

Many people helped me with this project directly or indirectly. I am listing them alphabetically: Alexander Abizaid, Andrea Abizaid, Javed Ahmed, Stephane Carlier, Marco Castagna, Michael Collins, Ricardo Costa, George Dangas, Esteban Escolar, Kenichi Fujii, Rainer Hoffmann, Myeong-Ki Hong, Kenneth Kent, Sang-Wook Kim, Jun-ichi Kotani, Yoshio Kobayashi, Ed Krebs, John Laird, Alexandra Lansky, Martin Leon, Roxana Mehran, Jeffrey Moses, Issam Moussa, Augusto Pichard, Jeffrey Popma, Lowell Satler, Gregg Stone, Satoru Sumitsuji, Hideo Takebayashi, Ron Waksman, Neil Weissman, and Takenori Yasuda. However, I would especially like to thank Akiko Maehara for her help with so many of the illustrations in this text. If I have forgotten someone, *mea culpa* – I apologize profusely.

Gary S Mintz

1
Basics

It is not necessary to understand ultrasound physics – even as it applies to IVUS imaging – in order to make good clinical use of IVUS information. In fact, most of this chapter can be skipped entirely. Its two most important parts are (1) understanding the basic imaging controls and the fact that only minimal "tweaking" of these controls is usually best and (2) recognition of artifacts and how they affect image interpretation and utility of the information.

TECHNOLOGIES

The first true IVUS system was designed by Bom and his associates in Rotterdam in 1971;[1,2] it was conceived as an improved technique for visualizing cardiac chambers and valves. The first transluminal images of human arteries were recorded by Yock and his associates in 1988.[3] Currently, there are two basic technical approaches to catheter-based ultrasound imaging: solid state and mechanical. There are advantages, disadvantages, and qualitative differences in image presentation with the mechanical versus the solid-state approach; however, current commercially available systems produce sufficient image quality, measurement accuracy, and catheter handling to be useful in almost any clinical setting.[4] That said, it is also now evident that there are measurement differences among the systems – even among different mechanical systems or among different catheters that interface with the same system.[5, 6] While these differences are not large enough to influence clinical decisions, they may be important in performing and interpreting serial studies. Therefore, when performing serial IVUS studies for assessment of progression/regression, restenosis, or transplant vasculopathy, only one system and catheter should be specified or the same equipment should be used for both index and follow-up studies in each individual patient.[7]

Solid-state technology

With solid-state technology, a cylindrical array of transducer elements is mounted on the tip of the catheter. By sequentially firing the multi-element array, a beam is created in a 360° arc to produce the tomographic image. The array can be programmed so that one set of elements transmits while a second set receives simultaneously. The coordinated beam generated by groups of elements is known as a synthetic aperture array. The image can be manipulated to focus optimally at a broad range of depths. The currently available electronic system provides simultaneous colorization of blood flow. As with all electronic ultrasound systems (including transcutaneous ultrasound or echocardiography), artifacts and imaging are especially problematic immediately adjacent to the transducer. Near-field ring-down subtraction is necessary prior to imaging. The catheter is a long monorail design. The entire catheter, not just the transducer, must be advanced or withdrawn to image the vessel.

Mechanical scanners

With mechanical technology, a single-element transducer is located within the tip of a polyethylene imaging catheter or sheath; using a flexible drive shaft, the transducer is then rotated "mechanically" to create the tomographic image. At approximately 1° increments, the transducer sends and receives ultrasound signals to provide 256 individual radial scan lines for each image. Mechanical transducer catheters require flushing with saline to provide a fluid pathway for the ultrasound beam; even small air bubbles can degrade image quality (high-frequency ultrasound does not transmit through air). Once the lesion is crossed with the stationary protective sheath, the transducer spins and is moved proximally and distally within the sheath to perform the imaging sequence. This facilitates smooth and uniform mechanical pullback to image the entire vessel. (An alternative approach to mechanical IVUS imaging is to attach the transducer to a micromotor and to position this assembly at the tip of the catheter, thereby eliminating the drive shaft. This variation of the mechanical technology is not currently in use.) The most commonly used catheter is a short-monorail design, although there is a design variation in which a long distal monorail can alternatively house the guidewire or the transducer, but not both; and there is a 16-cm long monorail design in development.

IMAGING PHYSICS

Ultrasound waves have a frequency > 20 000 cycles per second (i.e. above the audible range). For medical diagnostic purposes, ultrasound frequencies in the range of millions of cycles per second (megahertz = MHz) are used. The velocity at which sound travels through human soft tissue is fairly constant at approximately 1540 m/s. IVUS quantification should not require routine *calibration*. The accuracy of the measurements depends on the incorporation of the correct offset (which corrects for transducer, catheter, and sheath design) and estimated average speed of sound in blood and tissue into the scan-converting algorithm. However, correct system calibration should not be taken for granted.

Transducers are devices that convert one type of energy into another; IVUS transducers convert electrical energy into ultrasound energy and ultrasound energy back into electrical energy. An electrical impulse causes the transducer to emit an ultrasound pulse; afterwards, the transducer remains silent to detect reflected (or *backscattered*) ultrasound. Assuming that ultrasound travels through all tissues at a fixed speed, the time that it takes for the transmitted ultrasound impulse to be backscattered and returned to the transducer is a measure of distance. The intensity of the backscattered signal depends on a number of factors. These include (but are not limited to):

(1)   The intensity of the transmitted signal;
(2)   The attenuation (reduction) of the signal as it passes through tissue (all tissue attenuates ultrasound energy);
(3)   The distance from the transducer to the target (intensity is inversely related to distance);
(4)   The angle of the signal relative to the target (the closer the angle is to 90°, the more intense is the reflected signal);[8,9] and
(5)   The density (or reflectivity) of the tissue (which determines how much ultrasound energy passes through the tissue and how much is backscattered).

These factors affect not only the overall appearance of an image, but also the relative appearance of different sectors of the image throughout its 360° circumference. The reflected ultrasound is converted back into an electrical signal, and the reconverted electrical signal is sent to the ultrasound system to generate the planar image.

Echogenicity is the tendency of tissue to reflect ultrasound – the higher the echogenicity, the brighter the tissue appearance. The IVUS gray scale image is derived from the *amplitude* of the reflected signal, not its *radiofrequency* signature. Thus, much of the information in the reflected signal is not used. There is renewed interest in radiofrequency signal analysis for the purposes of tissue characterization. Frequency-domain analysis may allow detailed assessment of plaque composition.[10]

Current imaging techniques assume that vessels are circular, that the catheter is located in the center of the artery, and that the transducer is parallel to the long axis of the vessel. However, both transducer obliquity and vessel curvature can produce an image that incorrectly suggests that the vessel is elliptical. Transducer obliquity may be more of an issue in large vessels imaged with small catheters; it can result in an overestimation of dimensions and a reduction in image quality. However, in routine clinical coronary imaging, this error is relatively small.[11] Importantly, it is not possible to underestimate dimensions.

Resolution is the ability to discriminate two closely adjacent objects. Ultrasound cannot reliably detect or measure a structure that is smaller than the resolution of the device or differentiate between structures that are closer than the resolution of the device. Resolution affects the sharpness of an image, the distinctness of the borders, and, therefore, the reproducibility of the IVUS measurements. Because IVUS creates images in three-dimensional space, there are three spatial resolutions in each image slice: (1) axial resolution (the ability to discriminate two closely adjacent objects located along the axis of the ultrasound beam); (2) lateral resolution (the ability to discriminate two closely adjacent objects located along the length of the ultrasound catheter); and (3) angular or circumferential resolution (the ability to discriminate two closely adjacent objects located along the circumferential sweep of the ultrasound beam as it generates a planar image). These are listed here in order of the superiority of their resolution and are shown schematically in Figure 1.1. Axial resolution is typically 80–120 µm, and lateral resolution is typically 200–250 µm. Circumferential resolution is highly dependent on imaging artifacts such as NURD (non-uniform rotational distortion) and has not been quantified. Frequency is the number of sound cycles in a given time period, typically one second; wavelength is inversely related to frequency. Ultrasound waves with higher frequency (shorter wavelengths) are reflected from smaller objects. A higher-frequency beam has greater resolution; however, because a larger percentage of higher-frequency ultrasound is reflected, penetration decreases. In general, the higher the frequency, the greater is the resolution; and for a given frequency, the larger the size of the transducer aperture, the better the resolution. (The aperture is the face of the transducer that emits and/or receives ultrasound waves. Resolution and near-field depth are related to aperture size; with increasing aperture size, the near field is longer, thereby improving the overall axial resolution.) Focusing the transducer also improves resolution within the focused zone; however, the beam then diverges beyond the focal zone, and resolution suffers. Because ultrasound beams diverge, the optimal resolution is in the near field, closer to the transducer. The length of the near field is expressed by the equation $L = r^2/\lambda$, where L is the length of the near field, r is the radius of the transducer, and λ is the wavelength. Resolution suffers in the far field – particularly circumferential resolution. From a clinical standpoint, this causes far field structures to appear less distinct, their borders less clear, and the interpretation less certain. (See the examples of coronary aneurysms in Chapter 6.)

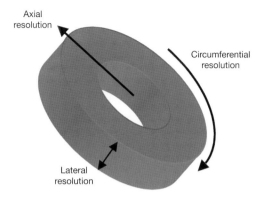

Figure 1.1 The three IVUS resolutions are shown: axial, lateral, and circumferential. Axial resolution – which is the best of the three resolutions – is along the beam of the IVUS transducer: hence the term axial. Lateral resolution is along the longitudinal axis of the artery and is determined by the width of the IVUS beam; it refers to the resolution of a single image slice and not to the accuracy of transducer pullback and length measurements. The third resolution – which, in truth, does not have a name, but which is termed here "circumferential" resolution – is along the sweep of the IVUS image. It is dramatically affected by NURD in mechanical systems

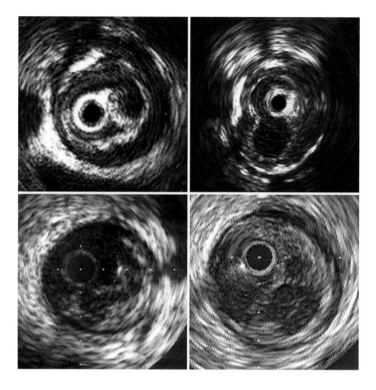

Figure 1.2 The top two examples have a poor dynamic range – the images are mostly black and white with few shades of gray. The bottom two examples have a wider dynamic range – i.e. more shades of gray

Penetration depends on a number of factors including the power output of the transducer (which is in part related to transducer design and aperture) and imaging frequency. Penetration is inversely related to frequency – the higher the frequency, the less the penetration. Larger transducers with lower frequencies are used for examination of large vessels because they create a deeper near field and have greater penetration.

Dynamic range is the number of gray scales that can be differentiated between the weakest and the strongest targets. It is usually expressed in decibels (dB). The dynamic range for IVUS is typically 17–55 dB. The greater the dynamic range, the broader the range of reflected signals (from weakest to strongest) that can be detected, displayed, and differentiated, and the greater the number shades of gray that are used to display the image. Therefore, the number of gray-scale levels is a measure of the dynamic range; and a large or broad dynamic range is a favorable image characteristic. An image with a wide dynamic range has many shades of gray. An image with a poor dynamic range has an exaggerated contrast and is mostly black and white. While a contrasty image may appear to be easier to interpret because borders are more distinct, in reality details are lost. Some systems have a variety of gray-scale curves – also called gamma curves – that can be selected depending on

operator preference. These control the relationship between the actual and the displayed gray scale, and are used primarily to present a more pleasing image. However, they also affect dynamic range and qualitative and quantitative characteristics and, if they are used excessively, may result in measurement inaccuracies. Dynamic range is also called *contrast resolution*. Examples are shown in Figure 1.2.

IMAGING ARTIFACTS

The recognition of imaging artifacts is critical in order to avoid image misinterpretation.

Ring-down refers to disorganization of the image closest to the face of the transducer or the surface of the catheter. Ring-down artifacts are usually observed as bright haloes of variable thickness surrounding the catheter that obscure the area immediately adjacent to the catheter. Ring-down artifacts are present in all medical ultrasound devices and create a zone of uncertainty adjacent to the transducer surface. Ring-down can be minimized by optimal transducer and/or sheath design, but suppression of ring-down using system controls can also eliminate tissue in the near field. Electronic-array systems tend to have more ring-down; therefore, ring-down is partially reduced by digital subtraction of a reference mask as well as by blanking out the extreme near field. However, this ring-down subtraction does not remain stable; and it should be repeated if IVUS is again performed later in the procedure. Otherwise, near-field artifacts can appear in the image. The steps that are used to reduce near-field ring-down can limit the ability of electronic array systems to image right up to the surface of the catheter. An unusual type of near-field artifact is shown in Figure 1.3.

NURD is an artifact unique to mechanical IVUS imaging systems; it stands for *non-uniform rotational distortion*. For optimal imaging, there must be a constant rotational velocity of the mechanical transducer. NURD is the consequence of asymmetric friction (or drag) along any part of the drive-shaft mechanism, causing the transducer to lag during one part of its rotation and whip through the other part of its 360° course, resulting in geometric distortion or smearing of the image (Figures 1.4 and 1.5). NURD affects angular (circumferential) resolution, precludes accurate cross-sectional measurements, and, for example, can distort the geometry of an implanted stent. NURD can occur for a number of reasons, including the presence of acute bends in the artery, tortuous guiding catheter shapes, variance in manufacturing of the hub or driveshaft, excessive tightening of a hemostatic valve, kinking of the imaging sheath, or an excessive small guide-catheter lumen. In an extreme situation, fracture of the drive cable can occur because of this friction. (Of interest, because there was no drive shaft, NURD was not seen with micromotor technology in which the motor was at the tip of the ultrasound catheter to rotate the transducer without a drive shaft.) A distinct motion artifact can result from an unstable catheter position. The vessel moves before a complete circumferential image can be created. This results in cyclic deformation of the image (Figure 1.6). Recognizing NURD is particularly important when quantifying information from mechanical IVUS imaging systems.[12]

Both mechanical and solid-state transducers can move as much as 5 mm longitudinally between diastole and systole.[13] This can preclude accurate assessment of arterial phenomena that depend on comparing systolic and diastolic images (i.e. arterial pulsation and compliance).

Side lobes are extraneous beams of ultrasound that are generated from the edges of the individual transducer elements (Figure 1.7). They follow the circumferential sweep of the beam. Side lobes are most prominent when imaging stents or other superstrong reflectors (e.g. calcium) and are also caused, in part, by high-gain settings. Side lobes may obscure the true lumen and stent borders,

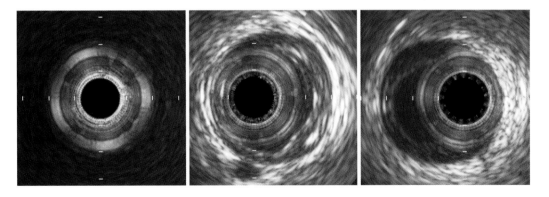

Figure 1.3 This exaggerated and unusual near-field artifact in an electronic-array system image was caused by an air gap between the PZT bond and the flex circuit

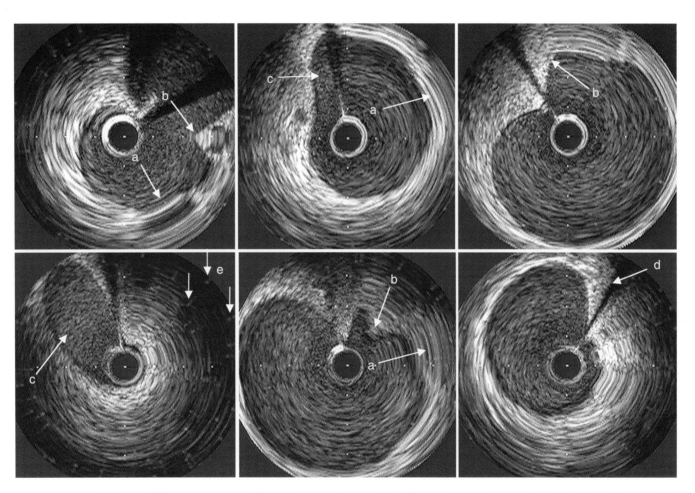

Figure 1.4 Six panels illustrate different appearances of NURD – non-uniform rotational distortion. NURD occurs only with mechanical systems. Part of the image is expanded in its circumferential sweep, and part is compressed. The image can appear smeared (a), lumpy (b), or very elliptical (c). Note how the guidewire artifact is also compressed (d). In addition, note the radiofrequency noise – the bursts of white dots – indicated by the white arrows (e).

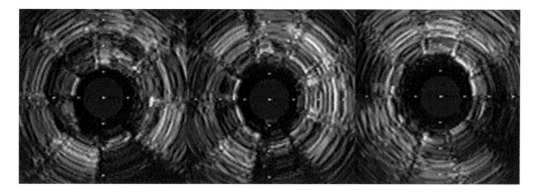

Figure 1.5 Another appearance of NURD; this pattern suggests an overly tight hemostatic valve

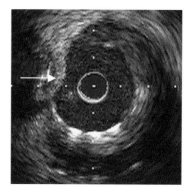

Figure 1.6 Deformation of the image (white arrow) was caused by a rapid, sharp motion of the catheter relative to the vessel before there was a complete 360° mechanical rotation of the transducer

interfere with area measurements, and affect the assessment of stent apposition, etc. In particular, it is especially important that side lobes from calcium should not be confused with intimal flaps of a dissection plane.

Reverberations are artifacts caused by secondary, false echoes of the same structure. They lie along the axial path of the ultrasound beam as it penetrates tissue. This gives the false impression of a second interface at multiples of the distance from the transducer to the first structure (Figure 1.8). Reverberations are more common from strong echoreflectors such as calcium, stent metal, guiding catheters, and guidewires.

Another type of stent artifacts are *"ghosts"* within the lumen (Figure 1.9).

IVUS is exquisitely sensitive to ambient radiofrequency *noise* or another ultrasound signal. This can appear as alternating spokes or random white dots within the image (Figures 1.4 and 1.10). Increasing overall gain will increase the brightness of any noise in the image.

While technically not an artifact, the guiding catheter can be mistaken for circumferential calcium at the aorto-ostial junction (Figures 1.11 and 1.12).

With short-monorail catheters, the guidewire appears in the image. The appearance and strength of the guidewire artifact depends on the motion of the IVUS catheter relative to the guidewire, the distance and spatial orientation between the transducer and the guidewire, and the composition of the guidewire and its tip (Figures 1.13–1.16). It is particularly important not to confuse the guidewire artifact with a stent strut because both are metallic reflectors. Guidewire artifacts can, at times, mask a significant part of the image. During bifurcation intervention, two guidewire artifacts are seen when using a short-monorail imaging catheter. Long-monorail catheters do not produce a

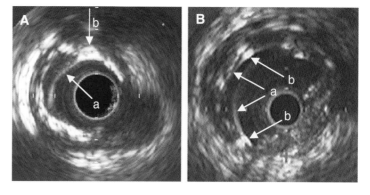

Figure 1.7 Side lobes (a) are intense reflections from the edges of strong echoreflectors – i.e. from calcium (b in Panel A) or stent metal (c in Panel B). Side lobes follow the circumferential sweep of the IVUS image, whether that sweep is created mechanically or electronically. In particular, it is important not to confuse side lobes with the flap of a dissection (Panel A); this confusion is more of an issue in non-stented arteries

guidewire artifact, except during bifurcation intervention, when a second guidewire is used and a single guidewire artifact is seen.

Even small air bubbles can degrade image quality. They can cause either a weak image (Figure 1.17) or a variety of artifacts (Figures 1.3 and 1.18–1.20). These are problems only with mechanical systems. Recent improvements in transducer housing design have made it more difficult to trap air bubbles.

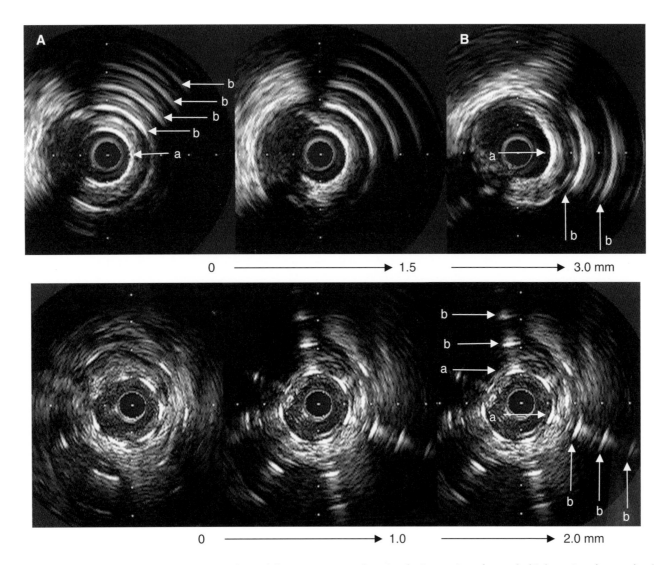

Figure 1.8 Reverberations are false, repetitive echoes of the same structure that give the impression of second, third, etc. interfaces at fixed-multiple distances from the transducer. In both examples, true structures are indicated by the arrows a; and the false structures (reverberations) are indicated by the arrows b. The reverberations follow the same contours as the true structures. The top example shows reverberations from calcium. In this example, the "true" calcium is closer to the transducer in Panel A compared with Panel B; this leads to more reverberations that are closer together in Panel A compared with Panel B. (Note that these strong, multiple reverberations are seen mostly after rotational atherectomy.) The bottom example shows reverberations from stent struts. Reverberations are analogous to looking in one mirror with another mirror behind you. Other examples of reverberations can be seen in Figure 1.12 (from guiding catheters), Figures 1.14 and 1.15 (from guidewires), and Figure 1.19 (from an air bubble)

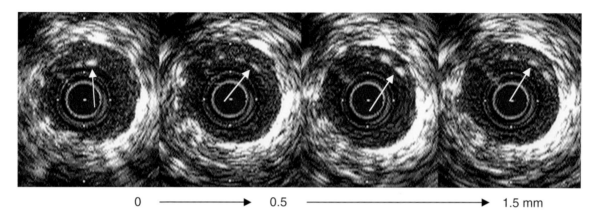

0 ⟶ 0.5 ⟶ 1.5 mm

Figure 1.9 Stent "ghosts" (white arrows) are reflections from stent metal on the opposite side from the true structure

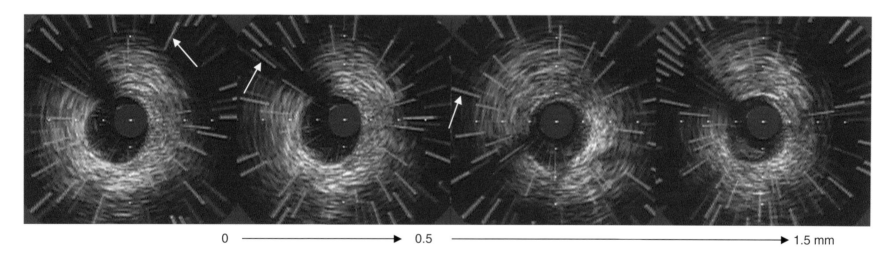

0 ⟶ 0.5 ⟶ 1.5 mm

Figure 1.10 Intense interference radiating from the center of the IVUS catheter (white arrows) is caused, in this case, by simultaneous activation of the Doppler FloWire

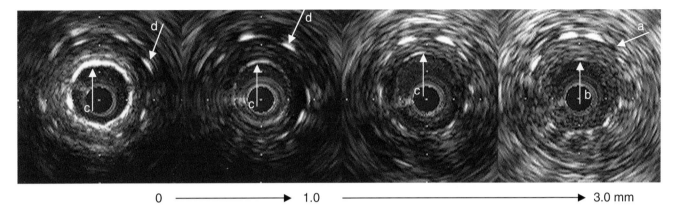

0 ————————➤ 1.0 ————————————————➤ 3.0 mm

Figure 1.11 In this example, the guiding catheter was deeply intubated into an ostial in-stent restenosis lesion. Note the stent (a), the intimal hyperplasia (b), and the guiding catheter (c). The stent (d) can be seen through the guiding catheter, as shown in this example, although its brightness is attenuated. Like calcium and metal, the material of the guiding catheter is intensely echogenic. Therefore, the deeper arterial structures are seen poorly because of attenuation and reflection of the ultrasound beam by the guide. Sometimes, there is complete shadowing caused by the guide. When imaging an aorto-ostial lesion, it is important to disengage the guiding catheter; otherwise, the guiding catheter can be mistaken for a calcified or fibrotic lesion with a minimum lumen diameter equal to the interior diameter (ID) of the catheter as shown in this example

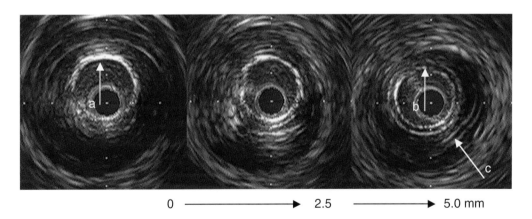

0 ————————➤ 2.5 ————————➤ 5.0 mm

Figure 1.12 Similar to Figure 1.11, the guiding catheter is also deeply intubated into this lesion to mimic anostial stenosis. However, in this case, the guiding catheter variably appears as a single-walled (a) or double-walled (b) structure. As in Figure 1.11, the deeper arterial structures are seen poorly because of attenuation and reflection of the ultrasound beam by the guide. Also notice the reverberations from the guiding catheter (c). Reverberations are secondary echoes – most often from an intensely reflective structure – that are produced at mathematically precise distances (in this case, double the distance) from the surface of the transducer to the structure

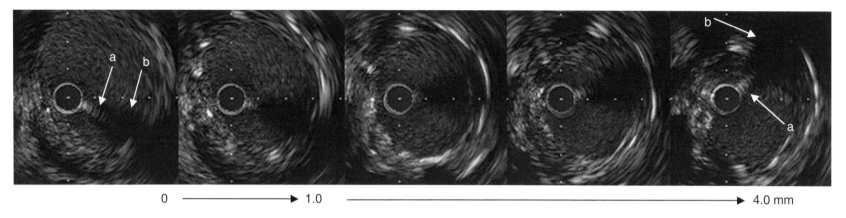

Figure 1.13 Guidewire artifact (a) with shadowing (b). Note that the guidewire appearance and location change during pullback. Guidewire artifacts are seen only with short-monorail IVUS catheters unless there is a second guidewire in the lumen

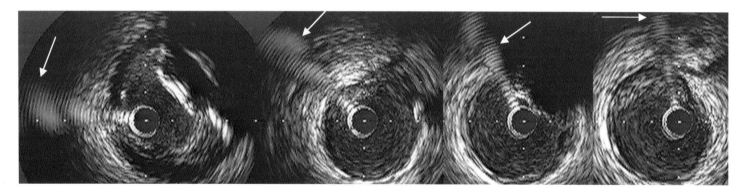

Figure 1.14 Note how the appearance and location of the guidewire (white arrows) changes during pullback. Guidewire artifacts are seen only with short-monorail IVUS catheters unless there is a second guidewire in the lumen. Unlike the guidewire in Figure 1.13, this guidewire produces many reverberations

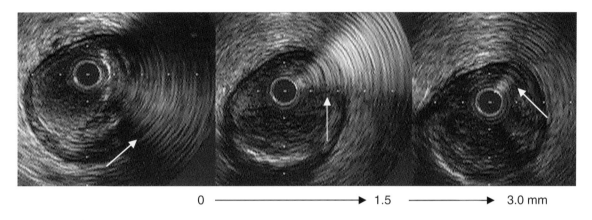

0 ——————————▶ 1.5 ——————▶ 3.0 mm

Figure 1.15 Although uncommon, the guidewire (white arrows) can obscure a significant percentage of the artery (see, in particular, the left-hand panel) as shown in this example. Guidewire artifacts are seen only with short-monorail IVUS catheters unless there is a second guidewire in the lumen

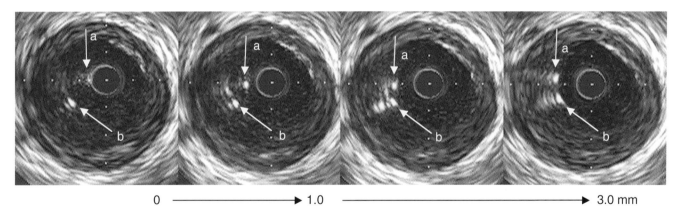

0 ——————————▶ 1.0 ————————————▶ 3.0 mm

Figure 1.16 With a short-monorail catheter, two guidewires (a and b) can be seen in the lumen of the proximal vessel when treating a bifurcation lesion and both branches are wired. Two guidewire artifacts are seen only with short-monorail IVUS catheters; with long-monorail catheters, only one guidewire artifact (the non-IVUS guidewire) is seen

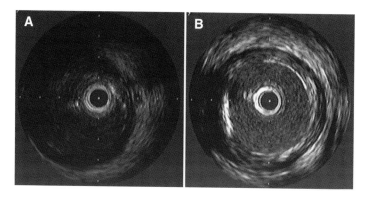

Figure 1.17 An air bubble is the most common cause of a weak image when using a mechanical scanner, and the most common manifestation of an air bubble is a weak image (Panel A). Flushing the catheter will expel the bubble and improve the image (Panel B). If the catheter contains a large amount of air, it is probably safer to remove and re-prep the catheter to avoid air embolization

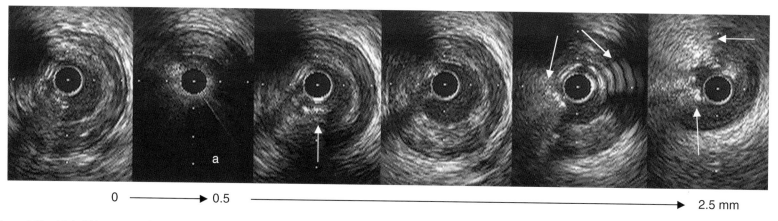

Figure 1.18 Air bubbles can produce a variety of image artifacts (white arrows), including total loss of image (a)

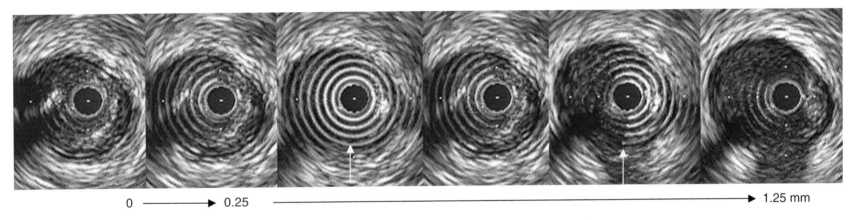

0 ⟶ 0.25 ⟶ 1.25 mm

Figure 1.19   In this example, a small air bubble produced a concentric circle artifact with multiple reverberations (white arrows)

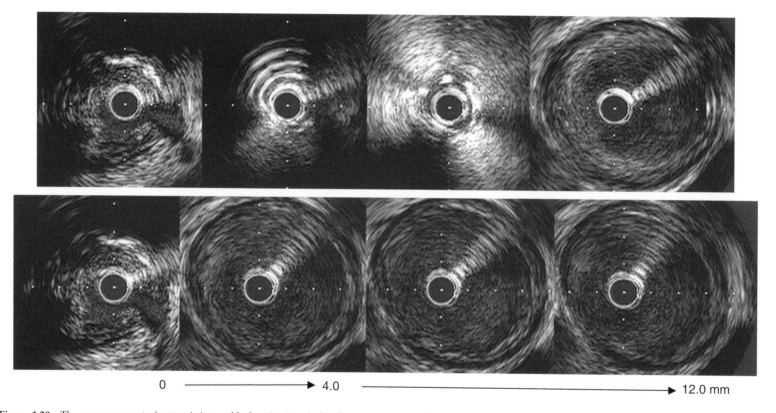

0 ——————————→ 4.0 ————————————————→ 12.0 mm

Figure 1.20 The same segment of artery is imaged before (top) and after (bottom) aggressively flushing the catheter to expel an air bubble

IMAGING CONTROLS

Appropriate use of system controls can improve an image, while misuse of the available controls can degrade an image. Other than the overall gain and zoom (or depth) settings, tweaking of these controls should be kept to a minimum. (The only exception is near-field subtraction with current solid-state systems.) In most cases, it is merely necessary to verify that the image is acceptable. In general, system settings should allow blood speckle to be visualized in the lumen. Because blood speckle is lower in reflectivity compared with tissue, seeing blood speckle means that it is less likely that near-field tissue will be blanked out. Some of these controls and their functions are as follows.

Increasing overall *gain* increases overall image brightness. Overall gain that is set too low limits the detection of low-amplitude signals. Overall gain that is set too high compresses the gray scale (narrowing the dynamic range and reducing the number of shades of gray) and causes all tissue to appear overly bright or echoreflective. Overall gain is useful in correcting for a transducer with low power output and in imaging a very large vessel with poor penetration. However, if the transducer is very weak, it is probably better to just get a new catheter and send the weak one back to the manufacturer.

The *TGC* (*time–gain compensation*) curve amplifies parts of the reflected signal and adjusts the image brightness at fixed distances from the catheter. The term TGC is derived from the fact that distance is measured as function of time – the time that it takes for the signal to be reflected back to the transducer. (A better term might be depth or distance–gain compensation.) Incorrect setting of the TGC curve can introduce significant artifacts into the images. For example, excessive reduction in near-field intensity (in an attempt to reduce blood speckle, ring-down, or other near-field artifacts) can also blank out tissue – notably echolucent tissue – and artificially produce a lumen. This is particularly important in assessing in-stent restenosis, since neointimal tissue is poorly echoreflective (Figure 1.21). If blood speckle can be seen in the lumen, it is less likely that near-field tissue will be blanked out. Slightly increasing the far-field intensity is useful in imaging large vessels. However, the best TGC curves are relatively flat. Certainly, there should be no abrupt changes in the TGC curve – i.e. in the intensity or amplification between adjacent parts of the TCG curve.

Reject eliminates low-amplitude signals; it is one way of removing noise from an image. However, when low-amplitude signals are eliminated, the dynamic range is truncated at its lower level, and echolucent tissue can be missed.

Compression regulates the dynamic compression and affects gray scale and overall gain to optimize differentiation between types of tissue. In general, the higher the compression setting, the more black and white the image.

Zoom or *depth* or *scale* adjusts the depth of the outer boundary of the image. It should be set so that the entire external elastic membrane is on the screen throughout the length of the vessel.

IMAGE PRESENTATION

There is no absolute (anterior versus posterior, left versus right) *rotational* orientation of the image. Instead, side branches are useful markers during clinical IVUS imaging, and the image is described as if viewing the face of a clock. Some authors also describe the use of perivascular landmarks as important references for both axial position and tomographic orientation within the vessel. These landmarks include the pericardium, muscle tissue, and the venous system. With some systems, images can be rotated electronically to produce a consistent orientation as an electronic aid to interpretation. It is theoretically possible to place an external ultrasound emitter that would create a fixed spatial reference by appearing as a "blip" on the IVUS image. It is also possible to track the transducer in three-dimensional space using a magnetic positioning sensor mounted on the transducer and an external reference; such a system is in current development.

An important limitation of "conventional" IVUS is that only single cross-sectional images of the coronary artery are displayed at any one time. Motorized transducer pullback and digital storage of cross-sectional images can be used to create longitudinal (L-mode, long-view, or longitudinal view) images. These images are typically displayed relative to the center of the transducer – rather than relative to the center of the artery. Longitudinal representation of IVUS images is useful for length measurements, for interpolation of shadowed deep arterial structures (such as the external elastic membrane behind calcium or stent metal), and for quickly identifying the minimal lumen area and reference segments of the vessel. However, lumen dimensions must still be measured from the appropriate cross-sectional image slices. There are major current limitations of L-mode display, including the obligate straight reconstruction of the artery, the ability to display only a single arbitrary cut plane, and catheter motion artifacts resulting in a "sawtooth" appearance because of movement of the transducer relative to the artery (Figure 1.22). True three-dimensional reconstruction or presentation of the longitudinal information is possible using a combination of angiography and IVUS or by tracking the path of the transducer in three dimensions using magnetic positioning technology.[14,15]

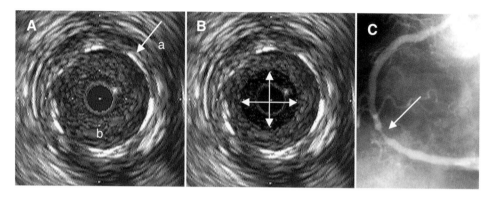

Figure 1.21 This patient presented with in-stent restenosis. In Panel A, acquired with correct TCG (time–gain compensation settings), note the stent a and the intimal hyperplasia b; intimal hyperplasia is packed around the IVUS catheter. Incorrect TGC curve settings in Panel B suppressed the neointimal tissue and created the false appearance of an adequate lumen measuring 2.3 mm × 2.3 mm (double-headed white arrows). Clues to this technical error are the following. (1) The lumen is perfectly circular, and the IVUS catheter is exactly in the center. This is because the tissue is suppressed for a specific distance from the surface of the transducer. (2) The in-stent restenosis lesion appears much less severe on the IVUS image than on the angiogram (white arrow in Panel C). (3) Blood speckle is not evident in the lumen; blood speckle is usually, but not always, less echogenic than neointimal tissue and is more easily suppressed. Correct TCG settings should not suppress blood speckle. A similar appearing loss of near-field tissue can also happen with electronic array systems, but for a different reason. In order to clean-up the near field, the electronic array systems impose a near-field blanking zone of approximately 2 mm; therefore, it is not possible to image down to the catheter, and the most central 2 mm × 2 mm area appears black and tissue-free

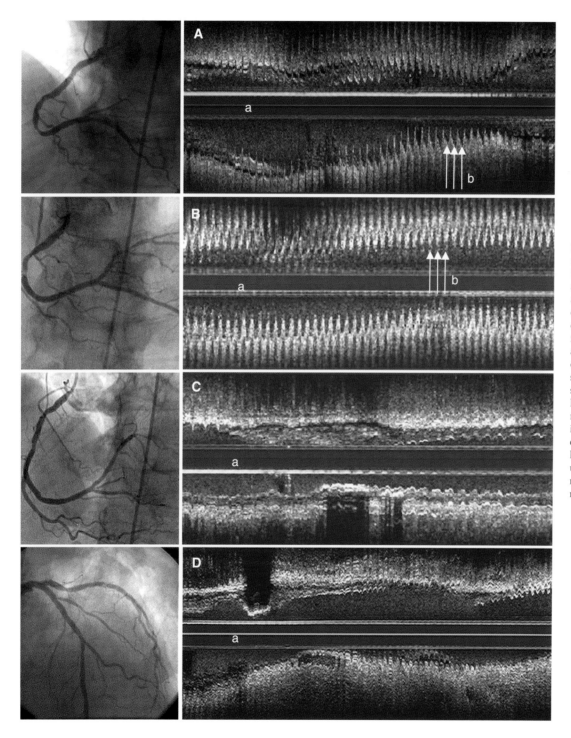

Figure 1.22 Four examples of longitudinal image reconstruction (or L-mode) are shown. The cross-sections are stacked relative to the path of the transducer (a), whose course is assumed to be in a straight line. Therefore, almost all curvature in the vessel is removed, and the vessel almost always appears as if it were a straight segment. In the top example (A), there is excessive motion of the transducer relative to the artery, causing a zigzag or sawtooth appearance (b). This is usually more of a problem with the right and circumflex arteries – because of their anterior and posterior atrioventricular groove courses, respectively – than with the left anterior descending (bottom example, D). The atrioventricular grooves move significantly between systole and diastole. Examples A and B are not suitable for analysis. Examples C and D, however, are analyzable. Other limitations to this display technique are that (1) the images are displayed relative to the IVUS catheter that is assumed to be the centerpoint of the image and (2) only one longitudinal reconstruction is usually seen at any one time. Accurate tomographic measurements – such as the minimum lumen area – are not possible; these measurements should always be made using the cross-sectional images. Nevertheless, this technique is useful in rapidly identifying the minimum lumen site and the proximal and distal references and in making length measurements

REFERENCES

1. Bom N, Lancee CT, van Egmond FC. An ultrasonic intracardiac scanner. Ultrasonics 1972; 10: 71–6

2. Bom N, ten Hoff H, Lancee CT, et al. Early and recent intraluminal ultrasound devices. Int J Card Imaging 1989; 4: 79–88

3. Yock PG, Johnson EL, Linker DT. Intravascular ultrasound: development and clinical potential. Am J Card Imag 1988; 2: 185–93

4. Fort S, Freeman NA, Johnston P, et al. In vitro and in vivo comparison of three different intravascular ultrasound catheter designs. Catheter Cardiovasc Interv 2001; 52: 382–92

5. Schoenhagen P, Sapp SK, Tuzcu EM, et al. Variability of area measurements obtained with different intravascular ultrasound catheter systems: impact on clinical trials and a method for accurate callibration. J Am Soc Echocardiogr 2003; 16: 277–84

6. Tardif JC, Bertrand OF, Mongrain R, et al. Reliability of mechanical and phased-array designs for serial intravascular ultrasound examinations – animal and clinical studies in stented and non-stented coronary arteries. Int J Card Imaging 2000; 16: 365–75

7. von Birgelen C, Hartmann M, Mintz GS, et al. Relation between progression and regression of atherosclerotic left main coronary artery disease and serum cholesterol levels as assessed with serial long-term ($\geq$ 12 months) follow-up intravascular ultrasound. Circulation 2003; 108: 2757–62

8. Picano E, Landini L, Distante A, et al. Angle dependence of ultrasounic backscatter in arterial tissues: a study in vitro. Circulation 1985; 72: 572–6.

9. DiMario C, Madretsma S, Linker D, et al. The angle of incidence of the ultrasonic beam: a critical factor for the image quality in intravascular ultrasonography. Am Heart J 1993; 125: 442–8

10. Nair A, Kuban BD, Tuzcu EM, et al. Coronary plaque classification with intravascular ultrasound radio-frequency data analysis. Circulation 2002; 2200–6

11. Stahr P, Voigtlander T, Rupprecht HJ, et al. Impact of vessel curvature on the accuracy of three-dimensional intravascular ultrasound: validatioin by phantoms and coronary segments. J Am Soc Echocardiogr 2002; 15: 823–30

12. Kimura BJ, Bhargava V, Palinski W, et al. Distortion of intravascular ultrasound images because of nonuniform angular velocity of mechanical-type transducers. Am Heart J 1996; 132: 328–36

13. Arbab-Zadeh A, DeMaria AN, Penny WF, et al. Axial movement of the intravascular ultrasound probe during the cardiac cycle: implications for three-dimensional reconstruction and measurements of coronary dimensions. Am Heart J 1999; 138: 865–72

14. Wahle A, Prause PM, DeJong SC, et al., Geometrically correct 3-D reconstruction of intravascular ultrasound images by fusion with biplane angiography – methods and validation. IEEE Trans Med Imaging 1999; 18: 686–99

15. Slager CJ, Wentzel JJ, Schuurbiers JC, et al. True 3-dimensional reconstruction of coronary arteries in patients by fusion of angiography and IVUS (ANGUS) and its quantitative validation. Circulation 2000; 102: 511–16

2
Quantitative and qualitative analyses

The IVUS image is not identical to a histologic image. Images are created when the ultrasound beam encounters an interface between tissues or structures of different density. A recent important publication is Standards for the acquisition, measurement, and reporting of intravascular ultrasound studies: a report of the American College of Cardiology Task Force on Clinical Expert Consensus Documents.[1] This consensus document is the current gold-standard for IVUS imaging. In general, this document contains the preferred nomenclature for describing an IVUS image. A similar report that should be mentioned is that of the Study Group on Intracoronary Imaging of the Working Group of Coronary Circulation and of the Subgroup on Intravascular Ultrasound of the Working Group of Echocardiography of the European Society of Cardiology.[2]

It is important for each laboratory to establish standards and have an acceptable inter- and intra-observer variability. This is true for both quantitative and qualitative analyses.

QUANTITATIVE ANALYSIS

IVUS measurements should be performed at the leading edge of each interface, never the trailing edge. With few exceptions, the location of the leading edge is accurate and reproducible, while measurements at the trailing edge are inconsistent and frequently yield erroneous results. Measurements should be performed relative to the center of mass of the lumen or external elastic membrane (EEM), not relative to the center of the catheter. IVUS acquisition hardware can be used to make measurements, but typically only with studies that have been performed on the same type of machine. Off-line measurement systems are available from a number of companies. However, public-domain software – NIH Image 1.62 (also called ImageJ) – can be downloaded and used on any personal computer.

Longitudinal representation of IVUS images is useful for length measurements, for interpolation of shadowed deep arterial structures (such as the EEM behind calcium or stent metal), and for quickly identifying the minimal lumen area and the proximal and distal reference image slices. However, area, diameter, and thickness measurements must be performed on the appropriate cross-sectional image slices.

During clinical IVUS imaging of non-stented lesions, there are only two distinct boundaries that have consistent histologic correlates: the lumen–intima (or lumen–plaque) interface and the media–adventitia interface. Thus, in non-stented vessels, there are only two cross-sectional area (CSA) measurements that can be reproducibly performed: EEM CSA (a reproducible measure of the area within the media–adventitia interface) and lumen CSA (a reproducible measure of the area within the intima). In stented vessels, there can be three boundaries: lumen CSA, stent CSA, and EEM CSA.

Lumen borders

The first "structure" that the IVUS beam sees is the blood-filled lumen. At the operational frequency of commercially available systems, blood has a speckled and continuously changing pattern that is distinct from tissue. The intensity of the blood speckle increases exponentially with (1) the frequency of the transducer (the higher the frequency, the greater the resolution, and the smaller the targets that are seen) and (2) stasis (because of red-cell clumping or rouleaux formation) which is most evident when the catheter is across a tight stenosis (Figure 2.1). In fact, static blood can be more echodense than the plaque (Figure 2.2). This can limit the ability to differentiate lumen from tissue (particularly soft plaque, neointima, and thrombus). Saline (or contrast) injection through the guiding catheter is useful in clearing blood (even static blood) from the lumen – thereby differentiating blood speckle from tissue and defining true lumen borders. Examples are shown in Figures 2.3 and 2.4. This technique should be used whenever the lumen border is unclear. Conversely, excessive manipulation of the TGC curve to suppress blood speckle should be avoided because it will suppress all structures in the near field – whether blood or tissue. It is also possible to design algorithms that will "filter out" the blood. Blood is constantly moving – even relatively static

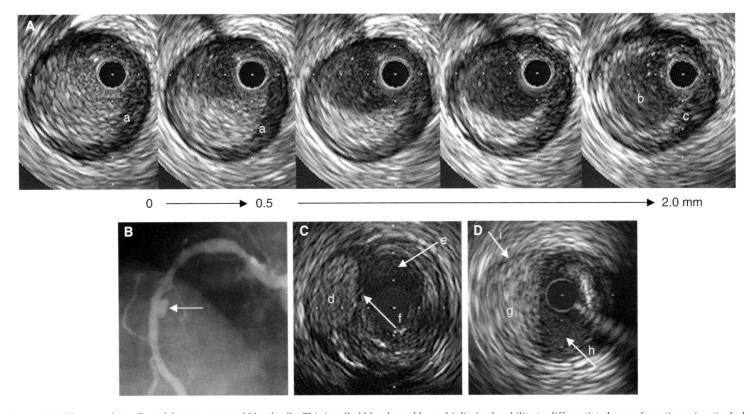

0 ⟶ 0.5 ⟶ 2.0 mm

Figure 2.1 Ultrasound is reflected from aggregated blood cells. This is called blood speckle, and it limits the ability to differentiate lumen from tissue (particularly hypoechoic structures such as soft plaque, neointima, and thrombus). The intensity of blood speckle increases exponentially as transducer frequency increases and as blood flow velocity decreases. Stasis leading to rouleaux formation and exaggerated blood speckle is most evident when the catheter is across a tight stenosis or when blood is trapped in a false lumen or cavitated structure. Panel A shows intraluminal blood stasis (a) where the intima is totally obscured. Moving the transducer reestablishes flow and "unmasks" the true lumen (b) and plaque (c). Compare the static blood speckle (a) with that of moving blood (b). A second example of blood stasis causing intense blood speckle is shown in the complex/ruptured plaque in Panel B (white arrow) and Panel C. Note that the evacuated plaque cavity (d) is filled with blood that is more echodense compared with the flowing blood (e) in the lumen. Presumably the IVUS catheter "sealed" the ruptured plaque cavity causing the trapped blood to aggregate and become intensely reflective. Note the thin flap of tissue (f) separating the cavity from the true lumen. A third example of blood stasis causing intense blood speckle is shown in Panel D. Post-intervention, blood accumulated with the blind pouch of a medial dissection, aggregated, and became intensely echoreflective (g) compared with flowing blood in the lumen (h). The trapped blood eliminated the echolucent appearance of the media, obscuring the media–adventia border (i). This phenomenon has been called an intramural hematoma

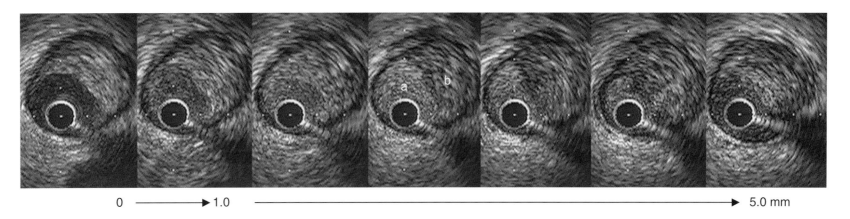

0 ——————►1.0 ———————————————————————————►5.0 mm

Figure 2.2 Blood (a) can be more echodense than plaque (b) – particularly across a tight stenosis (where stasis is exaggerated) in the absence of hyperechoic plaque

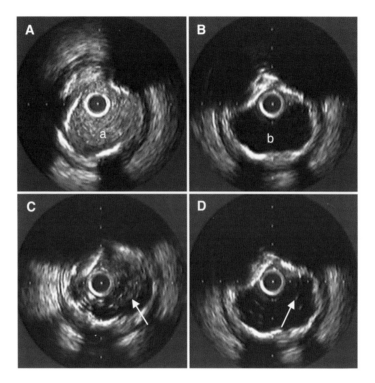

Figure 2.3 Panel A shows the lumen obscured by blood stasis (a). Flushing contrast or saline through the guiding catheter clears the lumen of the static blood. Contrast or saline is uniform in density; therefore, in its unagitated state, contrast or saline is black or entirely echolucent (b) as shown in Panel B. When contrast or saline is injected forcefully, it becomes agitated and mixed with blood to form clouds or bubbles as shown by the white arrows in Panels C and D, respectively. This is similar to echocardiographic contrast techniques

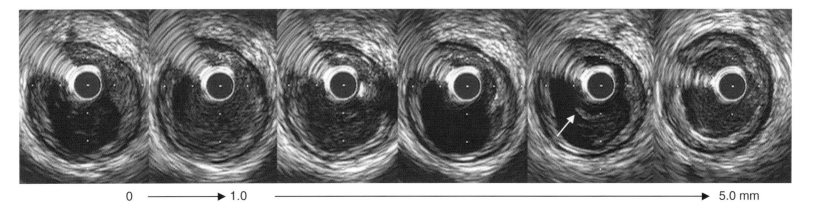

0 ⟶ 1.0 ⟶ 5.0 mm

Figure 2.4 An example of contrast injection used to clear the lumen of static blood is shown. Note that the effect is short-lived. When the effect starts to wear off, the contrast or saline again mixes with blood to form clouds or bubbles as shown by the white arrow

blood. If a "structure" changes between two consecutive sweeps of the scanner, then it is most probably blood. If this structure remains constant, then it is most probably tissue. This has been termed correlation. Since it is difficult to filter out blood speckle, manufacturers sometimes adopt an alternative approach of making blood speckle look different from plaque.

Lumen measurements are performed at the interface between the lumen and the leading edge of the intima relative to the center of mass of the lumen, not the center of the IVUS catheter, because the IVUS catheter may have an eccentric position. Measurements include lumen CSA, minimum lumen diameter (the shortest diameter through the center point of the lumen), and maximum lumen diameter (the longest diameter through the center point of the lumen).

Media

Truly normal coronary arteries are rare in the practice of interventional cardiology (Figure 2.5); only 160 μm (μm = microns) of intimal thickening are needed to consistently produce an intimal layer using current imaging frequencies.[3] (Whether normal arteries have distinct intimal, media, and adventitial layers during *in vivo* IVUS imaging and whether these layers can be measured accurately is the subject of some debate.[4,5]) In normal arteries, the material that most strongly reflects ultrasound is collagen. The reflectivity of collagen is 1000 times that of muscle. The adventitia of coronary arteries has a high collagen content and is, therefore, echoreflective. Conversely, the media of coronary arteries has a low collagen content, is mostly muscular, is typically echolucent, histologically averages a thickness of 200 μm in the absence of atherosclerosis, and becomes thinner in the presence of atherosclerotic disease.[6,7]

The internal elastic membrane separates the intima from the media. Although the internal elastic membrane is composed of strong echogenic elastic tissue, fibrous changes in the inner third of the media reduce the difference in acoustic impedance (reflectivity) between these adjacent layers, blurring the distinction between the internal elastic membrane and the inner border of the media.[6] In addition, normal intimal thickness increases with age from a single cell at birth to a mean of 60 μm at five years to 220–250 μm at 30–40 years of age.[8] With increasing atherosclerosis, the intima/plaque layer increases in thickness and tends to merge with the internal elastic lamina. All of these changes preclude reliable measurement or even estimation of media thickness.[9]

In some IVUS images, the media may appear erroneously thin because of an intense reflection from the intima or EEM. In other IVUS images, the media can appear "artifactually thick" because of signal attenuation and the weak reflectivity of the internal elastic membrane. One indication of a false or "exaggerated" medial thickness is that the media appears to be thicker under a thicker plaque layer than under a thinner plaque layer (Figure 2.6). A study comparing IVUS imaging before and after directional coronary atherectomy showed that cutting into this echolucent "media" zone resulted in media being identified in only 50% of histologic specimens.[10]

Plaque & media (P&M)

Because the media cannot be quantified accurately, IVUS measurements cannot determine the true histologic plaque area (the area bounded by the internal elastic membrane). Instead, IVUS studies use the EEM and lumen CSA measurements to create a surrogate for true plaque (or atheroma) CSA – the plaque plus media CSA; and the cross-sectional measurement of atherosclerotic plaque is reported as the plaque & media (or atheroma) CSA. This is calculated as EEM CSA minus lumen CSA and abbreviated as P&M CSA. In practice, the inclusion of the media into the atheroma area does not constitute a major limitation, because the media represents only a very small fraction of the P&M CSA. In addition, the percentage of media represented in the P&M complex does not change measurably during serial studies. IVUS measurement of maximum and minimum P&M thicknesses can be used to calculate an eccentricity index.

External elastic membrane (EEM)

The adventitia is composed of loose collagen and elastic tissue that merges with the surrounding peri-adventitia; it is 300–500 μm thick. A discrete interface exists at the border between the media and the adventitia; it is almost invariably present on an IVUS image and corresponds closely to the location of the EEM. This is sometimes also called the external elastic lamina (EEL). The EEM should be measured at the leading edge of the border between the media and the adventitia.

EEM circumference and CSA cannot be measured reliably at sites where large side-branches originate or in the setting of extensive calcification because of acoustic shadowing. If acoustic shadowing involves a relatively small arc (< 90°), planimetry of the EEM circumference can be performed by extrapolation from the closest identifiable EEM borders, although measurement accuracy and reproducibility will be reduced. The cross-sectional geometry of the coronary artery is more or less circular, and real-time axial movement of the transducer just proximal and distal to a calcific deposit (or to find the smallest arc of calcium within the deposit) may help to unmask and fill in continuous parts of the adventitia that are otherwise shadowed (Figure 2.7). The arc of calcium has been shown to vary significantly throughout the length of a lesion.[11] In addition, some stent designs may obscure the EEM; in these circumstances, a similar approach can be used to identify the EEM. Finally, longitudinal image reconstruction can identify the media–adventitia border just proximal or distal to calcium or stent metal and, therefore, aid in interpolation (Figure 2.8). Interpolating the EEM border will also allow calculation of P&M area, P&M thicknesses, plaque burden, etc. Because arteries decrease in size from immediately proximal to a large side branch to immediately distal to that branch, interpolation should not be used to "reconstruct" an EEM interrupted by a branch. The lesion site can be compared with the proximal and distal reference segments to generate a remodeling index (lesion EEM CSA divided by reference-segment EEM CSA).

Plaque burden and stenosis

The P&M CSA is often divided by the EEM CSA to generate a measurement called the plaque burden. This is also sometimes referred to as the percent atheroma area, percent plaque area, cross-sectional narrowing, or cross-sectional area obstruction. The latter two definitions (cross-sectional narrowing or cross-sectional area obstruction) should be avoided since this measurement does not indicate obstruction. Rather, as plaque accumulates and the EEM increases (positive remodeling) to maintain lumen dimensions, the P&M:EEM ratio also increases; but this is a measure of plaque accumulation, not of obstructive disease. A large plaque burden can occur in the absence of any obstruction. Conversely, lumen area stenosis (or diameter stenosis) is a measure of obstruction in which the lesion-site lumen CSA is compared with the reference lumen CSA; this is analogous to the calculation of the angiographic diameter stenosis.

A complete set of IVUS measurements of a non-stented lesion is shown in Figure 2.9.

Saphenous vein grafts

In situ veins do not have an EEM. However, saphenous vein grafts typically undergo "arterialization" with morphologic changes that include intimal fibrous thickening, medial hypertrophy, and lipid deposition to create an echolucent zone (Figure 2.10).[12] The "EEM" CSA – which is actually the vein-graft CSA – is measured by tracing the outer border of this echolucent zone (Figure 2.11). All other measurements, including "P&M" CSA (sometimes called the vein graft wall CSA) and plaque burden, are calculated in a similar manner to native coronary disease.[13–19]

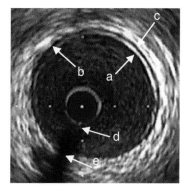

Figure 2.5 This is an example of a normal coronary artery with intima (a), media (b), and adventita (c). Note the thickness of the normal media. The maximum intimal/medial thickness (measured from the leading edge of the intima to the leading edge of the adventitia) is 0.15 mm. Also note the minimal guidewire artifact (d) with shadowing (e)

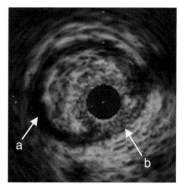

Figure 2.6 In this eccentric, hyperechoic, non-calcified plaque, the thickness of the media behind the thickest part of the plaque (a) measured 0.6 mm. This medial thickness is an artifact caused by attenuation of the beam as it passes through the hyperechoic plaque. In reality, anatomically, the media becomes thinner with increasing atherosclerosis. Compare this with the normal medial thickness in Figure 2.5 and with the medial thickness behind the thinnest part of the plaque in this image (< 0.1 mm, b). This finding is seen in other examples in this section

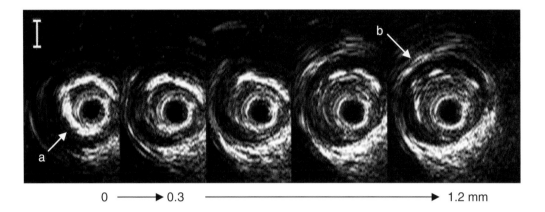

Figure 2.7   Calcium (a) shadows the deeper arterial structures, including the external elastic membrane (b). Moving the transducer proximally or, as in this example, distally – even just a small amount – can unmask the external elastic membrane

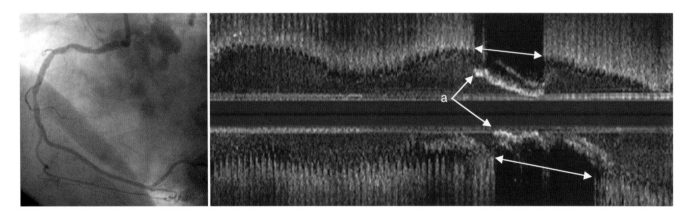

Figure 2.8   Longitudinal image reconstruction (also called L-mode) can be used to interpolate the external elastic membrane (double-headed white arrows) that is shadowed by calcium (a)

Proximal reference

Lesion
site

Distal reference

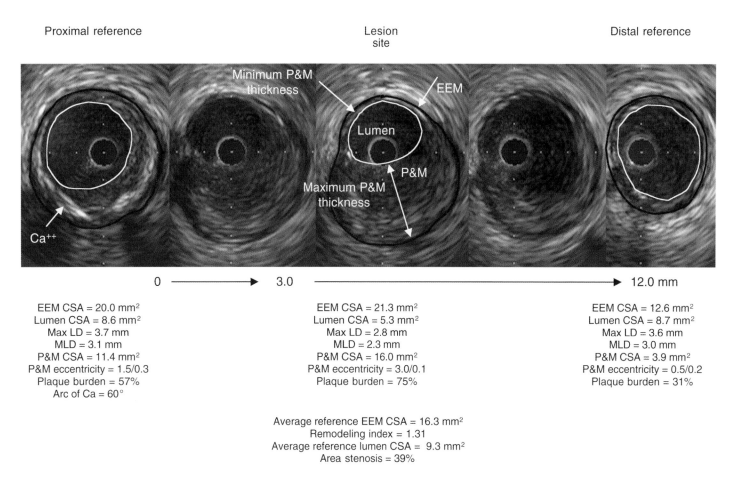

0 ——————▶ 3.0 ——————————————————▶ 12.0 mm

EEM CSA = 20.0 mm²
Lumen CSA = 8.6 mm²
Max LD = 3.7 mm
MLD = 3.1 mm
P&M CSA = 11.4 mm²
P&M eccentricity = 1.5/0.3
Plaque burden = 57%
Arc of Ca = 60°

EEM CSA = 21.3 mm²
Lumen CSA = 5.3 mm²
Max LD = 2.8 mm
MLD = 2.3 mm
P&M CSA = 16.0 mm²
P&M eccentricity = 3.0/0.1
Plaque burden = 75%

EEM CSA = 12.6 mm²
Lumen CSA = 8.7 mm²
Max LD = 3.6 mm
MLD = 3.0 mm
P&M CSA = 3.9 mm²
P&M eccentricity = 0.5/0.2
Plaque burden = 31%

Average reference EEM CSA = 16.3 mm²
Remodeling index = 1.31
Average reference lumen CSA = 9.3 mm²
Area stenosis = 39%

Figure 2.9 A complete set of IVUS measurements in a non-stented artery is shown. The black line highlights each external elastic membrane, and the white line indicates each image slice's lumen. Abbreviations: Max LD, maximum lumen diameter; MLD, minimum lumen diameter. The P&M CSA has also been called the atheroma CSA; and the plaque burden has also been called the atheroma burden

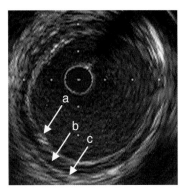

Figure 2.10 The normal, recently explanted saphenous vein has a monolayer appearance. An arterialized saphenous vein undergoes morphologic changes that include intimal thickening (a) and medial hypertrophy to create an echolucent zone (b) resulting in a reproducible outer border (c) that is analogous to the external elastic membrane in native arteries

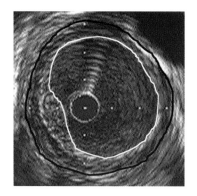

EEM CSA = 21.4 mm²
Lumen CSA = 12.1 mm²
Max LD = 4.2 mm
MLD = 3.2 mm
P&M CSA = 9.3 mm²
P&M eccentricity = 1.3/0.3
Plaque burden = 43%

Figure 2.11 Saphenous vein graft borders are traced just like a native artery, and similar measurements are made. Although there is no anatomic external elastic membrane, the outer border of the echolucent hypertrophied media is traced, and the measurements are often reported as external elastic membrane CSA or vein graft CSA (black line). The white line indicates the lumen

Stents

Endovascular stents are intensely echoreflective. The metallic prosthesis creates a third IVUS boundary between the lumen and the EEM. Stent CSA can be measured, and intimal hyperplasia (IH) CSA can be calculated as stent CSA minus lumen CSA. IH CSA is often reported as a percentage of stent CSA; it has been termed % IH or % IH (volume) obstruction. When tracing the stent, it is important not to mistake the guidewire for a stent strut; both are metallic reflectors.

The appearance of different stent designs and the ease or difficulty in measuring stent CSA can be seen in Figure 2.12. In general, most tubular-slotted or multicellular stents have a similar appearance. However, measurement of stent CSA is more reliable with tubular-slotted or multicellular stents (or coil stents that have a similar appearance) compared with the clam-shell design of the Gianturco–Roubin family of stents. Longitudinal reconstruction can aid in measuring an interpolated minimum stent CSA within a clam-shell stent design (Figure 2.13).

It is important to note that the endothelial layer that covers a stent has a thickness below the resolution of IVUS; therefore, re-endothelialization in the absence of IH accumulation appears as a stent without overlying tissue. When imaging stents, high-gain settings should be avoided because the metallic struts are strong ultrasound reflectors and easily create side lobes (Figure 1.7). If the media–adventitia border can be seen through the stent struts, the peri-stent P&M CSA can also be calculated as EEM CSA minus stent CSA.

Strut apposition refers to the proximity of stent struts to the arterial wall. Good apposition is defined as sufficiently close contact to preclude blood flow between any strut and the underlying wall. Malapposition (or incomplete apposition) is defined as separation of ≥1 stent struts from the intima, not overlapping a sidebranch, with evidence of blood flow behind the strut. Malapposed stent struts have a characteristic appearance that is seen in Figure 2.14. Documentation of malapposition can be enhanced by flushing saline or contrast from the guiding catheter to confirm the presence of flow behind the struts. Apposition is different from expansion, and the two terms should not be used interchangeably.

Post-intervention – in the absence of tissue prolapse or stent malapposition – the stent CSA will be equivalent to the lumen CSA. Measurements include stent CSA, minimum stent diameter (the shortest diameter through the center point of the stent), maximum stent diameter (the longest diameter through the center point of the stent), stent symmetry (ratio of minimum to maximum stent diameter),

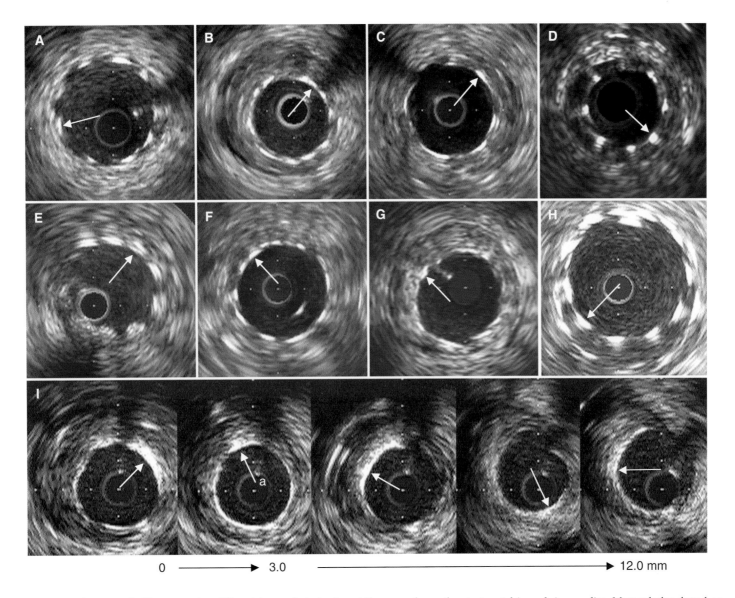

0 ——→ 3.0 ——————————————→ 12.0 mm

Figure 2.12 This example illustrates nine different types of stents; the white arrow shows the stent metal in each image slice. Most tubular-slotted or multicellular stents have a similar appearance: A = NIR, B = MultiLink, C = AVE GFX, D = Duet, E = Paragon, and F = Palmaz–Schatz. Some coiled stents – such as the CrossFlex (G) or the Wiktor stent – have an appearance that is like a tubular-slotted/muticellular stent. The mesh Wallstent (H) also has a similar appearance, but it has more stent metal. The design of the Gianturco–Roubin-II stent (I) results in an IVUS appearance that varies almost mm by mm over the length of the stent. With the exception of one cross-section (a), a complete stent circumference is usually not seen. Consequently, it is difficult to identify and measure the minimum stent CSA

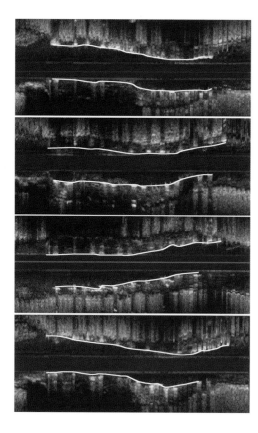

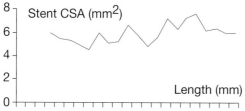

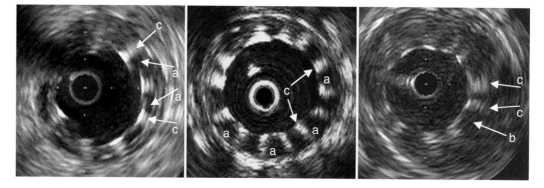

Figure 2.14 Three examples of acute stent malapposition are shown. Notice the space between the stent strut and the intima (a), the blood speckle behind the stent struts (b), and the multiple reflections from the malapposed stent struts that produce a characteristic rectangular appearance (c)

Figure 2.13 Longitudinal image reconstruction can be used to interpolate the minimum stent CSA within a Gianturco–Roubin stent, in which a complete stent circumference is rarely seen. Multiple longitudinal views are created, and the stent traced (white lines). The stent CSA is then calculated mm by mm along the stent length (bottom graph); and the minimum stent CSA is identified, in this case 4.5 mm² and stent expansion (the minimum stent CSA compared with a predefined reference, which can be the proximal, distal, largest, or average reference lumen CSA, or even the lesion or reference EEM CSA). Expansion is different from apposition, and the two terms should not be used interchangeably. A complete set of stented-segment IVUS measurements is shown in Figure 2.15.

Post-intervention, if there is tissue prolapse through the stent or thrombus formation within the stent, then the lumen CSA will be smaller than the stent CSA (Figure 2.16). Post-intervention, if there is stent–vessel wall malapposition, then the lumen CSA will be larger than the stent CSA; and the malapposition CSA (or number of malapposed struts) can be measured directly (Figure 2.17).

At follow-up, the lumen CSA is typically smaller than the stent CSA because of IH accumulation within the stent (Figure 2.18). It cannot be emphasized strongly enough that image controls must be appropriately set so as not to suppress the relatively echolucent neointimal tissue. Unless IVUS was performed at stent implantation, it is not possible to differentiate intimal hyperplasia from acute tissue prolapse. At follow-up in the presence of stent malapposition, the lumen CSA may be larger than the stent CSA; the malapposition CSA (or number of malapposed struts) should be measured directly (Figure 2.19).

Lengths and volumes

Motorized transducer pullback (ideally at 0.5 mm/s) yields accurate length measurements, particularly with mechanical systems, because the transducer is pulled through a stationary imaging sheath. Length is the number of seconds multiplied by the pullback speed. Lengths should not be measured with manual transducer pullback; they are not accurate. However, it is also theoretically possible to use spatial magnetic positioning technology to measure lengths without motorized transducer pullback. Known stent length serves as an internal validation of length measurements.[20] If, for example, at a pullback speed of 0.5 mm/s, it takes 45 s to image a 15-mm-long stent, then there is a technical problem with the pullback device, which must be corrected.

Motorized transducer pullback can also permit volumetric IVUS calculations using either Simpson's rule (in which multiple image slices acquired at a fixed interval – i.e. every 1 mm – are added) or multiple longitudinal views. A typical set of volumetric measurements will include EEM volume, lumen volume, stent volume, IH volume (stent volume minus lumen volume), % IH volume (IH volume divided by stent volume), P&M (or atheroma) volume (EEM minus stent volume in stented segments and EEM minus lumen volume in non-stented segments), and plaque burden (or percent atheroma volume) (P&M volume divided by EEM volume). The most accurate volumes are calculated from ECG-gated

motorized pullback; however, acquisition times are prolonged. Conversely, volumes should not be measured when using manual transducer pullback. They are not accurate.

Longer imaged segments, lesions, and stents will have larger volumes compared with shorter segments. Therefore, mean planar analysis (in which measured volumes are normalized for lesion length) should be reported together with actual volumes when comparing segments of unequal length. A typical set of mean planar (or cross-sectional area) measurements will include mean EEM CSA, mean lumen CSA, mean stent CSA, mean IH CSA (mean stent minus mean lumen CSA), % IH (mean IH CSA divided by mean stent CSA), mean P&M CSA (mean EEM minus stent CSA in stented segments and mean EEM minus lumen CSA in non-stented segments), and mean plaque burden (mean P&M CSA divided by mean EEM CSA).

Validation

The above cross-sectional, length, and volumetric IVUS measurements have been validated together with the inter-observer variability, intra-observer variability, and reproducibility.[9,21–30] Validation of volumetric measurements has been limited to studies performed using motorized transducer pullback, some of which have even incorporated ECG-triggered transducer pullback or image acquisition.[30–32]

PLAQUE COMPOSITION

The earliest changes that occur in the development of atherosclerosis (i.e. fatty streaks) do not change the ultrasonic appearance of the normal artery because they are below the resolution of IVUS. With further progression of atherosclerosis, IVUS detects an increase in intimal thickness. The threshold between normal and abnormal is the subject of some debate, but more than 0.3 mm of intimal thickening is probably abnormal and can be used to distinguish mild "physiologic" intimal thickening from atherosclerosis. It should also be noted that an artery that is normal in appearance may still respond abnormally to vasoactive stimuli.

Atherosclerotic lesions are heterogeneous and include varying amounts of calcium, dense fibrous tissue, lipid, smooth muscle cells, thrombus, etc. While IVUS cannot provide histologically accurate information regarding plaque composition, IVUS imaging can grossly separate lesions into subtypes according to echodensity and presence or absence of shadowing and reverberations.[33–35] The echointensity of

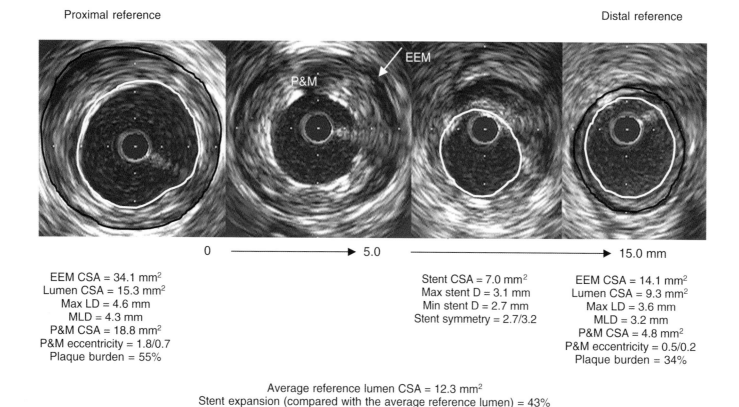

Proximal reference   Distal reference

0 ⟶ 5.0 ⟶ 15.0 mm

EEM CSA = 34.1 mm²
Lumen CSA = 15.3 mm²
Max LD = 4.6 mm
MLD = 4.3 mm
P&M CSA = 18.8 mm²
P&M eccentricity = 1.8/0.7
Plaque burden = 55%

Stent CSA = 7.0 mm²
Max stent D = 3.1 mm
Min stent D = 2.7 mm
Stent symmetry = 2.7/3.2

EEM CSA = 14.1 mm²
Lumen CSA = 9.3 mm²
Max LD = 3.6 mm
MLD = 3.2 mm
P&M CSA = 4.8 mm²
P&M eccentricity = 0.5/0.2
Plaque burden = 34%

Average reference lumen CSA = 12.3 mm²
Stent expansion (compared with the average reference lumen) = 43%

Figure 2.15 A complete set of IVUS measurement in a stented artery is shown. In addition, in this example, it is possible to indentify the external elastic membrane behind the stent and, therefore, to calculate the peri-stent plaque & media. The black line highlights each external elastic membrane, and the white line indicates each image slice's lumen or stent. Abbreviations: Max, maximum; D, diameter; LD, lumen diameter; MLD, minimum lumen diameter

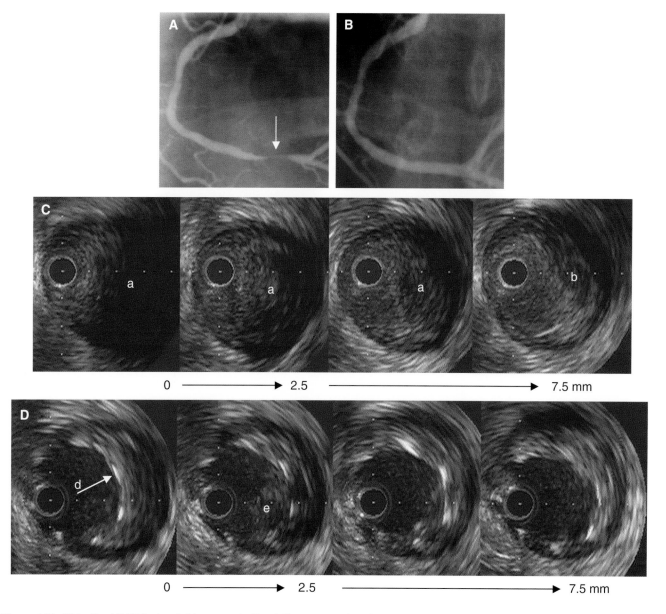

Figure 2.16 This distal RCA lesion (white arrow in Panel A) was treated with an NIR stent with a good angiographic result (Panel B). Pre-intervention IVUS imaging (Panel C) shows eccentric plaque with features of thrombus (a) and even a hypoechoic core (b). Of note, there is marked attenuation at the proximal end of this thrombotic lesion (c). Post-intervention IVUS imaging (Panel D) of the NIR stent (d) shows tissue prolapse (e) that reduces the lumen area from 9.0 mm^2 to 5.7 mm^2. Tissue prolapse post-stent implantation is more common in unstable and thrombus-containing lesions in native arteries and degenerated lesions in saphenous vein grafts

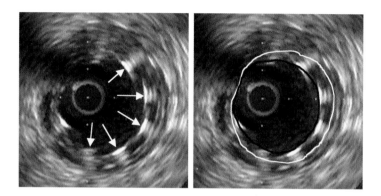

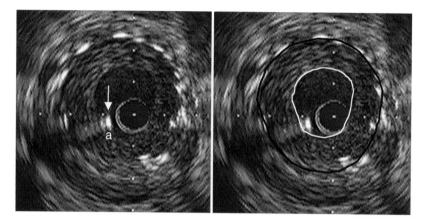

Figure 2.17   An example of stent malapposition at implantation is shown. Five stent struts are malapposed (white arrows). Because of stent malapposition, the lumen area (white line) is larger than the stent area (black line). The malapposition area measured 1.8 mm² and the maximum malapposition distance measured 0.6 mm

Figure 2.18   Because of intimal hyperplasia (a), the lumen area (white line) is smaller than the stent area (black line). The stent CSA measured 13.3 mm², the lumen CSA measured 3.7 mm², and intimal hyperplasia measured 9.6 mm². Note the guidewire artifact (white arrow); in stented lesions, it is particularly important not to mistake the guidewire artifact for a stent strut

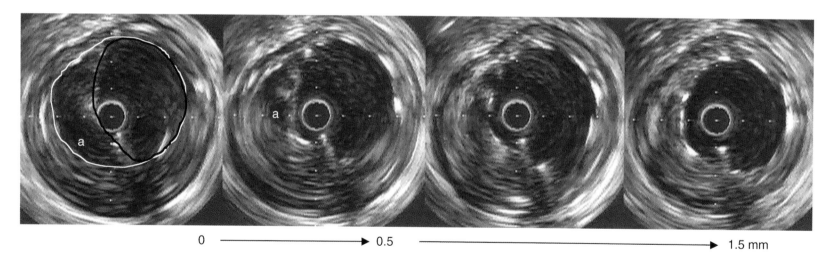

0 ⟶ 0.5 ⟶ 1.5 mm

Figure 2.19   An example of late stent malapposition (a) is shown. The lumen area (white line) is larger than the stent area (black line); the malapposition area measured 6.5 mm² and the maximum separation measured 1.4 mm. In general, late malapposed stent struts are free of significant intimal hyperplasia

different plaque components varies with the system settings and equipment used; it is for this reason that the collagen-rich adventitia is usually used as a reference.

The terminology used to describe specific plaque types is the subject of debate. Terms that have been used include calcific, echodense, fibrocalcific, fibrotic, hard, soft, echolucent, fatty, and fibrofatty. Because atherosclerosis is a heterogeneous process, many lesions are mixed and contain more than one plaque type. Regardless of the classification used, from the standpoint of therapeutic device responses, a calcific, fibrocalcific, or echodense plaque behaves differently from a soft, echolucent, or fibrofatty plaque.

The relatively large inter- and intra-observer variability in the qualitative IVUS gray-scale classification of plaque elements indicates the need for an improved analysis system. Computer-assisted techniques may facilitate gray-scale analysis and provide a more objective approach to plaque classification.[36] True histologic level plaque classification may be possible with IVUS tissue characterization that also employs radiofrequency domain information. While the *in vitro* validation data look promising, this technology – which has been dubbed "virtual histology" – is still in development.[37]

Calcium

Calcium is a powerful reflector of ultrasound; little of the beam penetrates through or even into the calcium. Thus, calcium casts a shadow over deeper arterial structures, only the leading edge of the calcific deposit can be seen, and even calcium thickness cannot be measured. (Shadowing represents the weakness or absence of signals beyond structures with high echoreflectivity such as calcium or stent struts. This artifact can hinder imaging beyond strong reflectors. However, because of diffraction – the bending of sound waves around edges, even edges of strong reflectors – a certain amount of ultrasound energy can "penetrate" a calcific deposit and thus provide useful information.)

In practice, the signature of calcium is echodense (hyperechoic) plaque (brighter than the reference adventitia) that shadows; however, dense fibrous tissue without calcium is also echodense and can sometimes cast a shadow. Occasionally, calcium (but not dense fibrous tissue) will produce reverberations: one or more equidistantly spaced rings at intervals that are a multiple of the distance from the transducer to the leading edge of the calcium. Reverberations are specific for calcium as opposed to dense fibrous tissue (although they can be produced by other strong echoreflectors) and are more common after calcium is treated with rotational atherectomy. Examples of calcium are shown in Figure 2.20.

Detection of lesion-associated calcium by IVUS also depends on the histologic pattern.[38,39] Small calcific deposits within a necrotic lipid core appear different from larger calcific elements, and microcalcifications can be missed entirely. Occasionally, shadowing without evident echoreflective plaque can occur just proximal or distal to a calcific deposit; moving the transducer proximally or distally will usually "unmask" the hyperechoic calcium (Figure 2.21). With the exception of microcalcifications, IVUS is sensitive and specific for detecting calcium within a plaque. However, it should be noted that while IVUS frequently shows a large block of calcium, pathologically this is an uncommon finding. Instead, on histopathology, there are more often multiple smaller fragments of calcium that probably coalesce on IVUS imaging.

Using IVUS, calcium can be localized to the lesion versus the reference segment; characterized as superficial (closer to the tissue–lumen interface, Figure 2.22) versus deep (closer to the media–adventitia junction, Figure 2.23); and quantified according to its arc and length. In addition, a volumetric index of calcium can be calculated by integrating the arc and length of calcium and determining the volume of the EEM that is shadowed.[40,41]

Fibrous plaques

Fibrous plaques represent the majority of atherosclerotic lesions. In general, the greater the fibrous tissue content, the greater the echogenicity of the tissue. Very dense fibrous plaques may produce sufficient attenuation to be misclassified as calcification with acoustic shadowing. Both calcified and fibrotic plaques are hyerpechoic. Examples of non-calcified echoreflective (or "hard") plaques are shown in Figure 2.24.

Soft plaques

Echolucent plaques are less bright compared with the reference adventitia (Figure 2.25). Some authorities do not like the term echolucent since it means that the structure does not reflect any ultrasound at all; an alternative term is hypoechoic. Although it has become common to refer to echolucent or hypoechoic plaques as "soft" (to differentiate them from echoreflective or hyperechoic plaques that are labeled "hard"), it is important to recognize that these plaques are not soft or compliant to the touch, but are as firm as "hard" plaques.[42] Furthermore, the compliance of a lesion – i.e. its response to balloon angioplasty or stent implantation – is dependent on more than just the ultrasound plaque classification. Other factors that influence the compliance of a lesion include patient age, plaque burden, compliance of the adventitia and peri-adventitial structures, and vessel size.[43]

Echolucent plaques contain varying amounts of fibrous and fatty tissue. Pure fat is much more echolucent than muscle. A lipid pool, therefore, should appear

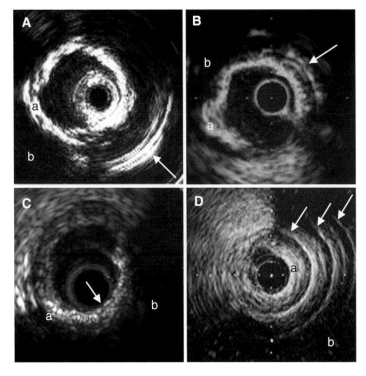

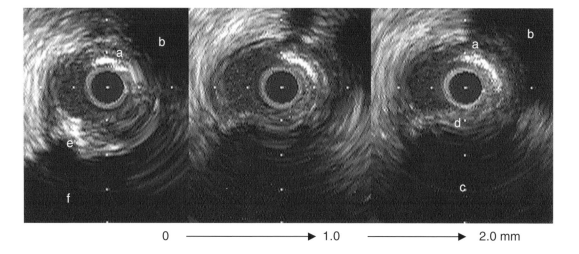

0 ——————————▶ 1.0 ——————————▶ 2.0 mm

Figure 2.20   Calcium, as imaged by four different IVUS machines, is shown. In each image slice, the plaque (a) is brighter than the adventitia with acoustic shadowing (b). Note the reverberations (white arrows) in Panels A, B and D. Panel D was imaged after rotational atherectomy. A = InterTherapy, B = Hewlett-Packard, C = Endosonics (now Volcano), and D = CVIS (now SciMed/Boston Scientific)

Figure 2.21   This lesion contains two arcs of calcium. In one arc of calcium (a), the typical IVUS features of hyperechoic plaque and acoustic shadowing (b) appeared simultaneously. In the other arc of calcium, there is a dissociation between these two typical IVUS findings. During the pullback from distal (right-hand panel) to proximal (left-hand panel), acoustic shadowing (c) appeared first while the plaque appeared hypoechoic. Eventually, a single image slice contains both hyperechoic plaque (e) and shadowing (f). When there is shadowing in the absence of hyperechoic plaque, movement of the transducer just proximal or distal often resolves the confusion

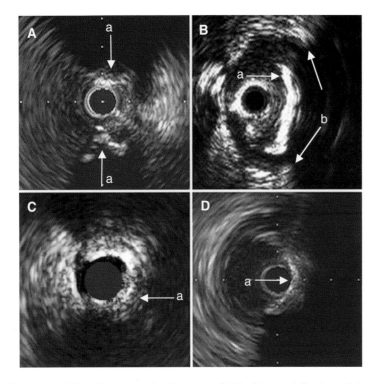

Figure 2.22 These four examples show superficial calcium – defined as calcium (a) that is closer to the intima than it is to the adventitia (b). Of course, when calcium occupies the intima (Panels A, C, and D), it is, by definition, superficial

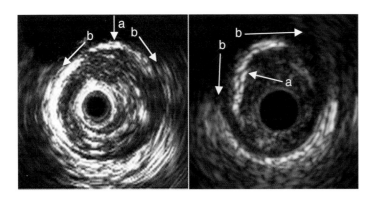

Figure 2.23 In each of these examples, deep calcium (a) is closer to the adventitia (b) than to the intima

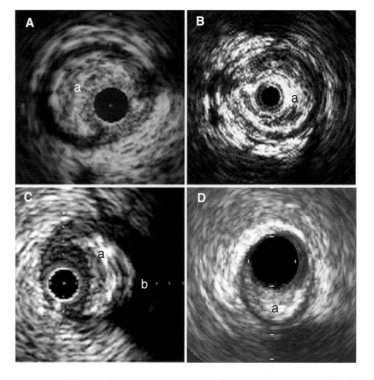

Figure 2.24 Fibrotic (hyperechoic, non-calcific) plaque as imaged by four different IVUS machines. In each of these examples, there is evidence of hyperechoic plaque (a) – plaque that is as bright or brighter than the adventitia. There is no shadowing in Panels A, B, and D. In Panel C, the shadowing (b) is either from deep calcium or from attenuation. A = Hewlett-Packard, B = InterTherapy, C = CVIS (now SciMed/Boston Scientific), and D = Endosonics (now Volcano)

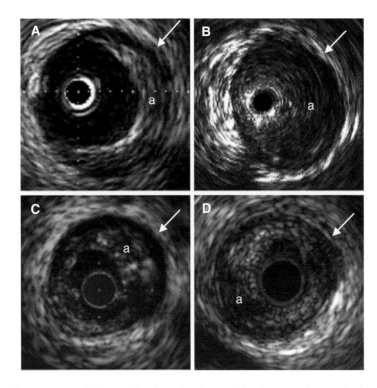

Figure 2.25 Soft plaque (a) – also called hypoechoic plaque – as imaged by four different IVUS machines. Soft plaque is a misnomer since it is not soft to the touch. Rather, it is "visually" soft. It is also called hypoechoic plaque, in that it is less echoreflective when compared with the adventitia (white arrows). A = CVIS (now SciMed/Boston Scientific), B = InterTherapy, C = Hewlett-Packard, and D = Endosonics (now Volcano)

as a dark or echolucent zone within a lesion; however, in practice, the *in vivo* identification of lipid pools (as well as of rupture-prone plaques or thin-capped atheromas) is beyond the limits of current technology. Reduced echogenicity may also result from a necrotic zone within the plaque, an intramural hemorrhage, or a thrombus. Most echolucent plaques contain minimal collagen and elastin.

Mixed plaques

Plaques frequently contain more than one acoustic subtype. In fact, atherosclerotic plaques are rarely homogeneous. If there is no one dominant plaque type, appropriate descriptions are "fibrocalcific", "fibrofatty", mixed, etc. Examples are shown in Figure 2.26.

Intimal hyperplasia

The neointimal hyperplasia that is characteristic of early in-stent restenosis often appears to have low echogenicity (Figure 2.27), even at times being less echogenic than blood speckle (Figure 2.28). Appropriate system settings are critical to avoid suppressing this relatively non-echogenic material. The intimal hyperplasia of late in-stent restenosis may appear more echogenic. Conversely, in some patients with brachytherapy failure, in-stent restenosis tissue can be truly echolucent – the so-called black hole or black wall phenomenon (Figure 2.29)

Thrombus

The identification of thrombus is one of the most difficult aspects of IVUS imaging.[44,45] Clues to the presence of thrombus include the following: (1) a sparkling "scintillating" appearance, (2) a lobulated mass projecting into the lumen, (3) a distinct interface between the suspected thrombus and underlying plaque, (4) identification of blood speckle within the thrombus indicating microchannels through the thrombus, and (5) mobility. An example is shown in Figure 2.30. While the combination of these features is, in general, specific, it is not sensitive, and the IVUS diagnosis of thrombus should be considered presumptive. It is important to emphasize that while the routine IVUS diagnosis of thrombus in native coronary arteries is difficult, the diagnosis of thrombus in saphenous vein grafts (where degenerated tissue can have all of these same features) is, frankly, totally unreliable.

LESION AND REFERENCE SELECTION

Reference segments

The proximal image slice is the site with the largest lumen proximal to a stenosis, but within the same segment (usually within 10 mm of the stenosis with no major intervening branches). This may not be the site with the least plaque. However, among slices with the same largest lumen area, the one with the least plaque should be selected. Ostial lesions and lesions immediately distal to a large sidebranch will not have a proximal reference.

Similarly, the distal reference is the site with the largest lumen distal to a stenosis, but within the same segment (usually within 10 mm of the stenosis with no intervening branches). Again, this may not be the site with the least plaque; however, among slices with the same largest lumen area, the one with the least plaque should be selected. It should be noted that the distal reference may be

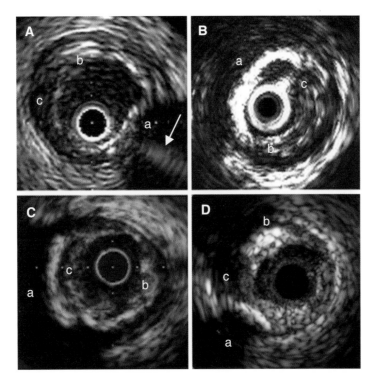

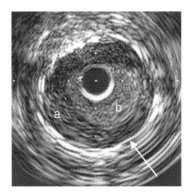

Figure 2.28 Intimal hyperplasia (a) can be less echodense than blood speckle (b). Stent CSA measured 12.9 mm², lumen CSA measured 4.8 mm², and intimal hyperplasia CSA measured 8.1 mm². The stent is indicated by the white arrow

Figure 2.26 Mixed plaque as imaged by four different IVUS machines. Each panel contains calcium (a), fibrotic plaque (b), and soft plaque (c) without any one dominant plaque type. A = CVIS (now SciMed/Boston Scientific), B = InterTherapy, C = Hewlett-Packard, and D = Endosonics (now Volcano). Note that the reverberations from the guidewire in Panel A (white arrow) continue even into the area shadowed by the calcium

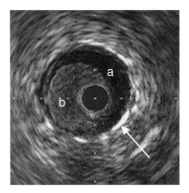

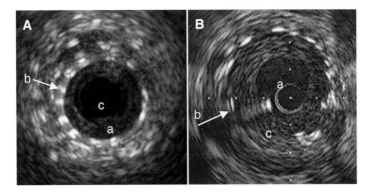

Figure 2.27 Two examples of in-stent restenosis with intimal hyperplasia (a). Note the stent (b) and the lumen (c). In these examples, intimal hyperplasia is more dense than blood speckle

Figure 2.29 Intimal hyperplasia (a) can be echolucent. This has been called a "black hole"; however, it is not a hole, because nothing is missing. Rather, it is merely echolucent neointimal tissue. This is more common after brachytherapy. Histology in some of these cases showed large myxoid areas with few interspersed smooth muscle cells that were scattered in an extracellular matrix containing mostly proteoglycan. (b indicates blood speckle.) Stent CSA measured 9.7 mm², lumen CSA measured 4.4 mm², and intimal hyperplasia CSA measured 5.3 mm². The stent is indicated by the white arrow

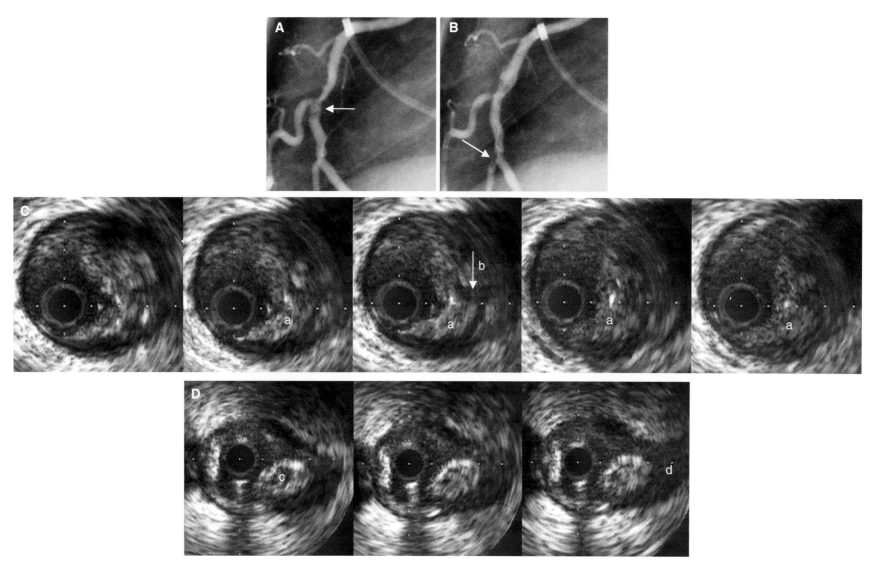

Figure 2.30   This example shows an unstable lesion before intervention (white arrow in Panel A) and after balloon angioplasty (Panel B); note the new, post-balloon angioplasty filling defect at the origin of the acute marginal branch in Panel B (white arrow). Pre-intervention IVUS (Panel C) shows many features of a thrombus: a lobulated, pedunculated mass (a); a distinct interface with the underlying vessel wall (b); and in real time, blood speckle within the lesion. Post-balloon angioplasty IVUS (Panel D) shows the thrombus (c) that has embolized into the acute marginal branch (d)

underperfused, especially during pre-intervention imaging, and may "grow" during an intervention as the stenosis is relieved. This change can be large when treating a chronic total occlusion, suggesting an element of negative remodeling secondary to chronic flow reduction as well as underperfusion. However, particularly in the setting of a chronic total occlusion, the distal reference may not "grow" to its steady state until days or weeks post-intervention.

Reference-segment volumes or mean reference-segment CSAs can be determined by measuring a fixed length of reference segment.

Lesion site

Within a segment, there will always be a worst stenosis, but there can be multiple secondary stenoses. In the case of multiple lesions within a single coronary segment, distinct stenoses require at least 5 mm of reference segment between them. If not, then the disease should be considered a single long lesion.

The worst stenosis should be the slice with the smallest lumen CSA. This may or may not represent the site with the largest P&M CSA. However, if there are multiple image slices with the same minimum lumen area, the one with the largest P&M CSA should be selected for quantitative analysis. This site may differ from its angiographic counterpart. In some cases, quantitative analysis of a single slice may describe the lesion adequately. In other cases, proper description may require analysis of an entire segment with quantitative analysis and measurement of a number of image slices. In either situation, the morphology of the lesion (i.e. the plaque composition, calcium, etc.) should be described by surveying the entire lesion or stenosis, not just the image slice with the smallest-lumen CSA. The many examples in this text illustrate how lesion morphology can vary from slice to slice.

Lesion-site volumes or mean lesion-site CSAs can be determined by measuring the entire length of the lesion.

For clinical purposes, pre- and post-intervention stenosis site selection and measurement begins by identifying the pre-intervention minimum lumen CSA, recognizing that the axial location of the worst stenosis may change during the intervention or at follow-up.

SERIAL STUDIES

It has become evident that there are measurement differences among the IVUS systems, including differences among the various mechanical systems and their different catheters. While these differences are not large enough to influence clin-

ical decision making, they are important in all mechanistic studies – particularly studies of progression/regression, transplant vasculopathy, and restenosis, where reproducibility, accuracy, and precision are more critical.

Ideally, for serial studies of device mechanisms, progression/regression, and restenosis, volumetric analyses should be performed. This will obviate the problem of image slice selection since the minimum lumen area can migrate significantly from pre-intervention to post-intervention to follow-up. Volumetric analysis requires motorized transducer pullback; this should be performed at 0.5 mm/s. The transducer should be placed at least 5–10 mm distal to the distal end of the segment of interest. It is important to begin imaging and recording prior to initiating motorized transducer pullback to avoid missing the distal end of the segment.

Planar analysis

However, if volumetric analysis is not performed, it is often advisable to measure several image slices to more completely describe the lesion: e.g. the anatomic locations of the slices with the smallest pre-intervention, post-intervention, and follow-up lumen areas. If only one image slice is to be measured, then it is important to compare image slice(s) with the same anatomic location; otherwise, the process (device effect, restenosis, etc.) cannot be separated from the axial variation in EEM, lumen, and P&M CSA. Image slice selection depends on the purpose of the analysis. For example, when studying the restenosis process, the anatomic location of the image slice with the smallest lumen CSA at follow-up should be selected for analysis; and the corresponding post-intervention (and pre-intervention) image slices should be identified and measured. When studying device mechanisms, then the anatomic location of the image slice with either the smallest pre-intervention minimum lumen CSA or the smallest post-intervention minimum lumen CSA should be used.

In this regard, motorized pullback is an important tool; it facilitates identification of the same anatomic section on multiple studies by measuring the distance to a reproducible fiduciary point (edge of a stent, branch, perivascular landmark, unusual calcium deposit, etc). The following sequence can be used to identify image slices on serial studies:

(1)   An image slice is selected from one study, and the distance from this image slice to the closest identifiable axial landmark (a fiduciary point) is measured (using seconds or frames of videotape);

(2)   Another study is screened to identify this fiduciary point, and the previously measured distance is used to identify the corresponding image slices on the second study;

(3) Vascular and perivascular markings (e.g. small side-branches, venous structures, and calcific and fibrotic deposits) are used to confirm slice identification. If necessary, the two studies are analyzed side-by-side and the imaging runs studied frame-by-frame to ensure that the anatomic slices correspond correctly.

Progression/regression

Nearly all IVUS studies of progression/regression employ volumetric IVUS methodology. A segment of a vessel is identified, and the ultrasound catheter is placed distal to a fiduciary point such as a coronary branch. Motorized pullback is performed, typically at 0.5 mm/s. Using the fiduciary side branch as the starting point, a long segment of vessel (25–50 mm) is analyzed, measuring the EEM, lumen, and P&M CSA at fixed intervals. Because a long pullback will contain at least 1000 frames, the analysis is routinely performed by making cross-sectional measurements at predefined intervals, typically every 1.0 mm or 0.5 mm. Nevertheless, some site matching is usually required because the fiduciary points

are often slightly different in sequences obtained at various time points. When calculating changes in P&M CSA and volume, the assumption is made that there is no change in media thickness, area, and volume. Volumetric as well as mean CSA analysis should be reported.

Restenosis

IVUS should be performed using motorized transducer pullback, and volumetric as well as mean CSA analysis should be reported. Protocols must be designed to image the entire treated segment, not just the lesion. This includes the lesion plus at least 5–10 mm proximal and distal to the lesion. Proximal and distal edges should be analyzed and reported separately. Understanding lesion effects – particularly intra-stent intimal hyperplasia – is more straightforward than understanding edge effects. Edge effects can be very focal and vary over short distances; therefore, it is preferable to analyze and report studies millimeter by millimeter over the length of the edge rather than merely averaging 5-mm-long edge segments. Averaging 5-mm-long edge segments can mask focal changes.

REFERENCES

1. Mintz GS, Nissen SE, Anderson WD, et al. Standards for the acquisition, measurement, and reporting of intravascular ultrasound studies: a report of the American College of Cardiology Task Force on Clinical Expert Consensus Documents. J Am Coll Cardiol 2001; 37: 1478–92
2. DiMario C, Gorge G, Peters R, et al. Clinical application and image interpretation in intracoronary ultrasound. Study Group on Intracoronary Imaging of the Working Group of Coronary Circulation and of the Subgroup on Intravascular Ultrasound of the Working Group of Echocardiography of the European Society of Cardiology. Eur Heart J 1998; 19: 207–29
3. Fitzgerald PJ, St. Goar FG, Connolly AJ, et al. Intravascular ultrasound imaging of coronary arteries. Is three layers the norm? Circulation 1992; 86: 154–8
4. Maheswaran B, Leung CY, Gutfinger DE, et al. Intravascular ultrasound appearance of normal and mildly diseased coronary arteries: correlation with histologic specimens. Am Heart J 1995; 130: 976–86
5. Porter TR, Radio SJ, Anderson JA, et al. Composition of coronary atherosclerotic plaque in the intima and media affects intravascular ultrasound measurements of media thickness. J Am Coll Cardiol 1994; 23: 1079–84
6. Isner J M, Donaldson RF, Fortin AH, et al. Attenuation of the media of coronary arteries in advanced atherosclerosis. Am J Cardiol 1986; 58: 937–9
7. Gussenhoven EJ, Frietman PAV, Tee SHK, et al. Assessment of medial thinning in atherosclerosis by intravascular ultrasound. Am J Cardiol 1991; 68: 1625–32
8. Velican D, Velican C. Comparative study on age-related changes and atherosclerosis involvement of the coronary arteries of male and female subjects up to 40 years of age. Atherosclerosis 1981; 38: 39–50
9. Mallery JA, Tobis JM, Griffith J, et al. Assessment of normal and atherosclerotic arterial wall thickness with an intravascular ultrasound imaging catheter. Am Heart J 1990; 119: 1392–400
10. Takagi A, Sumiyoshi T, Kawaguchi M, et al. Cutting into the sonolucent zone after coronary atherectomy: correlation between intravascular ultrasound images and histological findings. J Am Coll Cardiol 1996; 27: 199A (abstract)
11. Mintz GS, Douek P, Pichard AD, et al. Target lesion calcification in coronary artery disease: an intravascular ultrasound study. J Am Coll Cardiol 1992; 20: 1149–55
12. Spray TL, Roberts WC. Changes in saphenous veins used as aortocoronary bypass grafts. Am Heart J 1977; 500–16
13. Jain SP, Roubin GS, Nanda NC, et al. Intravascular ultrasound imaging of saphenous vein graft stenosis. Am J Cardiol 1992; 69: 133–6
14. Keren G, Douek P, Oblon C, et al. Atherosclerotic saphenous vein grafts treated with different interventional procedures assessed by intravascular ultrasound. Am Heart J 1992; 124: 198–206
15. Mendelsohn FO, Foster GP, Palacios I, et al. In vivo assessment by intravascular ultrasound of enlargement in saphenous vein bypass grafts. Am J Cardiol 1995; 76: 1066–9
16. Willard JE, Netto D, Demian SE, et al. Intravascular ultrasound imaging of saphenous vein grafts in vitro: comparison with histologic and quantitative angiographic findings. J Am Coll Cardiol 1992; 19: 759–64

17. Ge J, Liu F, Bhate R, et al. Does remodeling occur in the diseased human saphenous vein bypass grafts? An intravascular ultrasound study. Int J Card Imaging 1999; 15: 295–300
18. Hong M-K, Mintz GS, Hong MK, et al. Intravascular ultrasound assessment of the presence of vascular remodeling in diseased human saphenous vein bypass grafts. Am J Cardiol 1999; 84: 992–8
19. Nishioka T, Luo H, Berglund H, et al. Absence of focal compensatory enlargement or constriction in diseased human coronary saphenous vein bypass grafts. Circulation 1996; 93: 683–90
20. Fuessl RT, Mintz GS, Pichard AD, et al. In vivo validation of intravascular ultrasound length measurements using a motorized transducer pullback device. Am J Cardiol 1996; 77: 1115–18
21. Hodgson JMcB, Eberle M, Savakus A Validation of a new real time percutaneous intravascular ultrasound imaging catheter. Circulation 1988; 78: II-21 (abstract)
22. Hodgson JMcB, Graham SP, Sarakus AD, et al. Clinical percutaneous imaging of coronary anatomy using an over-the-wire ultrasound catheter system. Int J Card Imaging 1989; 4: 186–93
23. Gussenhoven EJ, Essed CE, Lancee CT, et al. Arterial wall characteristics determined by intravascular ultrasound imaging: an in vitro study. J Am Coll Cardiol 1989; 14: 947–52
24. Tobis JM, Mallery JA, Gessert J, et al. Intravascular ultrasound cross-sectional arterial imaging before and after balloon angioplasty in vitro. Circulation 1989; 80: 873–82
25. Potkin BN, Bartorelli AL, Gessert JM, et al. Coronary artery imaging with intravascular high-frequency ultrasound. Circulation 1990; 81: 1575–85
26. Nishimura RA, Edwards WD, Warnes CA, et al. Intravascular ultrasound imaging: in vitro validation and pathologic correlation. J Am Coll Cardiol 1990; 16: 145–54
27. Wenguang L, Gussenhoven WJ, Zhong Y, et al. Validation of quantitative analysis of intravascular ultrasound images. Int J Card Imaging 1991; 6: 247–53
28. DiMario C, The SH, Madretsma S, et al. Detection and characterization of vascular lesions by intravascular ultrasound: an in vitro study correlated with histology. J Am Soc Echocardiogr 1992; 5: 135–46
29. Matar FA, Mintz GS, Farb A, et al. The contribution of tissue removal to lumen improvement after directional coronary atherectomy. Am J Cardiol 1994; 74: 647–50
30. von Birgelen C, Kutryk MJB, Gil R, et al. Quantification of the minimal luminal cross-sectional area after coronary stenting by two- and three-dimensional intravascular ultrasound versus edge detection and videodensitometry. Am J Cardiol 1996; 78: 520–5
31. von Birgelen C, Mintz GS, de Feyter PJ, et al. Reconstruction and quantification with three-dimensional intracoronary ultrasound: an update on techniques, challenges, and future directions. Eur Heart J 1997; 18: 1056–67
32. von Birgelen C, van der Lugt A, Nicosia A, et al., Computerized assessment of coronary lumen and atherosclerotic plaque dimensions in three-dimensional intravascular ultrasound correlated with histomorphometry. Am J Cardiol 1996; 78: 1202–9
33. Tobis JM, Mallery J, Mahon D, et al. Intravascular ultrasound imaging of human coronary arteries in vivo. Analysis of tissue characterizations with comparison to in vitro histological specimens. Circulation 1991; 83: 913–26
34. Gussenhoven EJ, Essed CE, Frietman P, et al. Intravascular echographic assessment of vessel wall characteristics: a correlation with histology. Int J Cardiol Imaging 1989; 4: 105–16
35. Kimura BJ, Bhargava V, De Maria AN. Value and limitations of intravascular ultrasound imaging in characterizing coronary atherosclerotic plaque. Am Heart J 1995; 130: 386–96
36. de Winter SA, Heller I, Hamers R, et al. Computer-assisted three-dimensional plaque characterization in intracoronary ultrasound studies. Comput Cardiol 2003; 30: 73–6
37. Nair A, Kuban BD, Tuzcu EM, et al. Coronary plaque classification with intravascular ultrasound radiofrequency data analysis. Circulation 2002; 2200–6
38. Friedrich GJ, Moes NY, Muhlberger VA, et al. Detection of intralesional calcium by intracoronary ultrasound depends on the histologic pattern. Am Heart J 1994; 128: 434–41
39. Gutfinger DE, Leung CY, Hiro T, et al. In vitro atherosclerotic plaque and calcium quantitation by intravascular ultrasound and electron-beam computed tomography. Am Heart J 1996; 131: 899–906
40. Scott DS, Arora UK, Farb A, et al. Pathologic validation of a new method to quantify coronary calcific deposits in vivo using intravascular ultrasound. Am J Cardiol 2000; 85: 37–40
41. Tinana A, Mintz GS, Weissman NJ. Volumetric intravascular ultrasound quantification of the amount of atherosclerosis and calcium in nonstenotic arterial segments. Am J Cardiol 2002; 89: 757–60
42. Hiro T, Leung CY, de Guzman S, et al. Are "soft echoes" really soft? Ultrasound assessment of mechanical properties in human atherosclerotic tissue. Am Heart J 1977; 133: 1–7
43. Kok WE, Peters RJ, Prins MH, et al. Contribution of age and intimal lesion morphology to coronary artery wall mechanics in coronary artery disease. Clin Sci (Colch) 1995; 89: 239–46
44. Chemarin-Alibelli MJ, Pieraggi MT, Elbaz M, et al. Identification of coronary thrombus after myocardial infarction by intracoronary ultrasound compared with histology of tissues sampled by atherectomy. Am J Cardiol 1996; 77: 344–9
45. Frimerman A, Miller HI, Hallman M, et al. Intravascular ultrasound characterization of thrombi of different composition. Am J Cardiol 1994; 73: 1053–7

3
Practical considerations

Major resistances to the routine use of IVUS include procedural cost, physician education (both how to interpret the images and how to use the information), equipment complexity, and difficulties in integrating IVUS into a busy catheterization laboratory. IVUS will be used routinely only if it is quick to set up, easy to perform, and does not slow down the flow of the clinical cases. None of the past or current manufacturers has designed a product that is simple and fast. Therefore, an alternative approach – organizing the laboratory for efficiency – becomes necessary.

LABORATORY SET-UP

Each catheterization laboratory is set up differently. Even tasks performed by the same health-care professionals vary from laboratory to laboratory. The following are ideas and suggestions that have worked in one or more settings. With attention to detail, it is possible to integrate clinical IVUS imaging into a busy laboratory, maintain image acquisition standards, and not add significant time to the overall procedure (i.e. not add more than 5 min for an average of three runs: pre-intervention, at some time during the procedure, and post-intervention).

Director

There must also be a physician in charge. Integration of IVUS will be most successful if it is under the administrative structure of the Cardiac Catheterization Laboratory, not the Non-invasive Imaging (Echocardiographic) Laboratory. The temperament of the two environments is very different, interventional procedures cannot be put "on hold" waiting for arrival of equipment and/or personnel, and the individuals involved in IVUS imaging must have an understanding of coronary and vascular intervention.

Equipment

All currently available equipment provides clinically useful IVUS imaging information. That said, there are major subjective differences in image presentation, system design, system controls, and catheter handling among manufacturers. For example, electronic catheters are long-monorail designs; while slightly larger in diameter at the distal end compared with mechanical catheters, they maintain the same size along the rest of the shaft. Most mechanical catheters are short-monorail designs that do not easily negotiate tortuous arteries or stenoses just distal to a bend (e.g. ostial left circumflex stenosis). Short monorails are prone to prolapse; as a result, the tip should never be advanced over the floppy end of a guidewire. (An alternative mechanical catheter design is also available. This design has a long distal monorail section that alternatively can accommodate the guidewire or the transducer, but not both. The catheter is inserted over the guidewire into the distal vessel, the guidewire is withdrawn to its proximal "parked" position, the transducer is advanced into the distal section, imaging is performed, the transducer is withdrawn to its proximal "parked" position, the guidewire is advanced into the distal vessel, and the IVUS catheter is removed.)

Each laboratory must make its own decisions about equipment purchase. However, several recommendations apply to any major purchase:

- It is important to try out all of the available equipment before making a decision. Look at the images, handle the catheters, play with the system controls, etc.
- Establish a consensus among the operators.
- Any negotiation for purchase should include upgrades for a definable period because IVUS equipment is in a constant state of flux, with improvements always on the drawing board.
- Particularly in countries where IVUS technology is sold and serviced by distributors, it is important to evaluate the local organization as well as the actual technology.

- Depending on a laboratory's interventional and IVUS volume, it may make sense to purchase equipment from more than one manufacturer. However, it is better to be expert with one system than to be uncomfortable in the use of several.

Personnel

Even in a busy laboratory with constant IVUS use, it is difficult to train all laboratory personnel. This is particularly true if multiple IVUS imaging systems are used.

Many practical aspects of IVUS imaging (e.g. handling of videotapes) are foreign to traditional catheterization laboratory practices. IVUS imaging is facilitated by designating specific individuals who become responsible for all practical aspects of IVUS imaging:

(1) Equipment and catheter set-up;
(2) Image optimization;
(3) Proper recording of IVUS imaging runs;
(4) Accurate voice and onscreen alphanumeric documentation;
(5) Correct image interpretation and measurements;
(6) Patient and procedure logs;
(7) Equipment maintenance, etc.

These individuals can be fellows, nurses, or technologists depending on how a laboratory is staffed; but these individuals must be based in the catheterization laboratory, not just available if and when needed. For example, technologists can be trained to interpret images accurately, make measurements, provide the iterative feedback necessary for IVUS-based decision-making, and answer questions posed by the primary operators. Some authorities have criticized this approach, stating that IVUS technologists will become decision-makers and practice medicine. However, non-invasive technologists have analogous roles in the echocardiographic laboratory as do quantitative coronary angiographic technologists in the catheterization laboratory. Technologists can provide information to physicians who then make the clinical or procedural decisions. In fact, with time, particularly in a busy laboratory with many operators, technologists can become more expert at image interpretation than their physician counterparts – a parallel that exists in other clinical situations.

Off-line measurements

Measurements should be made off-line from replay of the videotape or hard drive after the imaging run is complete, not when the catheter is in the vessel. This saves procedure time and minimizes patient ischemia.

Angiographic monitors

The angiographic (e.g. "road-map") monitors can be "wired" to display the IVUS images. Angiographic monitors offer superior resolution, are convenient and visible to the operator, and allow the IVUS machine to be placed in a position away from the patient table and out of the way of the nurses providing patient care. The most up-to-date IVUS machines interface automatically with many different monitors. Older machines may require dedicated connections.

Procedural annotation

Accurate procedural information is critical. Even when recording verbal commentary, it is helpful if on-line procedural information is annotated onto the ultrasound system's video screen. The ideal on-screen labeling should contain three elements: (1) the timing of IVUS imaging (e.g. pre-intervention, etc.); (2) the procedure being performed (e.g. stent with information about size, length, and inflation pressure); and (3) the target vessel and location (e.g. proximal left anterior descending). It is often necessary to be creative with abbreviations in order to fit all of this into the small space that is allotted. Systems provide for voice annotation; however, voice annotation is no substitute for alphanumeric documentation, since the audio track can be erased, not copied, when duplicates are made, or fail.

All IVUS instruments have internal clocks, and the time is automatically recorded when the study is performed. It is helpful to note the time that corresponds to the center of the lesion. In the absence of systematic pre-intervention imaging, voice annotation or recording the time corresponding to the lesion may be the only way to identify the target lesion on subsequent review. It is important that these clocks be set to the correct local time.

IVUS imaging – with a notation of the vessel being imaged – should also be documented on the interventional procedure log or flow sheet.

Videotape and digital archiving

Good-quality videotapes are essential. It is recommended that virgin (never-used) broadcast-quality s-VHS tapes be used. There is a significant quality difference, and the cost differential is minimal. Videotapes should be stored in a secure place. Although they are not expensive, tapes become irresistible targets for petty thieves because they can be used in home or studio videocassette recorders. Back-up copies of each tape can be made by hooking two VCRs together. Both VCRs should be medical-grade s-VHS units with s-Video turned on, not "home theater" units that typically record and play at slower speeds that affect image quality. If there is voice annotation information, then the audio circuit must be linked as well. The first-generation copy loses some image quality, but is usually acceptable. The second-generation copy (copy of a copy) loses too much image information to be useful. Videotape storage can become unwieldy if each patient has a separate tape. In general, 20 studies can be recorded on each 120-min tape and numbered sequentially. Individual tapes (for each patient) should be reserved for multicenter studies in which the videotape must be sent away to a core laboratory. Video standards vary among continents; studies recorded in Europe (which uses the PAL standard) are incompatible with Western Hemisphere equipment that is based on the NTSC standard.

IVUS images are recorded at 72 pixels (lines) per inch, the video standard. This means that every pixel is approximately 0.35 mm; this also affects the resolution of IVUS. However, recording studies onto videotape superimposes the inherent problems of this medium onto the fundamental limitations of IVUS and video. For this and other reasons, manufacturers are moving to digital storage. Although the hard drive can handle only a limited number of studies (digitally recorded IVUS studies are large files), the studies can then be transferred to CDs that are now DICOM-compatible. Recalling studies from the hard drive or CDs can take a while. It is possible to store the digital IVUS studies together with the angiograms on a server. Unless IVUS studies are stored on a server, it is worthwhile to create copies of each CD. An unlimited number of copies can be made – even copies of copies – without image quality degradation.

Logbooks

Logbooks and simple databases are important for identifying patients who have been studied with IVUS and for locating the actual study. The minimum information is the patient's name, date of the study (and perhaps the time), vessel imaged, procedure, primary operator, and any unique findings. If videotapes are still being used, one page in a logbook should represent each videotape; and each patient should be recorded in the order that corresponds to the sequence of studies on the tape. This information should be entered into a simple database that can be easily searched. If only digital storage is used, then just a database (without a logbook) is necessary.

Noise

Many catheterization laboratories have excessive ambient electrical or radiofrequency noise that can produce artifacts on the ultrasound image. This paragraph is not meant to be a complete listing of these noisemakers, and troubleshooting becomes an art. Offenders include monitoring equipment, intraaortic balloon pumps, etc. Eliminating these problems requires working with both the IVUS and non-IVUS equipment vendors and in-house biomedical engineering. The Doppler FloWire can cause two types of interference: one is electrical, but the other is crosstalk between the two ultrasound instruments. Ultrasonic crosstalk is present whenever two sources of ultrasound are used simultaneously. In addition, in some hospitals, the paging system generates a radiofrequency signal that interferes with the IVUS image. Examples of noise are shown in Figures 1.4 and 1.10.

IMAGE ACQUISITION

In a busy laboratory with multiple operators, it is important to standardize image acquisition and analysis. Standardization facilitates off-line analysis and comparison of serial (pre- versus post-intervention or post-intervention versus follow-up) studies; it is *essential* for multicenter studies where imaging standards are dictated by the core laboratory.

There are two technical approaches to imaging: motorized or manual interrogation. Regardless of which approach is adopted, imaging should include careful uninterrupted imaging of (1) at least 10 mm of distal reference, (2) the lesion site(s), and (3) the entire proximal reference back to the aorta.

Motorized transducer pullback

The use of motorized transducer pullback aids (in fact, enforces) discipline and acquisition standards; there is no question of whether the transducer is being advanced or withdrawn. A pullback speed of 0.5 mm/s is preferable; by trial and error, this is the fastest rate at which the trained eye can assimilate the information. Faster pullback speeds have the disadvantage of imaging focal pathology too quickly, but they are commonly employed for longer extracardiac vessels in order to minimize imaging times. Important advantages of motorized pullback are:

(1) Controlled catheter withdrawal so that no segment of the vessel is skipped or imaged too quickly by pulling the catheter too rapidly;
(2) Ability to concentrate on the images without having to pay attention simultaneously to catheter manipulation;
(3) Length and volumetric measurements; and
(4) Uniform and reproducible image acquisition for multicenter and serial studies.

Disadvantages of motorized pullback are:

(1) Even at very slow pullback speeds, it is possible to skip over very focal lesions;
(2) Not enough attention may be paid to important regions of interest; and
(3) It is not possible to have the transducer "sit" at one specific site in the vessel.

Thus, with very focal stenoses, particularly ostial stenoses, a pullback speed of 0.25 mm/s is preferable if it is available. Motorized transducer pullback also does not preclude additional, careful manually controlled interrogation of the lesion or of a focal region of interest. When imaging stents, measured stent length (number of seconds multiplied by pullback speed) should closely equal the length of the implanted metal; this serves as an internal validation of motorized pullback image acquisition. Even with motorized pullback, there is axial motion of the catheter relative to the vessel between diastole and systole.

Manual transducer pullback

Manual transducer pullback should be performed slowly at a rate similar to motorized pullback. Advantages are the ability to concentrate on specific regions of interest by pausing the transducer at a specific location in the vessel. When left stationary, the spontaneous antegrade and retrograde motion of the transducer can be useful to study a lesion more closely. Disadvantages of manual transducer pullback include the possibility of skipping over significant pathology by pulling the transducer too quickly or unevenly and the inability to perform precise length and volume measurements. Furthermore, operators almost always tend to advance and withdraw the catheter when imaging interesting vessel segments; this seems to be irresistable and unavoidable and is confusing when the study is reviewed at a later date. Therefore, it is always important to perform one complete, uninterrupted imaging run from distal to proximal.

Special considerations for imaging aorto-ostial and left main lesions

In imaging an aorto-ostial lesion (ostial right coronary artery, ostial left main, or ostial vein graft), it is important to retract the guiding catheter back into the aorta. If not, the true aorto-ostial lesion will not be imaged, and the guiding catheter may be mistaken as a circumferentially calcified lesion whose lumen is the internal diameter of the guiding catheter (Figures 1.11 and 1.12). After backing-out the guiding catheter, it is important to verify that the path of the IVUS transducer will still be coaxial to the ostium of the vessel. Otherwise, the lumen will be imaged obliquely, and this is one of the situations where non-coaxial catheter alignment can result in an overestimation of lumen and other measurements –

particularly if the vessel has an upward take-off angle or if the lesion is short. (Conversely, non-coaxial catheter angulation cannot make even an aorto-ostial stenosis appear artificially severe.) Imaging of an aorto-ostial lesion should continue until there is visualization of the aorta. This is also important post-intervention to ensure that an ostial stent does, in fact, cover the ostium and is fully expanded. An example is shown in Figure 3.1 Figure 3.2. Many purported cases of ostial stent recoil are, in fact, stents that were never properly imaged post-implantation to verify correct placement (covering the ostial lesion with slight protrusion into the aorta) and full expansion.

When imaging the left main, it is important to put the guidewire and the IVUS catheter distally into the artery that is most co-axial with the left main – in most cases, the left anterior descending. This is another situation where non-coaxial catheter alignment and oblique vessel imaging can result in overestimation of lumen and other measurements (Figure 3.3). This is especially problematic if there is an acute angle into the distal vessel, if the left main stenosis is a distal location, or if the stenosis is short. Conversely, non-coaxial catheter angulation cannot make even a distal left main stenosis appear artificially severe. (In addition, when imaging the left anterior descending or left circumflex, it is always advisable to image the left main during at least one imaging run. It is a "free" look at the vessel that most influences patient outcome.)

SAFETY

Operator training

IVUS imaging should be considered an interventional technique. All IVUS operators should be trained in percutaneous coronary interventions. While uncommon, complications do occur – even when just engaging the guiding catheter (Figures 3.4 and 3.5) or advancing the guidewire (Figure 3.6). Each catheterization laboratory should establish its own credentials for catheter handling and image interpretation.

Adjunct pharmacology

Today most diagnostic coronary angiograms are performed without anticoagulation. When converting from a diagnostic angiogram to IVUS imaging, it is important to give the patient an anticoagulant (unfractionated or low-molecular-weight heparin, bivalrudin, etc.) before inserting the IVUS catheter into a coronary artery. Otherwise, there is a risk of thrombosis (Figure 3.7). For example, most of the time, 3500 units of unfractionated heparin will prolong the PTT (but not the ACT), provide adequate protection, and still allow the sheaths to be removed promptly with or without an access closure device. Most of the current catheters are 6-Fr compatible which facilitates hemostasis. IVUS imaging can, therefore, be performed on an outpatient basis just like a diagnostic angiogram.

It is also advisable to give intracoronary nitroglycerine (100–200 μg) before imaging to avoid catheter-induced spasm and minimize ischemia. This is particularly important with pre-intervention and diagnostic imaging. If the patient has already received nitroglycerine or is on a nitroglycerine drip, additional intracoronary nitroglycerine is still important. The dose should be limited only by the patient's blood pressure.

Technical issues

Care must be used in crossing stents immediately after placement, particularly if wire position has been lost and the stent recrossed. The wire may enter the stent through a cell rather than through the end. This is also a potential concern when imaging a side branch that has been jailed by a main-vessel stent or after bifurcation stenting. In these cases, it may be more prudent to use a long-monorail catheter design.

The relatively short monorail tip of the mechanical catheters can easily bend or kink, particularly in tortuous segments – a "shepherd's crook" right coronary artery or acute take-off of the left circumflex from the left main – and especially if there is a tight stenosis just distal to the bend or tortuous segment. If a wire loop develops, it may be prudent to remove the IVUS catheter, guidewire, and guiding catheter as a single unit. Short-monorail catheter issues should become less of a problem if the 16-cm long-monorail mechanical catheter design is available.

With mechanical systems, if the catheter was not flushed prior to insertion into the coronary artery, or with older catheter designs that may trap a considerable amount of air in the transducer, flushing the catheter in the coronary artery may lead to air embolization. A small amount of air is well tolerated. A large amount may lead to chest pain, ST segment elevation, and diminished flow, no-reflow, or vessel cut-off. Therapy includes the administration of vasodilators, analgesics, and 100% oxygen via mask.

Ischemia

Despite miniaturization of ultrasound catheters, pre-intervention imaging can result in lumen occlusion and, occasionally, ischemia. However, the amount of ischemia is usually modest, is reduced by administration of intracoronary

nitroglycerin prior to introducing the IVUS catheter, and is usually well tolerated. Common sense should prevail. Excessively long imaging runs should be avoided (i.e. it is not necessary to start in the distal left anterior descending when the lesion is in the left main), and the catheter should be removed in the setting of significant angina with ECG changes. Ischemia can also be minimized by making measurements from the recorded study, not during live imaging.

Published studies

The above examples and issues not withstanding, there have been three large pre-1996 studies of the safety of IVUS. Other than transient spasm, acute complications appear to be rare, and long-term sequelae are not different from controls.

Hausman et al.[1] reported 2207 patients from 28 centers (including 915 patients studied for diagnostic purposes). There were no complications in 2034 patients (92.2%). In 87 patients (3.9%), complications were judged to be unrelated to IVUS imaging. In 63 patients (2.9%), transient spasm occurred during imaging. In 9 patients (0.4%), complications were judged to have a "certain" relationship to IVUS (5 acute occlusions, 2 dissections, 1 embolism, and 1 dissection). In 14 patients (0.6%), complications were judged to have an "uncertain" relationship to IVUS (5 acute occlusions, 3 dissections, and 1 arrhythmia). Major events (acute myocardial infarction or emergency bypass surgery) occurred in 3 of 9 and 5 of 14 of these patients, respectively. The complication rate was higher in patients with unstable angina or acute myocardial infarction and in patients undergoing intervention (as apposed to just diagnostic imaging).

Batkoff and Linker[2] reported 718 IVUS "examinations" performed at 12 centers. There were 8 events (1.1%), but no adverse clinical consequences; all occurred in patients with unstable angina undergoing percutaneous intervention. There were 4 cases of transient vessel spasm, 2 cases of dissection, and 2 cases of wire entrapment.

Gorge et al.[3] reported 7085 IVUS studies from 51 centers. Spasm occurred in 3% of all studies. Major complications (dissection, thrombosis, ventricular fibrillation, and refractory spasm) occurred in 10 cases (0.14%). There was only one major event.

The Hausman, Batkoft, and Gorge studies,[1-3] however, did not address the potential long-term harm of IVUS imaging – i.e. progression of disease from trauma to the vessel wall. In the first such report using older-generation 5-Fr IVUS catheters, Pinto et al.[4] studied 58 cardiac transplant recipients and compared 49 IVUS-imaged vessels with 61 non-imaged vessels. At one year, there was no difference in the change in vessel diameters as assessed by quantitative coronary angiography. Two subsequent reports studied larger numbers of patients using

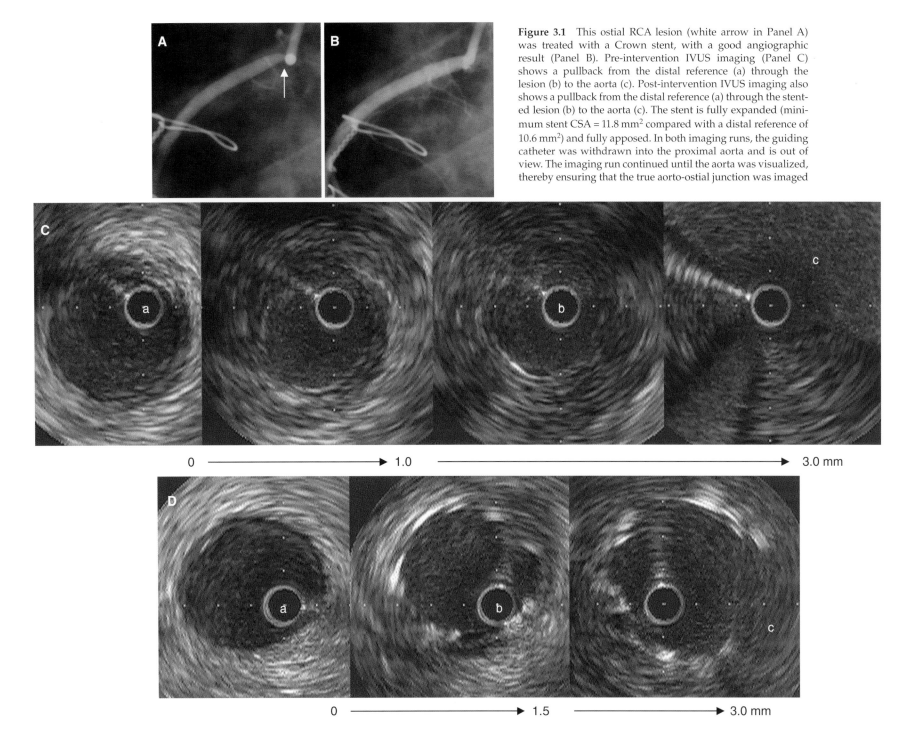

Figure 3.1 This ostial RCA lesion (white arrow in Panel A) was treated with a Crown stent, with a good angiographic result (Panel B). Pre-intervention IVUS imaging (Panel C) shows a pullback from the distal reference (a) through the lesion (b) to the aorta (c). Post-intervention IVUS imaging also shows a pullback from the distal reference (a) through the stented lesion (b) to the aorta (c). The stent is fully expanded (minimum stent CSA = 11.8 mm^2 compared with a distal reference of 10.6 mm^2) and fully apposed. In both imaging runs, the guiding catheter was withdrawn into the proximal aorta and is out of view. The imaging run continued until the aorta was visualized, thereby ensuring that the true aorto-ostial junction was imaged

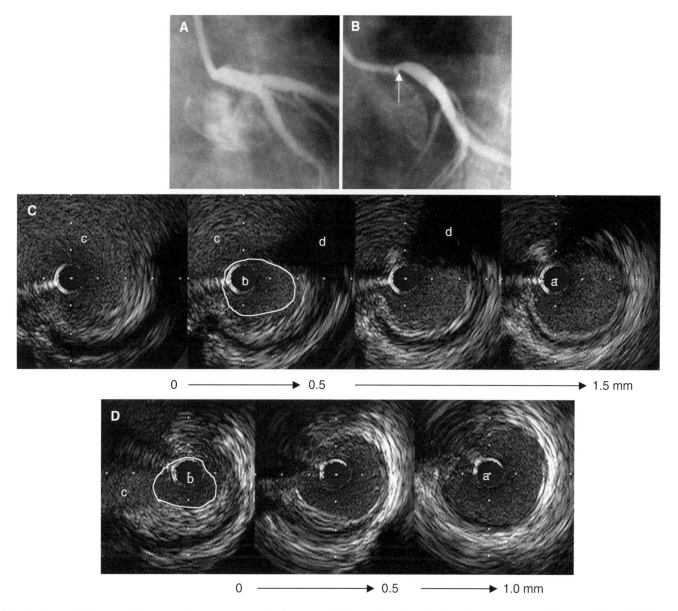

Figure 3.2 Guiding catheter orientation can affect measurements of aorto-ostial stenosis by changing transducer alignment. This eccentric ostial left main lesion (Panel A and white arrow in Panel B), was imaged twice using IVUS (Panels C and D) – from the distal reference (a) through the lesion (b) to the aorta (c). After the first imaging run (Panel C), the guiding catheter was realigned to be more coaxial with the left main ostium, and the imaging run was repeated (Panel D). In the first imaging run, where the guiding catheter was not aligned and the IVUS catheter was not coaxial, the minimum lumen CSA measured 5.5 mm^2. When the guiding and IVUS catheters were readjusted, the minimum lumen CSA measured 3.8 mm^2. The transducer angle in Panel A was also responsible for the oblique cut through the aorta in Panel C, causing acoustic shadowing (d). Transducer angulation can artifactually increase, but not decrease cross-sectional measurements

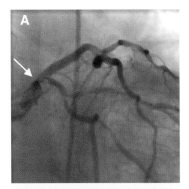

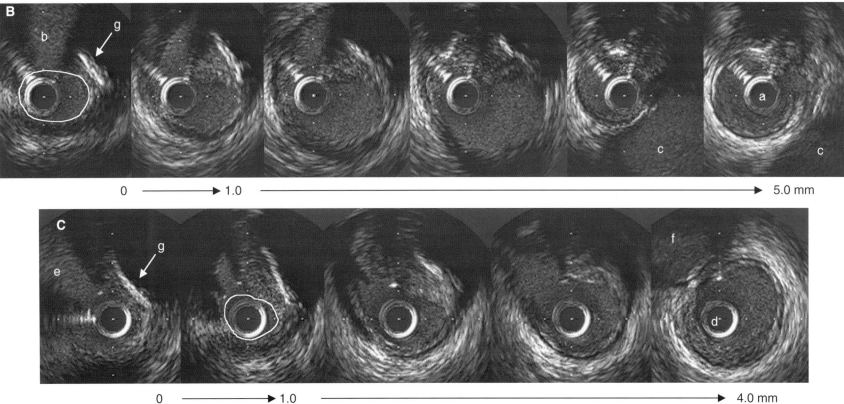

Figure 3.3 This patient presented with left circumflex in-stent restenosis and an intermediate stenosis in a short left main artery (white arrow in Panel A). IVUS imaging was first performed from the circumflex (a) to the aorta (b) because of the circumflex disease (Panel B). Note the origin of the left anterior descending (c); the left main measured 4.0 mm^2. IVUS was then repeated from the left anterior descending (d) to the aorta (e) as shown in Panel C. Note the origin of the left circumflex (f); the left main measured 1.9 mm^2. Compared with the left circumflex, the orientation of the left anterior descending is more coaxial to the left main. Note the calcium (g) in both imaging runs. Transducer angulation can artifactually increase, but not decrease cross-sectional measurements

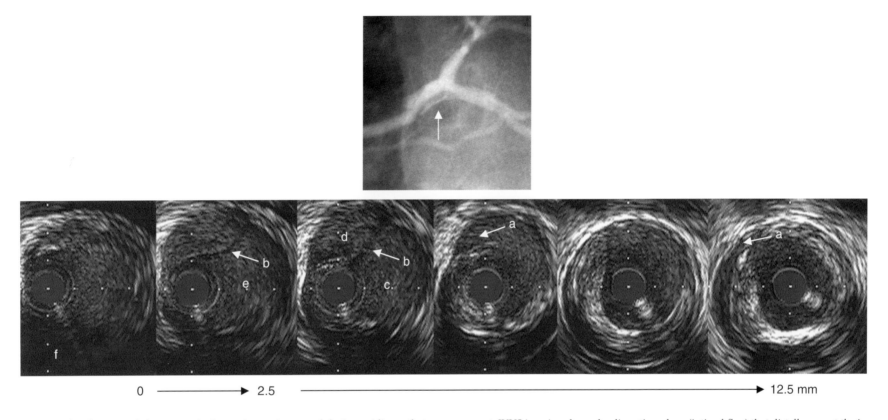

Figure 3.4 This dissection (white arrow in the angiogram) occurred during guiding catheter engagement. IVUS imaging showed a dissection plane (intimal flap) that distally was at the junction of plaque and normal vessel wall (a) while proximally was a thin membrane (b) separating true lumen (c) from false lumen (d). The true minimum lumen CSA (e) measured 8.1 mm². The thin proximal intimal flap looked echolucent compared with the blood speckle in the true and false lumina because of the reduced echogenicity of the intimal flap and because its thickness was near or below the resolution of the transducer. Notice that the pullback continued until the aorta (f) was seen

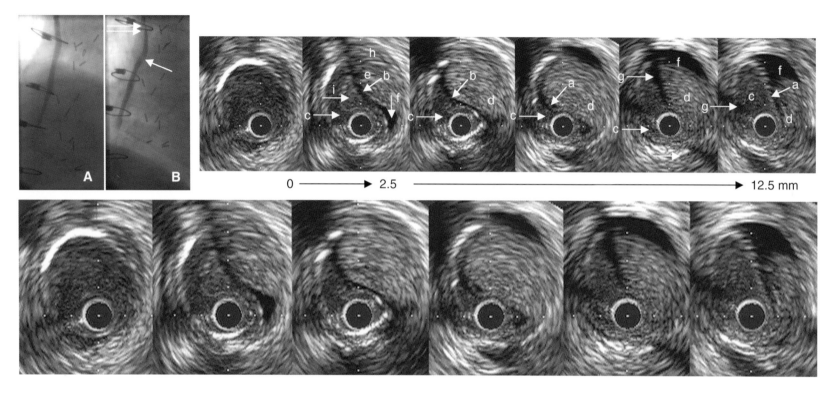

Figure 3.5 During engagement of this saphenous vein graft to the right coronary artery (Panel A), there was an abrupt decrease in lumen caliber (double white arrow in Panel B) with slow flow and suggestion of a filling defect (single white arrow in Panel B). IVUS imaging shows a flap that appears echoreflective distally (a) and echolucent proximally (b). The true lumen (c) measured 1.4 mm² at its smallest location. The false lumen was occupied by both echoreflective blood stasis (d and e) and echolucent static contrast or saline (f). The thin proximal flap looked echolucent (b) compared with the true and false lumen blood speckle (c, d, and e) because of its reduced echogenicity and because its thickness was near or below the resolution of the transducer. The guidewire artifact is indicated by the white arrow (g). These are typical features of an intramural hematoma. Intramural hematomas are a variant of a dissection. They tend to occur in normal arcs of vessel wall. The external elastic membrane expands outwards, and the internal elastic membrane is pushed inwards to become the flap (a and b) that separates the true lumen from the false lumen and causes lumen compromise. Blood accumulates in the false lumen caused by the split in the media to become static and echogenic, if not completely thrombotic. When contrast also accumulates within the split in the media, a layering of echolucent contrast or saline (f) and echogeneic blood (d) takes place. In real time, there is often evidence of "to-and-fro" motion of the blood–contrast–saline interface. The hematoma in the false lumen tends to obscure the interface between the external elastic membrane and the adventitia to create a homogeneous visual structure that includes the false lumen (e), the periadventitial structures (h), and the external elastic membrane between them. Intramural hematomas are one of the causes of filling defects during an intervention. Note the plaque (i) was pushed inwards

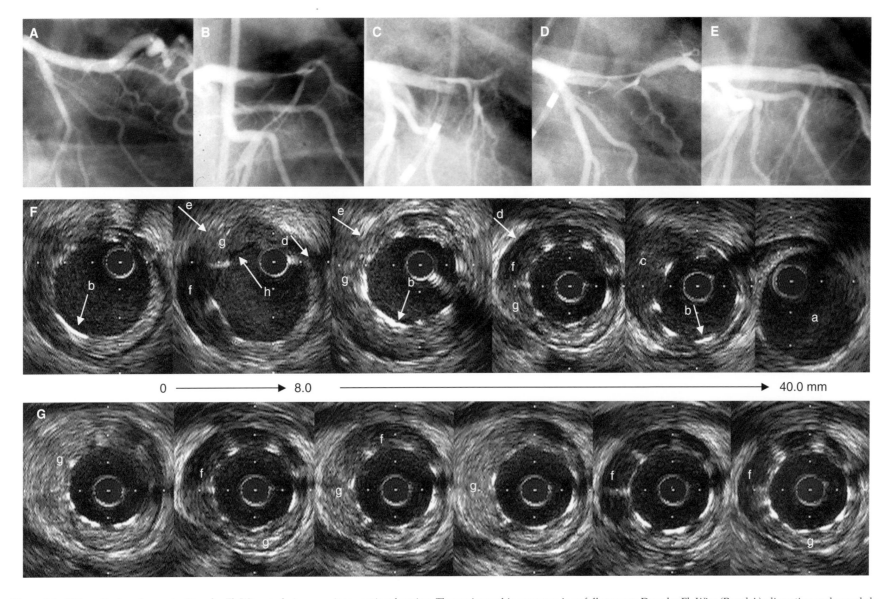

Figure 3.6 This patient underwent a Doppler FloWire study in a non-interventional setting. The angiographic sequence is as follows: pre-Doppler FloWire (Panel A); dissection and vessel closure caused during advance of the FloWire (Panel B); transfer to an interventional facility (Panel C); after crossing the dissection and balloon predilation (Panel D); and after placement of two NIR stents (Panel E). The IVUS imaging run was performed at the end of the procedure. Note that the distal vessel (a) was normal. The stent (b) crosses the major diagonal branch distally (c). Between the stent (b) and the external elastic membrane (d and e), there is retained contrast or saline (f) and blood stasis (g) that often obscures the external elastic membrane (see, in particular, e). The internal elastic membrane (h) is supported and mostly obscured by the stent, but can be seen in one of the frames. Like Figure 3.5, these are the typical features of an intramural hematoma. Intramural hematomas tend to occur in segments of normal vessel. In this case, the Doppler FloWire split the non-atherosclerotic media. The external elastic membrane bulged outwards and the internal elastic membrane collapsed inwards as blood accumulated within the media. The vessel is presumed to be normal because the distal vessel is normal and there is only contrast, saline, blood stasis, or hematoma between the stent and the external elastic membrane. In real time, retained contrast or saline (f) and blood stasis (g) could be seen to mix in a to-and-fro fashion (Panel G)

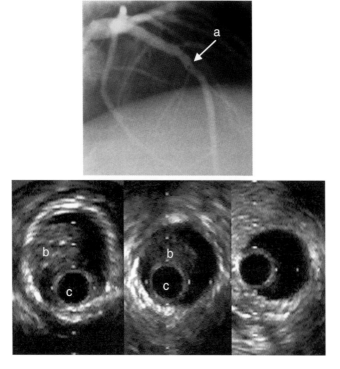

Figure 3.7 While performing an IVUS study, a small filling defect was noted in the LAD (a). In the IVUS study, notice the thrombus (b) attached to the IVUS catheter (c). Also, notice that there is no guidewire artifact when using the long-monorail solid-state catheter

Patient and Lesion Demographics

Name		Vessel	
Date		Location	
Age			
Record #		Procedure	
Physician		Indication	

Reference Segment Quantification

	Pre	Post	Final	F/U
Proximal				
EEM CSA				
Lumen CSA				
Distal				
EEM CSA				
Lumen CSA				

Lesion Pre-intervention

Plaque composition		Calcium	
Thrombus		Superficial	
Soft		Deep	
Fibrotic		Mixed	
Calcified		Arc	
Mixed		Length	
Other			
		Lesion length	

Lesion Post-intervention

Complications	
Dissection	
Hematoma	
Perforation	
Other	

Lesion Quantification

	Pre	Post	Final	F/U
Device				
EEM CSA				
Stent CSA				
Lumen CSA				

Comments

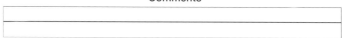

Figure 3.8 A comprehensive lesion-based IVUS report is shown. There is place for recording the main measurements for each image slice; the derived calculations (i.e. the plaque & media CSA, the area stenosis, and the plaque burden) can be determined from these measurements. In a multi-lesion study, one report should be completed for each lesion. The addition of a small drawing of the location of the lesion would also enhance this report

modern IVUS equipment (smaller catheters, etc.). Son *et al.*[5] divided 86 transplant recipients into three groups: no IVUS, IVUS of the left anterior descending performed only at the end of the first post-operative year, and IVUS of the left anterior performed both at baseline and at one year post-transplant. Angiographically, there were no differences between instrumented and non-instrumented arteries (i.e. the left circumflex) at baseline, during the first post-operative year, or additional changes in the second post-operative year.

Recently, Ramasubbu *et al.*[6] reported a study of 226 transplant recipients in whom 548 arteries were imaged and 130 arteries were not imaged. On subsequent angiograms, stenoses were observed in 19.5% of imaged arteries and 16.2% of non-imaged arteries ($p = 0.4$). Regardless of the number of IVUS studies and the duration of follow-up, late arterial diameters of imaged and non-imaged arteries were similar, and there was a significant, but similar, decrease in arterial diameters of imaged and non-imaged arteries. Thus, IVUS imaging does not appear to be associated with any long-term sequelae – at least as studied in transplant recipients.

STEPS

The following are the basic steps required in performing an IVUS study.

- Position the guidewire in the distal vessel.
- Make sure that the patient is adequately anticoagulated.
- Administer intracoronary nitroglycerin.
- (If using the solid-state system, position the IVUS catheter outside the guiding catheter in the aorta and perform catheter near-field subtraction, if necessary.)
- Advance the IVUS catheter distal to the target site.
- Begin imaging and verify that the image is acceptable or, if necessary, tweak the overall gain to compensate for a weak catheter and adjust the zoom (depth) for large vessels.
- If imaging an aorto-ostial lesion, retract the guiding catheter back into the aorta and verify that the path of the IVUS transducer will still be coaxial to the ostial segment of the vessel.
- Begin recording.
- Withdraw the transducer or catheter to a point proximal to the target site – ideally, back to the aorta at least once during the procedure.
- When imaging, the transducer can be seen fluoroscopically and its position relative to the angiographic anatomy checked using small amounts of contrast injection; contrast or saline flush injection will also help delineate lumen borders (Figure 2.3 and 2.4).
- Remove the catheter and review the recorded study to make the necessary measurements.
- If the quality of the images is poor, repeat the study. If the catheter malfunctions, select a new one and send the malfunctioning catheter back to the manufacturer.

REPORT

A written report for the IVUS examination should be generated. The report helps to communicate relevant information and becomes an important part of the patient's medical record. Although the length and complexity of the report will vary greatly depending on the needs of different operators and institutions, at a minimum content should include:[7]

- Patient demographic information;
- Lesion demographic information;
- Date;
- Physician;
- Indication;
- Brief description of the IVUS procedure – for example, the equipment used, the level of anticoagulation achieved, and the coronary arteries imaged;
- Basic findings, including any measurements that were performed and any notable morphologic plaque/lesion features;
- Changes in therapy that resulted from the information provided by IVUS;
- IVUS-related complications and any consequent therapy.

In addition, a more complete report should also include the analysis of three cardinal image slices – a distal reference segment, lesion site, and a proximal reference segment (unless the lesion is ostial or just distal to a large side branch). Lumen and external elastic membrane (EEM) cross-sectional areas (CSA), calculated plaque & media (P&M) CSA, calculated plaque burden, and calculated area stenosis should be reported. If a stent is present, minimum stent CSA, expansion, and a description of strut apposition should be included. An example of a complete report form is shown in Figure 3.8. In this example, the P&M CSA, plaque burden, and area stenosis are not listed; however, the primary source numbers (lesion and reference EEM and lumen CSA) can be used to calculate these variables.

REFERENCES

1. Hausmann D, Erbel R, Alibelli-Chemarin M-J, et al. The safety of intracoronary ultrasound: a multicenter survey of 2207 examinations. Circulation 1995; 91: 623–30
2. Batkoff BW, Linker DT. The safety of intracoronary ultrasound: data from a multicenter European registry. Cathet Cardiovasc Diagn 1996; 38: 238–41
3. Gorge G, Peters RJG, Pinto F, et al. Intravascular ultrasound: safety and indications for use in 7085 consecutive patients studied in 32 centers in Europe and Israel. J Am Coll Cardiol 1996; 27: 155A (abstract)
4. Pinto FJ, St Goar FG, Gao SZ, et al. Immediate and one-year safety of intracoronary ultrasound imaging. Evaluation with serial quantitative angiography. Circulation 1993; 88: 1709–14
5. Son R, Tobis JM, Yeatman LA, et al. Does use of intravascular ultrasound accelerate arteriopathy in heart transplant recipients? Am Heart J 1999; 138: 358–63
6. Ramasubbu K, Schoenhagen P, Balghith MA, et al. Repeated intravascular ultrasound imaging in cardiac transplant recipients does not accelerate transplant coronary artery disease. J Am Coll Cardiol 2003; 41: 1739–43
7. Mintz GS, Nissen SE, Anderson WD, et al. Standards for the acquisition, measurement, and reporting of intravascular ultrasound studies: a report of the American College of Cardiology Task Force on Clinical Expert Consensus Documents. J Am Coll Cardiol 2001; 37: 1478–92

4

Quantitative and qualitative IVUS data and their angiographic correlations

There are more differences between IVUS and coronary angiography than there are similarities. Atherosclerosis is a disease of the arterial wall; angiography visualizes the arterial lumen. Coronary arteries are complex three-dimensional structures with branch points, tortuous segments, and bends; IVUS provides tomographic imaging while coronary angiography is a shadowgraph technique that visualizes the lumen in multiple projected longitudinal "silhouettes". Atherosclerosis is a diffuse process involving entire arterial segments; angiography assesses coronary artery disease by comparing stenotic with supposedly "normal" segments. This chapter describes the differences between IVUS and angiography that have been described by multiple investigators and that are important to understanding the clinical uses of IVUS. The figures and tables are based on a single-center analysis of over 3000 unselected patients – stable and unstable, interventional and diagnostic, etc.

ANGIOGRAPHICALLY NORMAL CORONARY ARTERIES

Angiograms appear normal in 10–15% of patients undergoing coronary angiography for suspected coronary artery disease. Using IVUS, plaque formation can be demonstrated in approximately half of the patients with normal angiograms.[1] Furthermore, when endothelium-mediated vasodilation is also tested, less than 40% are truly normal. This suggests the need for revision of our understanding and classification of syndrome X – true angina with normal coronary angiograms.

In support of this, IVUS studies in cardiac transplant recipients performed an average of one month post-operatively showed at least one atherosclerotic lesion (defined as intimal thickness > 0.5 mm) in approximately half of the 262 patients studied. This reflects donor atherosclerosis and is important since these donors were not thought to have coronary artery disease. The frequency of at least one

lesion using this definition was 17% in donors < 20 years, 37% in donors 20–29 years, 60% in donors 30–39 years, 71% in donors 40–49 years, and 85% in donors ≥ 50 years of age.[2,3]

REFERENCE-SEGMENT DISEASE

IVUS routinely shows significant atherosclerosis in angiographically "normal" reference segments in patients with significant stenoses undergoing intervention. In a study of 884 such patients, only 6.8% of the angiographically "normal" reference segments were disease-free, and the average plaque burden of the most normal-looking reference segment was $51 \pm 13\%$.[4] The explanation for angiographically "silent" atherosclerosis is as follows. Positive remodeling of the diseased arterial wall (increase in external elastic membrane (EEM)) occurs to compensate for the accumulation of atherosclerotic plaque. The magnitude of the increase in EEM cross-sectional area (CSA) is in direct relationship to the amount of accumulated plaque; this preserves lumen dimensions. Pathologic studies have shown that, on average, lumen compromise is delayed until the lesion occupies more than an estimated 40–50% of the potential area within the internal elastic lamina (equivalent to a 40–50% plaque burden).[5,6] However, there is a wide variation in the reference-segment plaque burden among different arterial segments, even in the same patient, depending on the amount of plaque accumulation and the degree of remodeling. In a series of over 3000 patients, the frequency distribution of the proximal and distal reference-segment plaque burdens is shown in Figure 4.1. Reference-segment plaque burdens of 70% or more in the absence of lumen compromise are not unusual and should not be equated with obstructive disease. Independent predictors of reference-segment plaque burden that have been reported include male gender, patient age, diabetes mellitus, hypercholesterolemia, and presence of multivessel disease.[4]

REFERENCE-SEGMENT MEASUREMENTS

IVUS reference-segment measurements are usually larger than angiography; however, in individual patients this difference is very variable, and some IVUS reference-segment measurements are actually smaller than angiography. In our analysis of over 3000 patients, the mean IVUS reference-segment lumen dimensions measured 0.41 ± 0.60 mm or $17 \pm 23\%$ larger than the mean angiographic reference. The difference was:

- Greatest in the left anterior descending coronary artery ($+0.48 \pm 0.56$ mm), the right coronary artery ($+0.44 \pm 0.60$ mm), and saphenous vein grafts ($+0.42 \pm 0.64$ mm); intermediate in the left circumflex ($+0.35 \pm 0.55$ mm); and least in the left main ($+0.01 \pm 0.76$ mm);
- Approximately twice as great when comparing the maximum IVUS reference-segment lumen diameter with angiography ($+0.73 \pm 0.65$ mm);
- Proportionately greater in smaller vessels, decreasing asymptotically with increasing vessel size to approach zero at an angiographic reference of approximately 3.75 mm.

A comparison of the IVUS and angiographic reference-segment lumen dimensions is shown in Figures 4.2 and 4.3. Some authorities have advocated the use of IVUS "true vessel", "media-to-media", or midwall reference-segment dimensions for device sizing; the comparisons with angiography are shown in Figures 4.4 and 4.5. These larger differences reflect reference-segment plaque accumulation and remodeling. Finally, other authorities have advocated "true vessel" or "media-to-media" lesion-site dimensions for device sizing. A comparison of IVUS lesion EEM dimensions versus angiographic dimensions is shown in Figure 4.6. Because there are many possible reference measurements, it is critically important to specify what is being compared and/or used for device sizing. For example, each vessel has a proximal and distal reference and a lesion; and each has a maximum, minimum, and mean lumen, midwall, and EEM diameter.

Tapering

Coronary arteries taper.[7] The reference-segment lumen CSA tapers 1.1 ± 1.2 mm^2 ($9 \pm 10\%$) for every 10 mm of arterial length. Lumen tapering is greater in the left anterior descending than in the right coronary or left circumflex artery. The EEM CSA tapers 2.1 ± 1.5 mm^2 ($10 \pm 6\%$) for every 10 mm of arterial length. EEM tapering tends to be greater in the left anterior descending and left circumflex than the right coronary arteries.

Lumen tapering depends both on EEM tapering and on the amount of distal versus proximal plaque accumulation. However, this varies with lesion location.

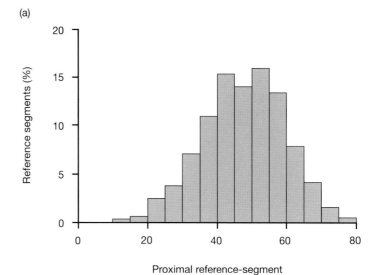

(a)

Proximal reference-segment plaque burden (%)

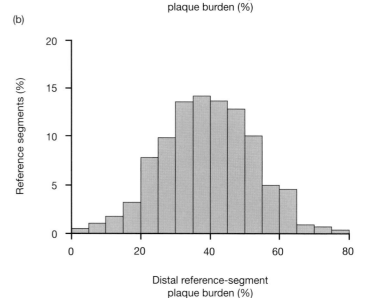

(b)

Distal reference-segment plaque burden (%)

Figure 4.1 The frequency distributions of the plaque burden in the proximal (Panel (a)) and distal (Panel (b)) angiographically normal reference segments are shown. Plaque burden is calculated as plaque & media area divided by external elastic membrane area. The mean proximal reference-segment plaque burden was $46 \pm 12\%$ and the mean distal reference-segment plaque burden was $38 \pm 17\%$

(a)

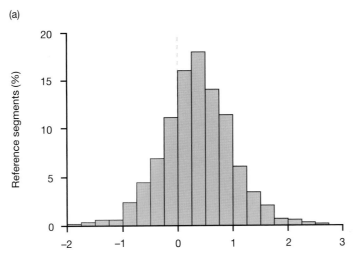

(b)

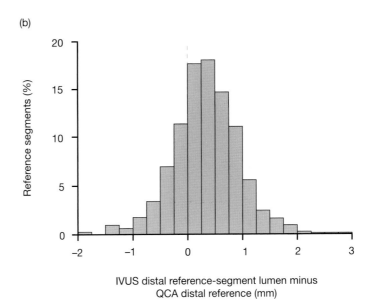

(c)

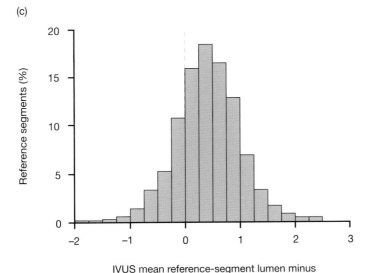

Figure 4.2 The frequency distributions of the difference between the IVUS reference-segment lumen dimensions and the angiographic reference-segment dimensions are shown. Panel (a) compares the IVUS mean proximal reference-segment lumen diameter with the proximal angiographic reference; the difference was 0.36 ± 0.64 mm. Panel (b) compares the IVUS mean distal reference-segment lumen diameter with the distal angiographic reference; the difference was 0.36 ± 0.64 mm. Panel (c) compares the IVUS mean reference-segment lumen (mean of the proximal and distal references) with the mean angiographic reference; the difference was 0.41 ± 0.60 mm. The angiographic reference was calculated using quantitative coronary angiography (QCA). The IVUS reference-segment lumen dimensions were calculated mathematically from the lumen CSAs

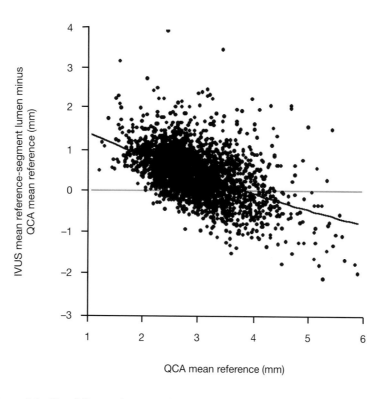

Figure 4.3 The difference between the IVUS and angiographic mean reference-segment lumen dimensions is greatest in the smallest vessels, with increasing angiographic reference diameter, and is "zero" at approximately 3.75 mm. The "zero point" was approximately the same (3.5–4.0 mm) for all vessels: left main, left anterior descending, left circumflex, and saphenous vein grafts. Angiographic measurements were calculated using quantitative coronary angiography (QCA). The IVUS reference-segment lumen dimensions were calculated mathematically from the lumen CSAs

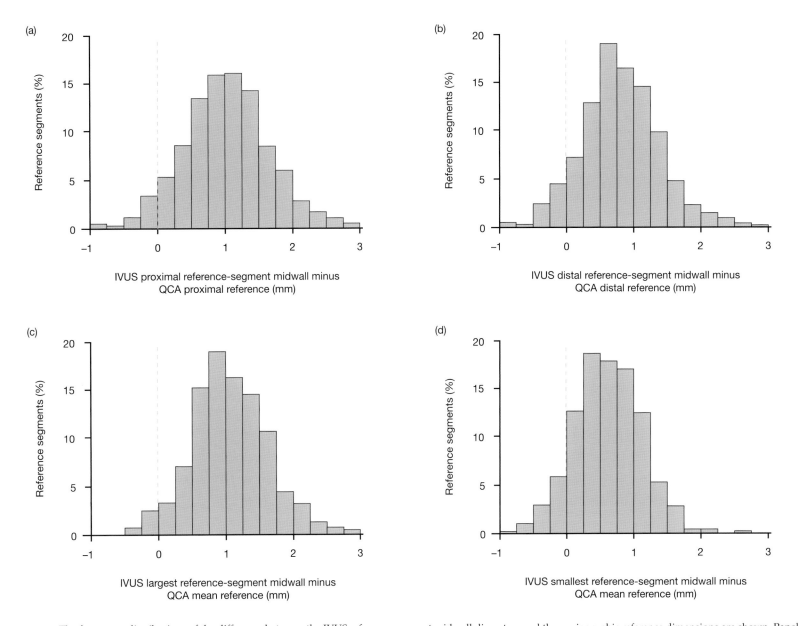

Figure 4.4 The frequency distributions of the difference between the IVUS reference-segment midwall diameters and the angiographic reference dimensions are shown. Panel (a) compares the IVUS mean proximal reference-segment midwall diameter with the proximal angiographic reference; the difference was 1.03 ± 0.65 mm. Panel (b) compares the IVUS mean distal reference-segment midwall diameter with the distal angiographic reference; the difference was 0.82 ± 0.64 mm. Panel (c) compares the IVUS maximum reference-segment midwall diameter (larger of the proximal and distal mean midwall diameters) with the mean angiographic reference; the difference was 1.08 ± 0.60 mm. Panel (d) compares the IVUS minimum reference-segment midwall diameter (smaller of the proximal and distal mean midwall diameters) with the mean angiographic reference; the difference was 0.60 ± 0.52 mm. Angiographic measurements were calculated using quantitative coronary angiography (QCA). The IVUS reference-segment midwall dimensions were calculated mathematically from the lumen and external elastic membrane CSAs

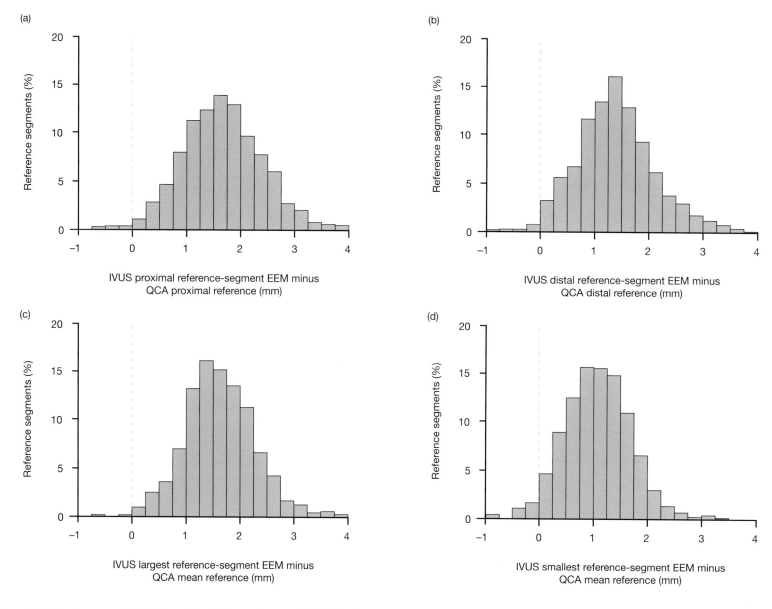

Figure 4.5 The frequency distributions of the difference between the IVUS reference-segment EEM diameters and the angiographic reference dimensions are shown. Panel (a) compares the IVUS mean proximal reference-segment EEM diameter with the proximal angiographic reference; the difference was 1.68 ± 0.76 mm. Panel (b) compares the IVUS mean distal reference-segment EEM diameter with the distal angiographic reference; the difference was 1.41 ± 0.83 mm. Panel (c) compares the IVUS maximum reference-segment EEM diameter (larger of the proximal and distal mean EEM diameters) with the mean angiographic reference; the difference was 1.66 ± 0.75 mm. Panel (d) compares the IVUS minimum reference-segment EEM diameter (smaller of the proximal and distal mean EEM diameters) with the mean angiographic reference; the difference was 1.07 ± 0.62 mm. Angiographic measurements were calculated using quantitative coronary angiography (QCA). The IVUS reference-segment EEM dimensions were calculated mathematically from EEM CSAs

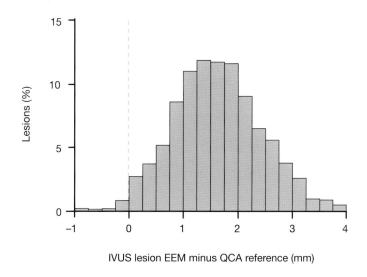

Figure 4.6 The frequency distribution of the difference between the IVUS mean lesion EEM diameter and the angiographic mean reference dimension is shown. The difference measured 1.64 ± 0.91 mm. Angiographic measurements were calculated using quantitative coronary angiography (QCA). The IVUS lesion EEM dimensions were calculated mathematically from the lesion EEM CSA

For example, lumen tapering is dependent solely on EEM tapering in the left anterior descending artery, but on both EEM tapering and distal versus proximal plaque accumulation in the right coronary artery.

Reverse lumen tapering (defined as a distal lumen that is greater than the proximal lumen) is more common in the right (19%) and the left circumflex (18%) coronary arteries than in the left anterior descending artery (2%). This is the result of more distal reference-segment plaque accumulation compared with the proximal reference.

LESION SEVERITY

Several studies have compared IVUS with quantitative coronary angiography (QCA) in the measurement of lesion-site lumen dimensions. Pre-intervention, the correlation ranges from 0.77 to 0.98.[8–11] However, this correlation is worse with intermediate lesions.[12] Coronary angiography underestimates stenosis severity most markedly in vessels with a 50–75% plaque burden and in patients with multivessel disease. In addition, IVUS shows that approximately 25% of lesions with a lumen area < 4.0 mm^2 (the IVUS criterion for a significant stenosis) have an

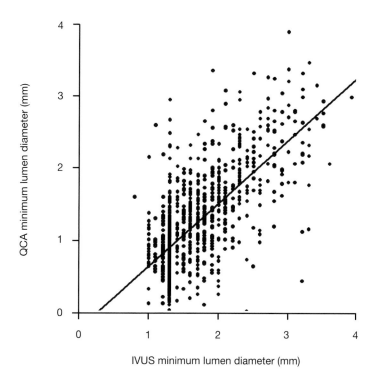

Figure 4.7 Pre-intervention, the correlation between QCA and IVUS minimum lumen diameters was $r = 0.70$, $p < 0.0001$. Note that IVUS cannot measure dimensions smaller than the physical size of the catheter (approximately 1.0 mm). Therefore, the scatter plot is truncated at approximately 1.0 mm

angiographic diameter stenosis $< 50\%$; that is, they are angiographically not significant. These "insignificant" lesions tend to be more common in the right coronary artery and in arteries with one angiographically significant stenosis.[13]

Post-balloon angioplasty, the correlation between IVUS and angiography falls to 0.28–0.42.[14,15] Nakamura *et al.*[16] indicated that, post-balloon angioplasty, the discrepancy is greater in the presence of deep-vessel injury ($n = 39$, $r = 0.05$, $p = 0.74$) than in the presence of superficial lesion injury ($n = 37$, $r = 0.67$, $p = 0.001$).

We compared the measurement of minimum lumen diameters by both IVUS and QCA pre-intervention (including IVUS studies performed for diagnostic purposes) and/or post-intervention. These correlations are shown in Figures 4.7 and 4.8.

Suboptimal angiographic visualization also impairs accurate assessment of stenosis severity. Aorto-ostial stenoses, bifurcation stenoses (particularly at the bifurcation of the left main), and lesions at the ostial of the left anterior descend-

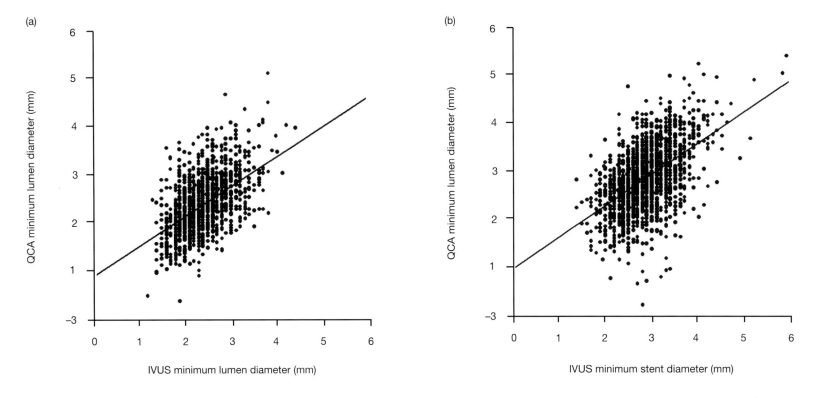

Figure 4.8   The correlation between the QCA and IVUS minimum lumen diameters post-intervention is shown. Panel (a) shows non-stent interventions and Panel (b) shows stent implantation. The correlation was almost identical regardless of the type of intervention ($r = 0.53$ and $r = 0.54$, respectively, $p < 0.0001$)

ing are often poorly seen because of guiding catheter wedging, vessel overlap, angulation, foreshortening, etc. Out-of-plane projections do not always solve the problem. Obesity, emphysema, and chest deformities can affect angiographic quality. Extreme lumen eccentricity (i.e. a slit-like lumen) can also be confusing. The ideal angulation for determining the angiographic minimum lumen diameter may be difficult in certain anatomic lesion subsets. Additional or out-of-plane angiographic projections do not always solve the problem, but can result in the use of a larger than optimum amount of radiographic contrast medium. IVUS does not suffer from these common angiographic limitations and can rapidly "decipher" an ambiguous angiographic study.

Left main disease

Hermiller *et al.*[17] showed that a very high percentage (89%) of patients with angiographically normal left main coronary arteries had disease by IVUS. These findings were confirmed in studies by Yamagishi, Gerber, Ge and colleagues.[18–20] Hermiller *et al.* also reported no correlation between IVUS and angiographic lumen dimensions in patients with angiographically detectable left main disease, a finding confirmed by Abizaid *et al.*[21] in moderate left main stenoses.

Reasons for the discrepancy between angiography and IVUS (or necropsy) assessment of left main coronary artery disease include:

(1) Diffuse atherosclerotic involvement affecting the angiographic diameter stenosis calculation because there is no normal reference segment (creating the so-called small left main);

(2) A short left main which also makes identification of a normal reference segment difficult;

(3) Unique geometric issues in left main coronary artery disease because the correlation between angiography and IVUS (or necropsy) appears to be somewhat better in non-left main coronary artery stenoses and

(4) Significant inter- and intra-observer variability in the angiographic assessment of left main coronary artery disease[22–29] (in fact, taken together, these studies indicate that the left main coronary artery is the arterial segment with the greatest inter- and intra-observer variability in angiographic assessment).

CALCIUM

IVUS routinely detects target lesion calcification that is angiographically "silent". In a study of 1155 native-vessel target lesions, IVUS detected calcium in 73% (ver-

sus 38% by angiography).[30] The arc of lesion calcium measured $115 \pm 110°$, with an arc of superficial calcium of $85 \pm 108°$ and a length of lesion calcium of 3.5 ± 3.7 mm. Conversely, 373/1155 reference segments (32%) contained calcium ($p < 0.0001$ compared with the target lesion). The arc of reference segment-calcium measured $42 \pm 80°$, and the length of reference-segment calcium measured 1.7 ± 3.6 mm (both $p < 0.0001$ compared with target-lesion calcium). Only 44 (4%) native arteries had reference-segment calcium in the absence of lesion calcium. Coronary angiography detected superficial calcium more often than deep calcium, presumably because superficial calcium was, potentially, thicker than deep calcium. The sensitivity of angiography was 25% in lesions with one-quadrant calcium, approximately 50% in lesions with two-quadrant calcium, 60% in lesions with three-quadrant calcium, and 85% in lesions with four-quadrant calcium. The false-positive rate of any angiographic calcium was 11%; however, the false-positive rate of angiographic "severe" calcium was only 2%. There was no clear explanation for angiographic calcium in the absence of IVUS calcium. These results are shown in Figures 4.9 and 4.10 and Table 4.1.

In another study of 183 native-vessel lesions, Tuzcu *et al.*[31] reported that IVUS detected calcium in 138 (75%) while angiography detected calcium in 63 (34%). In patients with angiographically visible calcium, the IVUS arc of calcium was greater than in patients without angiographically invisible calcium ($175 \pm 85°$ versus $108 \pm 71°$, $p = 0.0001$). In this study, the most important predictor of lesion-associated calcium was angiographic calcium elsewhere in the coronary tree, which leads to important implications in the assessment of angiographic filling defects.

Lesions in small arteries are also more calcified than those in larger arteries.[32] The frequency of lesion-associated calcium reached 86% in arteries with an angiographic reference-segment lumen dimension < 2.0 mm. This greater frequency of lesion-associated calcium was associated with larger arcs and lengths of calcium as well. However, there was no relationship between vessel size and reference-segment calcium.

Independent predictors of reference-segment calcification were patient age and serum creatinine levels.[4] More recently, it has been suggested that the transition from azotemia to dialysis not pre-dialysis renal insufficiency,[33] leads to increased arterial calcium.

Both pathologic and IVUS studies have shown that arterial calcification is a marker for and an index of the overall arterial atherosclerotic plaque burden.[34–36]

Saphenous vein grafts

Calcium is less common in saphenous vein grafts than in native coronary arteries, and the patterns of calcium in vein grafts are different. In native arteries,

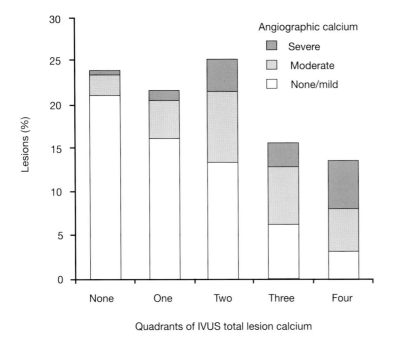

Quadrants of IVUS total lesion calcium

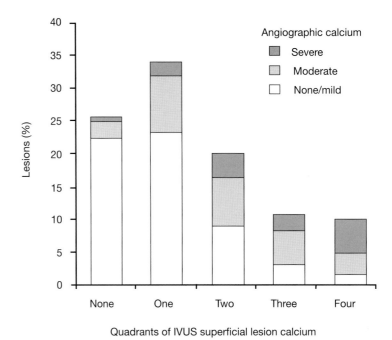

Quadrants of IVUS superficial lesion calcium

Figure 4.9 Angiographic calcification can be classified as none/mild, moderate (radio-pacities noted only during the cardiac cycle prior to contrast injection), and severe (radio-pacities noted without cardiac motion prior to contrast injection, generally compromising both sides of the arterial lumen). This figure shows the frequency distribution of the number of quadrants of IVUS-lesion calcium (whether this calcium is superficial, deep, or both) as well as a comparison with the angiographic classification of lesions into none/mild, moderate, and severe calcium. Note that the sensitivity of angiography does not exceed 50% until there are at least three quadrants of calcium (>180°). Also note the small false-positive rate of angiography

Figure 4.10 Angiographic calcification can be classified as none/mild, moderate (radiopacities noted only during the cardiac cycle prior to contrast injection), and severe (radiopacities noted without cardiac motion prior to contrast injection, generally compromising both sides of the arterial lumen). This figure shows the frequency distribution of the number of quadrants of IVUS superficial-lesion calcium as well as a comparison with the angiographic classification of lesions into none/mild, moderate, and severe calcium. By comparing this with Figure 4.9, it can be seen that the sensitivity of angiography is better when detecting superficial calcium. The sensitivity of angiography exceeds 50% even in two quadrants of superficial calcium, and the sensitivity of angiography exceeds 75% in detecting three or more quadrants of superficial calcium

Table 4.1 Angiographic versus IVUS calcium

| | Angiographic calcium | | | |
	None/Mild	*Moderate*	*Severe*	*p*
Lesion				
Arc of calcium (°)	65 ± 85	160 ± 104	219 ± 108	< 0.0001
Arc of superficial calcium (°)	41 ± 76	122 ± 111	203 ± 119	< 0.0001
Length of calcium (mm)	2.2 ± 3.1	4.1 ± 3.1	6.4 ± 4.9	< 0.0001
Length of superficial calcium (mm)	1.3 ± 2.5	3.0 ± 2.9	5.6 ± 4.9	< 0.0001
Reference				
Arc of calcium (°)	21 ± 57	53 ± 87	83 ± 92	< 0.0001
Length of calcium (mm)	1.0 ± 2.6	2.5 ± 4.5	3.9 ± 4.5	< 0.0001
Total length of calcium (mm)	3.1 ± 4.5	6.6 ± 5.5	10.3 ± 6.6	< 0.0001

Table 4.2 Angiographic versus IVUS eccentricity

| | Angiographic eccentricity | | |
	No	*Yes*	*p*
Lesion			
Maximum P&M thickness (mm)	2.2 ± 6.1	2.2 ± 0.6	1.0
Minimum P&M thickness (mm)	0.9 ± 4.6	0.7 ± 1.9	0.3
Maximum/minimum P&M thickness	4.1 ± 6.9	4.1 ± 3.4	0.9
Reference			
Maximum P&M thickness (mm)	1.1 ± 0.5	1.1 ± 0.8	0.5
Minimum P&M thickness (mm)	0.4 ± 0.2	0.4 ± 0.2	0.6
Maximum/minimum P&M thickness	4.2 ± 5.5	4.0 ± 8.2	0.5

calcium is mostly lesion-associated, while in saphenous vein grafts, calcium is equally common in lesions and reference segments. In a recent analysis of 133 saphenous vein grafts, calcium was found in 40%: 14% in the lesion, 13% in the proximal reference, and 13% in the distal reference.[37] Therefore, two-thirds of vein-graft calcium was outside of the lesion site. Importantly, more of the calcium was in the wall of the graft (i.e. deep) rather than in the plaque, and calcium-containing grafts were older and more common in insulin-treated diabetics. This suggested that calcium was the result of vein-graft wall degeneration rather than lesion formation and maturation.

ECCENTRICITY

Few lesions are truly concentric (eccentricity index = 1, where the eccentricity index = maximum/minimum, plaque & media thickness), and although almost all lesions show some degree of eccentric plaque distribution, there is no consensus as to the exact IVUS definition of an eccentric plaque. In a large series of 1446 native-vessel lesions, only 198/995 (19.9%) lesions had a normal arc of arterial wall within the lesion (equivalent to the pathologic definition of lesion eccentricity).[38] In this study, as well as in reports by Braden *et al.*[39] and Ito *et al.*,[40] the angiographic classification of lesions as eccentric versus concentric was not relat-

ed to plaque distribution (as measured by the IVUS eccentricity index. This is shown in Figure 4.11 and Table 4.2. Furthermore, using similar angiographic and IVUS criteria (three times as much plaque on one side of the lesion as on the other), the concordance rate between IVUS and angiography was only 53.8%. The angiographic classification of a lesion as concentric or eccentric is determined, in part, by the lesion length. Angiographic classification requires a visual interpolation of the course of the normal coronary artery, its lumen, and its vessel wall to assess plaque thickness; interpolation is more difficult in longer lesions and in those with more atherosclerotic plaque.[38] This is also true for saphenous vein grafts.

Bifurcations

IVUS studies have related plaque distribution to side-branches and bifurcation lesions. These studies have shown that, regardless of the angiographic appearance, plaque is deposited preferentially opposite to the major branch. (Using the analogy of a pair of pants, bifurcation plaque is typically located at the hips and spares the inseam.) Kimura *et al.*[41] studied lesions located in the very proximal left anterior descending and found that the plaque was located opposite the circumflex, spared the flow divider, and maintained eccentricity across a wide range of vessel stenoses. An example is shown in Figure 4.12. This is also true of the flow dividers in a trifurcation (Figure 4.13).

Another study, recently reported by Badak et al,[42] showed that the side-branch take-off angle in the cross-sectional plane influenced plaque distribution in bifurcation lesions. Plaque accumulated directly opposite a side branch with a perpendicular take-off angle. In the setting of non-perpendicular side branch take-off, the plaque was still deposited opposite the side-branch, but it tended to accumulate preferentially toward the acute angle between the main vessel and its branch and away from the obtuse angle.

These studies indicate that the flow-divider or carina between the main vessel and the side branch (the inseam in the pants analogy) is almost always spared. Thus, there is a need to revise the conventional angiographic classifications of bifurcation lesions since many of them show carinal (or flow-divider) involvement (Figure 4.14).[43]

The ideal IVUS assessment of a bifurcation requires imaging both the main vessel and its side branch. While a qualitative determination of the presence or absence of side-branch disease is possible from the main branch, assessment of lumen compromise is not accurate.

LESION LENGTH

Angiography measures lesion length from shoulder to shoulder in the least foreshortened projection. However, it is not always possible to eliminate foreshortening, and a single projection cannot deal with vessel tortuosity or bendpoints. IVUS measures lesion length by tracking the transducer through the coronary artery regardless of bend points or tortuosity, and, of course, foreshortening is not an issue. In addition, lesion length determination requires identification of the ends of the lesion – a process that can be difficult because these ends are rarely disease-free. A comparison of IVUS versus angiographic lesion length measurements is shown in Figure 4.15.

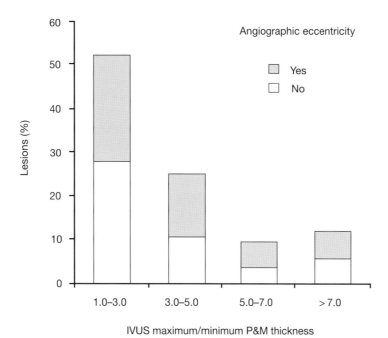

Figure 4.11 *Angiographic eccentricity* is identified as a lesion having one of its edges in the outer one-quarter of the apparently normal lumen. This figure compares the angiographic classification of lesions as eccentric or concentric to the ratio of the maximum/minimum IVUS plaque & media (P&M) thickness. Note that the sensitivity of angiography is the same for lesions regardless of the ratio of the maximum/minimum P&M thickness

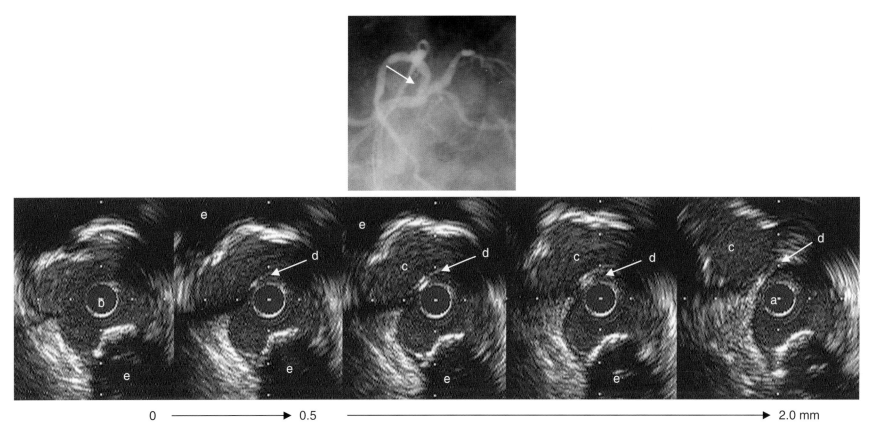

Figure 4.12 The bifurcation of the left main into the left anterior descending and left circumflex were imaged in this example (white arrow in the angiogram). On pullback from the left anterior descending (a) to the very distal left main at the level of its bifurcation (b), the left circumflex (c) and carina (d) are seen. The carina is free of disease throughout. Note the fibrocalcific disease with shadowing (e) in the left anterior descending and the left circumflex. The minimum lumen CSA in the left anterior descending measures 3.7 mm^2. However, while tangential IVUS imaging of the left circumflex shows that it is abnormal, the actual minimum lumen area cannot be measured

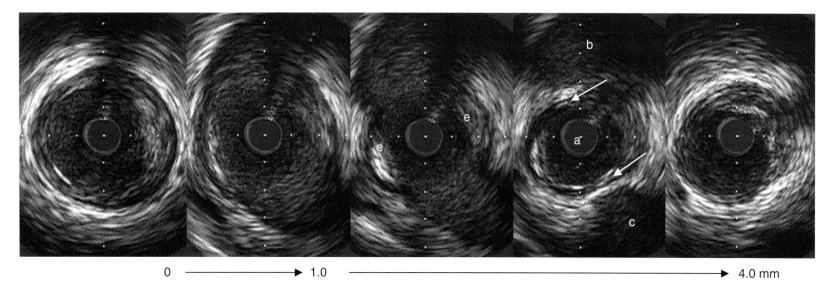

Figure 4.13 This example shows a trifurcation of the left anterior descending (a) at the origin of a diagonal (b) and (a) septal (c) branch. Note that both carinae are free of disease (white arrows) and that plaque is deposited perpendicular to the two carinae (e)

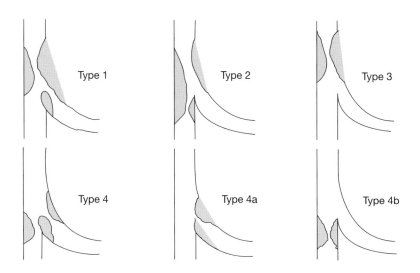

Figure 4.14 A popular angiographic classification of bifurcation lesions is shown. Note that in each type – with the notable exception of Type 3 – the carina is shown to have plaque accumulation. IVUS imaging consistently shows that the carina is spared

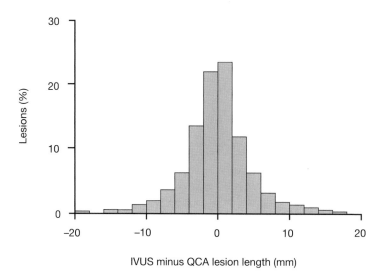

Figure 4.15 Angiographic lesion length is measured from shoulder to shoulder in the view with the least foreshortening. This figure shows the frequency distribution of the difference between the IVUS and quantitative coronary angiographic (QCA) lesion length measurements

REFERENCES

1. Erbel R, Ge J, Bockisch A, et al. Value of intracoronary ultrasound and Doppler in the differentiation of angiographically normal coronary arteries: a prospective study in patients with angina pectoris. Eur Heart J 1996; 17: 880–9

2. Tuzcu EM, Hobbs RE, Rincon G, et al. Occult and frequent transmission of atherosclerotic coronary disease with cardiac transplantation: insights from intravascular ultrasound. Circulation 1995; 91: 1706–13

3. Tuzcu EM, Kapadia SR, Tutar E, et al. High prevalence of coronary atherosclerosis in asymptomatic teenagers and young adults. Evidence from intravascular ultrasound. Circulation 2001; 103: 2705–10

4. Mintz GS, Painter JA, Pichard AD, et al. Atherosclerosis in angiographically "normal" coronary artery reference segments: an intravascular ultrasound study with clinical correlations. J Am Coll Cardiol 1995; 25: 1479–85

5. Glagov S, Weisenberg E, Zarins CK, et al. Compensatory enlargement of human atherosclerotic coronary arteries. N Engl J Med 1987; 316: 1371–5

6. Stiel GM, Stiel LSG, Schofer J, et al. Impact of compensatory enlargement of atherosclerotic coronary arteries on angiographic assessment of coronary heart disease. Circulation 1989; 80: 1603–9

7. Javier SP, Mintz GS, Popma JJ, et al. Intravascular ultrasound assessment of the magnitude and mechanism of coronary artery and lumen tapering. Am J Cardiol 1995; 75: 177–80

8. Nissen SE, Gurley JC, Grines CL, et al. Intravascular ultrasound assessment of lumen size and wall morphology in normal subjects and patients with coronary artery disease. Circulation 1991; 84: 1087–99

9. Davidson CJ, Sheikh KH, Harrison JK, et al. Intravascular ultrasonography versus digital subtraction angiography: a human in vivo comparison of vessel size and morphology. J Am Coll Cardiol 1990; 16: 633–6

10. Nissen SE, Grines CL, Gurley JC, et al. Application of a new phased-array ultrasound imaging catheter in the assessment of vascular dimensions. In vivo comparison to cineangiography. Circulation 1990; 81: 660–6

11. De Scheerder I, De Man F, Herregods MC, et al. Intravascular ultrasound versus angiography for measurement of luminal diameters in normal and diseased coronary arteries. Am Heart J 1994; 127: 243–51

12. Abizaid AS, Mintz GS, Mehran R, et al. One year follow-up after percutaneous transluminal angioplasty was not performed based on intravascular ultrasound findings. Importance of lumen dimensions. Circulation 1999; 100: 256–61

13. Maehara A, Mintz GS, Bui AB, et al. Determinants of angiographically silent stenoses in patients with coronary artery disease. Am J Cardiol 2003; 91: 1335–8

14. Tobis JM, Mahon DJ, Honye J, et al. Intravascular ultrasound imaging following balloon angioplasty. Int J Card Imaging 1991; 6: 191–205

15. Davidson CJ, Sheikh KH, Kisslo KB, et al. Intracoronary ultrasound evaluation of interventional technologies. Am J Cardiol 1991; 68: 1305–9

16. Nakamura S, Mahon DJ, Maheswaran B, et al. An explanation for discrepancy between angiographic and intravascular ultrasound measurements after percutaneous transluminal coronary angioplasty. J Am Coll Cardiol 1995; 25: 633–9

17. Hermiller JB, Buller CE, Tenaglia AN, et al. Unrecognized left main coronary artery disease in patients undergoing interventional procedures. Am J Cardiol 1993; 71: 173–6

18. Yamagishi M, Hongo Y, Goto Y, et al. Intravascular ultrasound evidence of angiographically undetected left main coronary artery disease and associated trauma during interventional procedures. Heart Vessels 1996; 11: 262–8

19. Gerber TC, Erbel R, Gorge G, et al. Extent of atherosclerosis and remodeling of the left main coronary artery determined by intravascular ultrasound. Am J Cardiol 1994; 73: 666–71

20. Ge J, Liu F, Gorge G, et al. Angiographically "silent" plaque in the left main coronary artery detected by intravascular ultrasound. Coron Artery Dis 1995; 6: 805–10

21. Abizaid AS, Mintz GS, Abizaid A, et al. One year follow-up after intravascular ultrasound assessment of moderate left main coronary artery disease in patients with ambiguous angiograms. J Am Coll Cardiol 1999; 34: 707–15

22. Fisher LD, Judkins MP, Lesperance J, et al. Reproducibility of coronary arteriographic reading in the coronary artery surgery study (CASS). Cathet Cardiovasc Diagn 1982; 8: 565–75

23. Isner JM, Kishel J, Kent KM, et al. Accuracy of angiographic determination of left main coronary narrowing. Circulation 1981; 63: 1056–64

24. Detre KM, Wright E, Murphy ML, et al. Observer agreement in evaluating coronary angiograms. Circulation 1975; 52: 979–86

25. DeRouen T A, Murray J A, Owen W. Variability in the analysis of coronary arteriograms. Circulation 1977; 55: 324–8

26. Zir LM, Miller SW, Dinsmore RE, et al. Interobserver variability in coronary angiography. Circulation 1976; 53: 627–32

27. Sanmarco ME, Brooks SH, Blankenhorn DH. Reproducibility of a consensus panel in the interpretation of coronary angiograms. Am Heart J 1978; 96: 430–7

28. Cameron A, Kemp HG Jr, Fisher LD, et al. Left main coronary artery stenosis: angiographic determination. Circulation 1983; 68: 484–9

29. Flemming RM, Kirkeeide RL, Smalling RW, et al. Patterns in visual interpretation of coronary arteriograms as detected by quantitative coronary arteriography. J Am Coll Cardiol 1991; 18: 945–51

30. Mintz GS, Popma JJ, Pichard AD, et al. Patterns of calcification in coronary artery disease. A statistical analysis of intravascular ultrasound and coronary angiography in 1155 lesions. Circulation 1995; 91: 1969–5

31. Tuzcu EM, Berkalp B, De Franco AC, et al. The dilemma of diagnosing coronary calcification: angiography versus intravascular ultrasound. J Am Coll Cardiol 1996; 27: 832–8

32. Mintz GS, Pichard AD, Kent KM, et al. Interrelation of coronary angiographic reference lumen size and intravascular ultrasound target lesion calcium. Am J Cardiol 1998; 81: 387–91

33. Gruberg L, Kim SG, Mintz GS, et al. Renal function and coronary artery disease: an intravascular ultrasound study. Circulation 2003; 106: II-586

34. Mintz GS, Pichard AD, Popma JJ, et al. Determinants and correlates of target lesion calcium in coronary artery disease: a clinical, angiographic, and intravascular ultrasound study. J Am Coll Cardiol 1997; 29: 268–74

35. Sangiorgi G, Rumberger JA, Severson A, et al. Arterial calcification and not lumen stenosis is highly correlated with atherosclerotic plaque burden in humans: a histologic study of 723 coronary artery segments using nondecalcifying methodology. J Am Coll Cardiol 1998; 31: 126–33.

36. Tinana A, Mintz GS, Weissman NJ. Volumetric intravascular ultrasound quantification of the amount of atherosclerosis and calcium in nonstenotic arterial segments. Am J Cardiol 2002; 89: 757–60.

37. Castagna MT, Mintz GS, Weissman NJ, et al. Calcification in saphenous vein grafts: clinical correlated and intravascular ultrasound findings. J Am Coll Cardiol 2002; 39: 36A

38. Mintz GS, Popma JJ, Pichard AD, et al. Limitation of angiography in the assessment of plaque distribution in coronary artery disease. A systematic study of target lesion eccentricity in 1446 lesions. Circulation 1996; 93: 924–31

39. Braden G A, Herrington D M, Kerensky R A, et al. Angiography poorly predicts actual lesion eccentricity in severe coronary stenoses: confirmation by intracoronary ultrasound. J Am Coll Cardiol 1994; 23: 413A

40. Ito K, Yamagishi M, Yasumura Y, et al. Impact of coronary artery remodeling on misinterpretation of angiogrpahic disease eccentricity: evidence from intravascular ultrasound. Int J Cardiol 1999; 70: 275–82

41. Kimura BJ, Russo RJ, Bhargava V, et al. Atheroma morphology and distribution in proximal left anterior descending coronary artery: in vivo observations. J Am Coll Cardiol 1996; 27: 825–31

42. Badak O, Schoenhagen P, Tsunoda T, et al. Characteristics of atherosclerotic plaque distribution in coronary artey bifurcations: an intravascular ultrasound analysis. Coron Artery Dis 2003; 14: 309–16

43. Lefèvre T, Louvard Y, Morice M-C, et al. Stenting of bifurcation lesions: classification, treatment, and results. Catheter Cardiovasc Interv 2000; 49: 274–83

5

Remodeling, acute coronary syndromes, vulnerable plaques, plaque rupture, stenosis formation, and progression/regression

The authors of an important recent consensus document recommended the term "vulnerable plaque" to identify all thrombosis-prone plaques and plaques with a high probability of undergoing rapidprogression.[1] They proposed a list of vulnerable plaque types: (1) rupture-prone plaques with a large lipid core and a thin fibrous cap infiltrated by macrophages; (2) ruptured plaques with subocclusive thrombi and early organization; (3) erosion-prone plaques with proteoglycan matrix in a smooth muscle cell-rich plaque; (4) eroded plaques with subocclusive thrombi; (5) intraplaque hemorrhage secondary to leaking vasa vasorum; (6) calcific nodules protruding into the vessel lumen; and (7) chronically stenotic plaques with severe calcification, old thrombus, and eccentric lumens.

Of these, plaque ruptures are the most common type of plaque-related complication leading to thrombosis; they account for approximately 70% of fatal acute myocardial infarctions and/or sudden coronary deaths. Most techniques for detecting vulnerable plaques are being developed to identify rupture-prone plaques. Rupture-prone plaques are more often non-stenotic than stenotic. In cases of non-ruptured plaques, plaque erosion or nodular calcification usually underlies the luminal thrombus.

Anatomic (as apposed to functional) markers of vulnerability at the plaque/arterial level include plaque cap thickness, plaque lipid core size, luminal narrowing, expansive (versus constrictive) remodeling, color, lipid content (versus collagen content, which influences mechanical stability), pattern of calcium (nodule versus scattered, superficial versus deep, etc.), and total arterial calcium and plaque burden. IVUS lacks the ability to identify many of these markers of vulnerability. Conversely, IVUS observations have importance beyond just the identification of vulnerable plaques. To date, most of the IVUS analyses have compared stable versus unstable patients, ruptured versus unruptured plaques, and lesions versus reference segments. (Only one IVUS study has attempted to predict plaque instability.[2]) While statistical differences are common and important, the diagnostic value of the various IVUS findings tends to be low in individual lesions or patients.

REMODELING

During the development and progression of atherosclerosis, the external elastic membrane (EEM) cross-sectional area (CSA) may increase. This is termed "positive" or "outward" or "expansive" remodeling. Conversely, the EEM CSA may decrease. This has been termed "negative" or "inward" or "constrictive" remodeling.

To digress for a moment, during the follow-up period after an intervention, the EEM CSA can also change. Unfortunately, this has also been called "remodeling", leading to the erroneous conclusion that the two types of EEM changes are the same – which is probably not correct. Chronic post-interventional changes in EEM CSA may merely reflect perivascular trauma, hematoma formation, and scar contraction. Therefore, in this chapter and throughout this text, the term "remodeling" will be reserved for changes to coronary arterial wall dimensions that occur during the development and progression of atherosclerosis, not as a consequence of intervention.

The ideal natural history study of atherosclerosis and remodeling requires serial observations, perhaps multiple studies, over a span of years. The slope of the line relating the change in EEM CSA to the change in plaque & media (P&M) CSA would indicate the direction and magnitude of remodeling (Figure 5.1).[3]

- A slope >1.0 would indicate positive remodeling with overcompensation (resulting in net lumen increase).

- A slope = 1.0 would indicate perfect positive remodeling, where the increase in plaque was exactly balanced by the increase in EEM CSA leading to no lumen change.

- A slope < 1.0 would indicate inadequate positive remodeling (incomplete compensation).

- A slope < 0 (or reduction in EEM CSA) would indicate negative or constrictive remodeling.

In fact, as shown in a small number of IVUS studies, changes in EEM CSA in patients with established atherosclerosis may be more responsible for changes in lumen dimensions than plaque accumulation.[4,5]

Atherosclerotic plaque and remodeling in non-stenotic segments

Remodeling was described first by Glagov *et al.*[6] in autopsied hearts (primarily non-stenotic segments) by correlating EEM CSA with plaque CSA and plaque burden. Positive (or outward) remodeling was postulated to explain the finding of atherosclerosis that did not encroach on the arterial lumen. These observations were confirmed *in vivo* during routine clinical IVUS imaging, which showed ubiquitous and diffuse atherosclerosis within angiographically normal (non-obstructive) reference segments.[7] In fact, approximately 75% of the total atherosclerotic plaque volume is contained in non-stentotic reference segments.[8]

Positive remodeling occurs to some degree within almost all atherosclerotic reference segments, although the amount of disease and the magnitude of remodeling may vary from segment to segment and from patient to patient. Regardless of the plaque burden – which can exceed 75% in some patients (Figure 5.2) – these reference segments are not stenotic and do not warrant interventional treatment.

Disease-free coronary arteries are circular. However, atherosclerotic arteries with eccentric plaque accumulation may remodel into a non-circular configuration (Figure 5.3).

Definitions of lesion-site remodeling using observations at a single time point

Most IVUS reports of remodeling have been based on IVUS studies performed at a single point in time. Lesion remodeling is most often studied by comparing the lesion with proximal and/or distal reference segments – even though these reference segments have also remodeled. Reference segment(s) should be within the same coronary segment (to minimize the effect of vessel tapering), contain as little disease as possible (to minimize the effect of reference-segment remodeling), and avoid any major intervening side branches because arterial dimensions decrease immediately distal to a side branch. A number of definitions of remodeling have been proposed:

- Lesion EEM CSA/reference-segment EEM CSA. If the lesion EEM CSA is greater than the reference-segment EEM CSA (index > 1.0), there is positive remodeling. If the lesion EEM CSA is smaller than the reference-segment EEM CSA (index < 1.0), there is intermediate/negative remodeling.[3,9]

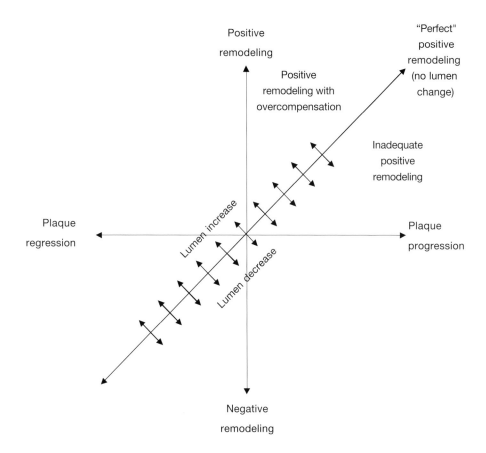

Figure 5.1 This schematic diagram illustrates the concepts of remodeling and plaque progression and their impact on lumen dimensions. This schematic diagram also illustrates the potential interaction of the changes in lumen, external elastic membrane (remodeling), and plaque during regression studies

- Some authors set the above threshold higher. Thus, positive remodeling has also been defined as a remodeling index > 1.05, negative remodeling as a remodeling index < 0.95, and intermediate (or no) remodeling as a remodeling index between 0.95 and 1.05.[10]

- Nishioka *et al.*[11] proposed the following classification: positive remodeling (lesion EEM CSA greater than the proximal reference, seen in 54%), negative remodeling (lesion EEM CSA smaller than the distal reference, seen in 26%), and intermediate remodeling (lesion EEM CSA intermediate between the proximal and distal references, seen in 20%).

Examples of positive, intermediate, and negative remodeling are shown in Figure 5.4.

Is negative remodeling merely an artifact in which the lesion EEM CSA appears smaller compared with the diseased, positively remodeling reference segments? Apparently not – because in a study of patients with minimal reference-segment disease, negative remodeling was seen in approximately half of the lesions.[12]

It is always important to define the reference segment used for any comparison. The distal reference segment may be underperfused and artificially small prior to an intervention, particularly if the catheter is tight across the stenosis. Therefore, some authors have compared the lesion with only the proximal reference.[10,13] Coronary arteries taper, and lesions have a variable axial location between the proximal and distal references. Therefore, other authors have calculated a "theoretical interpolated" lesion EEM CSA, based on the size of the proximal and distal reference EEM, tapering, and the axial location of the lesion relative to the two references. Positive remodeling is where the lesion EEM CSA is greater than the "theoretical interpolated" EEM CSA.[14,15] This approach – shown in Figure 5.5 – is particularly useful in studying longer lesions, diffuse segments, or tapered arteries. The right coronary artery tapers the least and has the fewest branches. Therefore, it has proved unusually suitable for studying remodeling in various clinical and anatomic situations.

IVUS can also assess remodeling by measuring the consequence of lesion-site versus reference-segment plaque accumulation: (reference-segment lumen CSA minus lesion-site lumen CSA) divided by (lesion P&M CSA minus reference P&M CSA). With perfect lesion-site remodeling, excess lesion P&M CSA (compared with the reference) would not decrease the lumen compared with the reference.[16] Almost by definition, negatively remodeled stenoses tend to have less plaque compared with positively remodeled stenoses in a similar-sized artery.

One confusing aspect of these various definitions is that they can result in an individual lesion being classified as positive remodeling by one definition, but not by another. In part, this is because of the limitations resulting from reference-site selection, reference-site plaque burden, vessel tapering, etc.[13–17] Nevertheless, remodeling tends to be normally distributed;[13] and any one of these definitions is useful in comparing populations and in assessing clinical pathophysiologic correlations of remodeling. Furthermore, lesions with the greatest positive or negative remodeling tend to be classified as such by all of the above definitions, while the greatest disagreement occurs in lesions with intermediate remodeling (those with a remodeling index close to 1.0).

Recently, in an as yet unpublished study by von Birgelen *et al.*, the remodeling index was validated using serial IVUS assessment of 46 non-stenotic left main lesions imaged at least 12 months apart. The follow-up remodeling index could be correlated with the baseline remodeling index ($r = 0.58$, $p < 0.001$); the classification of lesions into positive versus intermediate/negative remodeling did not change in three-quarters of the lesions; and 89% of lesions with a follow-up remodeling index > 1.0 had prior documented increases in EEM CSA. In particular, almost all positively remodeled lesions continued to increase their EEM CSA, while intermediate/negatively remodeled lesions could either increase or decrease their EEM CSA.

Positive remodeling in unstable lesions

In pathologic and angioscopic studies, positive remodeling is strongly associated with plaque rupture, yellow plaque color, and thrombus formation.[18–20] There is also consistent IVUS data indicating that acute coronary syndrome (ACS) lesions more often have positive remodeling characteristics (Figures 5.6 and 5.7) compared with either chronic stable angina lesions or with control plaques elsewhere in the coronary tree.[10,21–24] Nevertheless, not all culprit lesions in ACS patients – even in these aforementioned clinical studies – are positively remodeled (Figure 5.8). The absence of positive remodeling in an acute setting may indicate that the culprit-lesion morphology is one of plaque erosion rather than rupture, particularly if there are no IVUS features of a ruptured plaque.

Intermediate/negative remodeling in stable plaques

Stable plaques more often have intermediate or negative remodeling characteristics. Negative remodeling may be related to the amount of calcium (Figure 5.9), may be more common in patients who smoke, and is strongly associated with angioscopic white plaques.[13,20,25,26] Negative remodeling is seen in patients with coronary spasm (Figure 5.10) and at ostial and bifurcation stenoses (Figures 5.11 and 5.12).[27,28] In the setting of aorto-ostial lesions, negative remodeling may be associated with stenosis formation without any atherosclerotic plaque (Figure 5.13).[29]

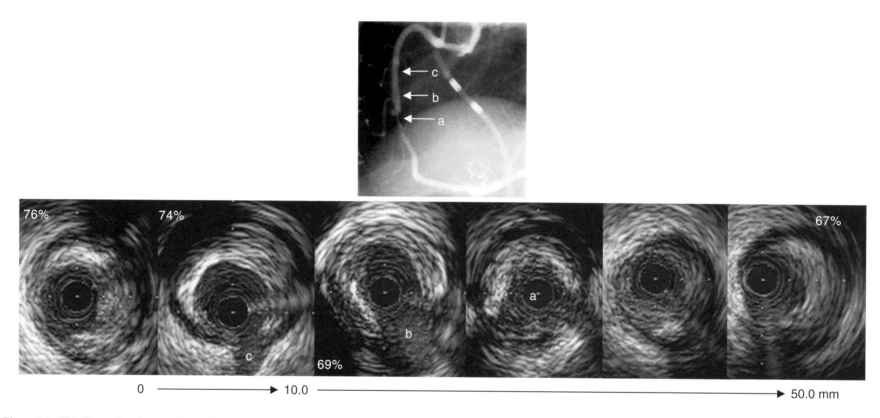

Figure 5.2   This illustration shows a 50-mm long segment of a right coronary artery with a large plaque burden in the non-stenotic, angiographically normal reference segments. The lesion (a) and two small right ventricular branches (b and c) are shown in both the angiogram and the IVUS image. The plaque burdens of the four non-stenotic IVUS cross-sections, which ranged from 67% to 76%, are shown in each image slice. Notice that the plaque accumulated opposite each of the right ventricular branches

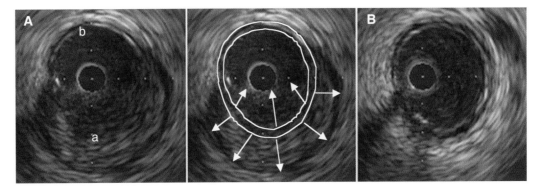

Figure 5.3   This illustration shows how eccentric plaque accumulation leads to eccentric remodeling. Panel A is a lesion with eccentric plaque accumulation (a) opposite normal arc of vessel wall (b). Panel B is the corresponding nearly disease-free reference segment. The external elastic membrane and the lumen of the reference segment were traced and then superimposed on the lesion (outer and inner white lines) in the middle panel. Notice how eccentric plaque accumulation (a) was accompanied by eccentric positive remodeling (outer white arrows). Conversely, the arc of disease-free arterial wall within the lesion (b) did not remodel. Nevertheless, the eccentric positive remodeling was inadequate because of the reduction in lumen dimensions compared with the reference (8.7 vs. 5.3 mm^2, inner white arrows)

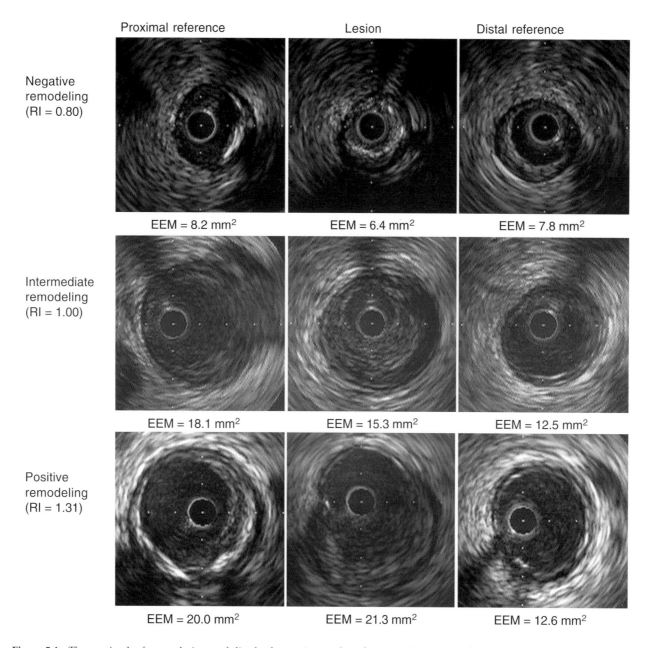

Proximal reference   Lesion   Distal reference

Negative remodeling (RI = 0.80)

EEM = 8.2 mm²   EEM = 6.4 mm²   EEM = 7.8 mm²

Intermediate remodeling (RI = 1.00)

EEM = 18.1 mm²   EEM = 15.3 mm²   EEM = 12.5 mm²

Positive remodeling (RI = 1.31)

EEM = 20.0 mm²   EEM = 21.3 mm²   EEM = 12.6 mm²

Figure 5.4 The proximal reference, lesion, and distal reference image slices from negative, intermediate, and positive remodeling lesions are shown. The external elastic membrane (EEM) CSA measurement is shown on each slice. The remodeling index (RI) was calculated using the mean of the proximal and distal reference EEM CSA

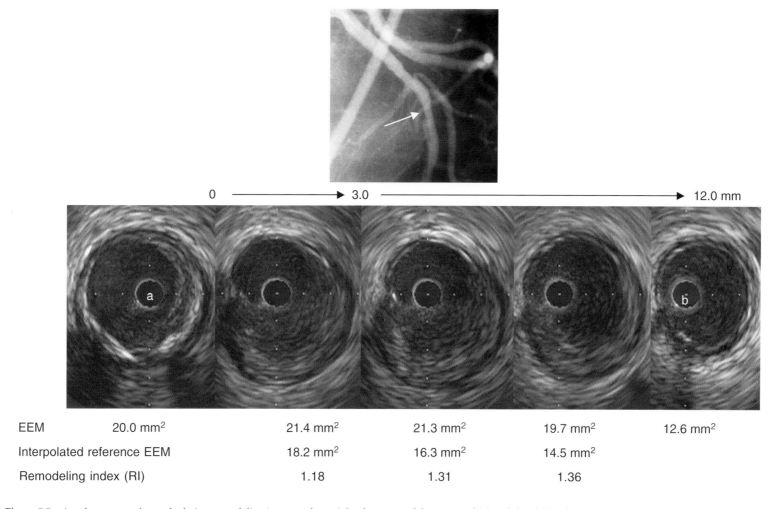

EEM	20.0 mm²		21.4 mm²	21.3 mm²	19.7 mm²	12.6 mm²
Interpolated reference EEM			18.2 mm²	16.3 mm²	14.5 mm²	
Remodeling index (RI)			1.18	1.31	1.36	

Figure 5.5 Another approach to calculating remodeling is to use the weighted average of the proximal (a) and distal (b) references to calculate an interpolated reference external elastic membrane (EEM). The remodeling index (RI) is then calculated as lesion divided by the interpolated reference EEM. This patient presented with an acute coronary syndrome and a culprit lesion in the left anterior descending coronary artery (white arrow in the angiogram)

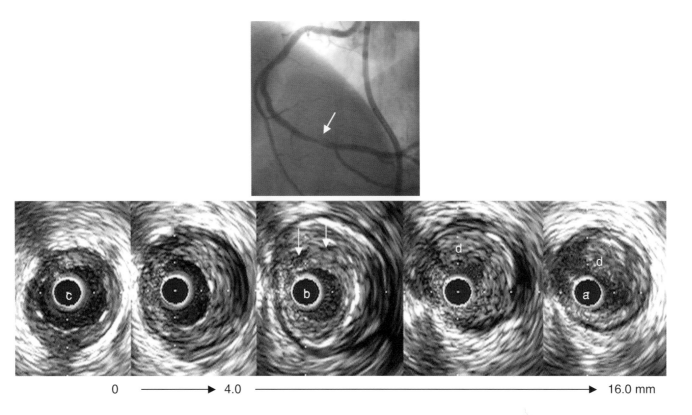

Figure 5.6 This patient presented with an acute coronary syndrome and a culprit lesion in the right coronary artery (white arrow in the angiogram). The IVUS pullback is from the distal reference (a) through the lesion (b) to the proximal reference (c). The distal reference external elastic membrane (EEM) CSA measured $11.3\,mm^2$, the lesion EEM measured $19.5\,mm^2$, and the proximal reference measured $10.7\,mm^2$. The remodeling index was calculated to be 1.77. Note the distal intraluminal mass (d) as well as the microchannels within the plaque (white arrows) consistent with thrombus. The minimum lumen CSA measured $2.8\,mm^2$

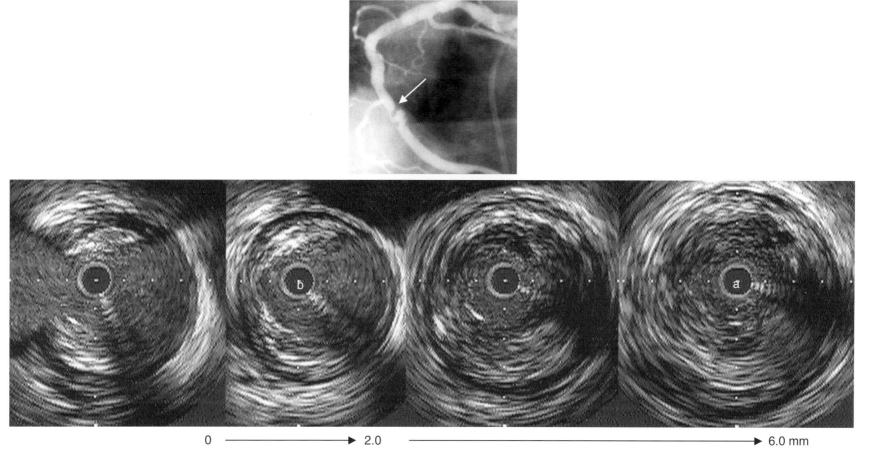

0 ⟶ 2.0 ⟶ 6.0 mm

Figure 5.7   This patient presented with an acute coronary syndrome and a culprit lesion in the right coronary artery (white arrow in the angiogram). The IVUS catheter did not cross the lesion; therefore, the pre-intervention pullback began with the lesion (a) and continued to the proximal reference (b). Despite the lack of a distal reference, the lesion has clear positive remodeling characteristics: the lesion external elastic membrane (EEM) CSA measured 48.8 mm², which, when compared with the proximal reference EEM CSA of 26.9 mm², resulted in a calculated remodeling index of 1.81. The minimum lumen CSA measured 1.9 mm²

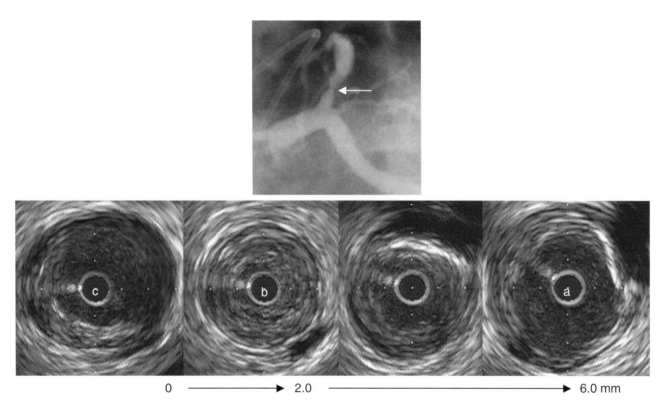

Figure 5.8 This patient presented with an acute coronary syndrome (non-Q myocardial infarction) and a culprit lesion in the left anterior descending artery (white arrow in the angiogram). The IVUS pullback is from the distal reference (a) through the lesion (b) to the proximal reference (c). The remodeling index was calculated as 0.61 (lesion and mean reference external elastic membrane CSA measured 14.9 mm^2 and 24.4 mm^2, respectively)

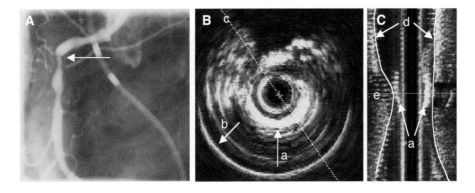

Figure 5.9 This patient with chronic stable angina presented for a percutaneous intervention of a calcified, angulated right coronary artery stenosis (white arrow in Panel A). The cross-sectional IVUS image in the center of the lesion (Panel B) shows near-circumferential calcification (a) with reverberations (the strongest of which is shown by the arrow b) and complete shadowing of the external elastic membrane (EEM). The line (c) in Panel B represents the cut-plane of the longitudinal view shown in Panel C. The longitudinal view artificially straightens the angulated stenosis, but still shows the classic hour-glass configuration of a negatively remodeled, calcified stenosis. The longitudinal view allows interpolation of the EEM (d) even behind the calcium (a). The line (e) indicates the axial location of the cross-sectional image in Panel B

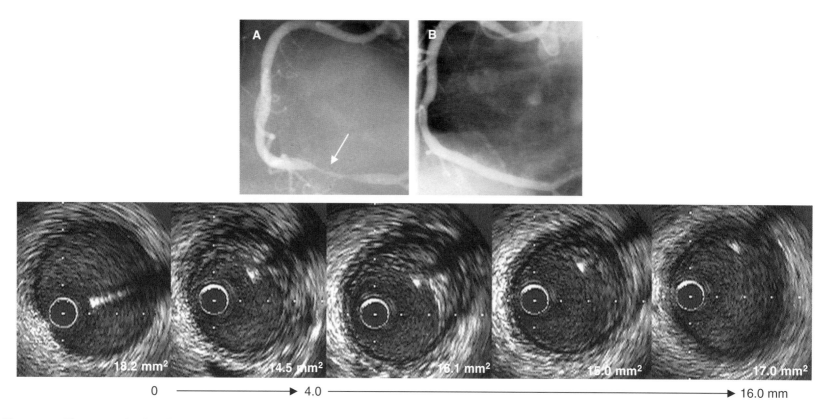

Figure 5.10   This patient developed spontaneous coronary spasm of the right coronary artery (white arrow in Panel A), which was relieved by intracoronary nitroglycerin (Panel B). Afterwards, the IVUS imaging run shows moderate eccentric plaque accumulation with a lesion plaque burden of 47% (a). The external elastic membrane of each image slice is shown. The remodeling index at the site of maximum plaque accumulation (centre image slice) was 0.91

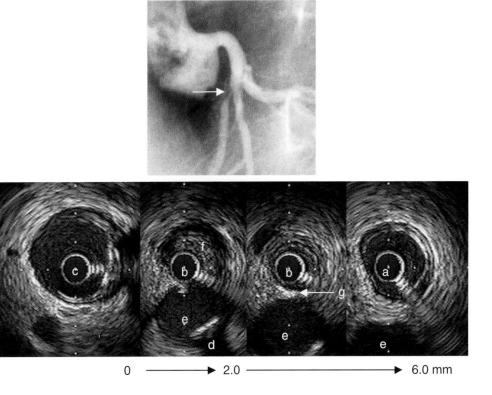

Figure 5.11 This patient presented with a left anterior descending stenosis just distal to the major diagonal (white arrow in the angiogram). According to a popular angiographic classification (Figure 4.14), this would be a Type 4b bifurcation stenosis. The IVUS imaging run from distal (a) through the lesion (b) to the proximal reference (c) shows several notable findings. First, there is mild calcium (d) in the diagonal (e). Second, there is eccentric plaque accumulation (f) opposite this diagonal with typical sparing of the carina (g). Third, the distal reference external elastic membrane is much smaller than the proximal reference (6.2 mm^2 vs. 9.6 mm^2) because of distal vessel underperfusion and/or a stepdown in vessel size distal to the diagonal. Fourth, there is negative remodeling with a remodeling index of 0.64 compared with the distal reference. (The intervening diagonal branch makes the proximal reference an inappropriate comparison when calculating a remodeling index. The distal reference plaque burden measures 38%.) An intermediate right coronary stenosis in this same patient, also with negative remodeling, is shown in Figure 5.12

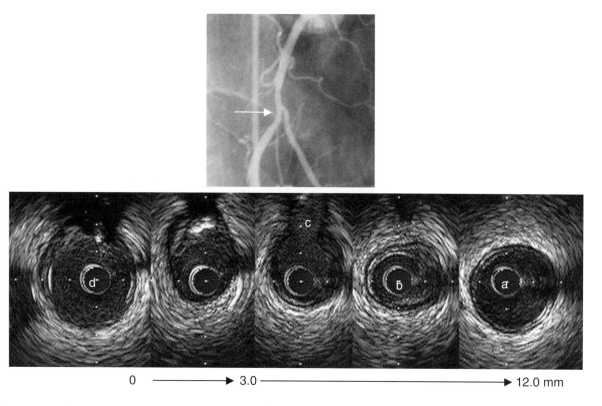

0 ⟶ 3.0 ⟶ 12.0 mm

Figure 5.12 The patient in Figure 5.11 also had this intermediate stenosis in the right coronary artery at the level of the right ventricular branch (white arrow in the angiogram). The IVUS imaging run from distal (a) through the lesion (b) across the ostial of the right ventricular branch (c) to the proximal reference (d) shows negative remodeling. The distal reference external elastic membrane (EEM) measures 8.2 mm^2 with less than 0.3 mm of intimal thickening, the proximal reference EEM measures 11.0 mm^2, and the lesion-site EEM measures 5.7 mm^2, giving a remodeling index of 0.59. There are both lesion-specific and patient-related variables that determine positive versus negative remodeling. Note the minimal reference-segment disease in this example

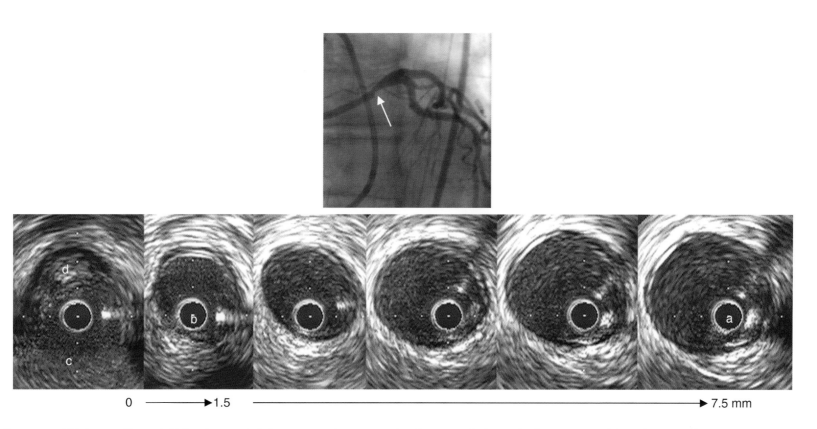

Figure 5.13 This intermediate ostial left main stenosis (white arrow in the angiogram) is almost entirely the result of negative remodeling. The distal reference (a) external elastic membrane (EEM) CSA measured 16.8 mm^2 compared with the lesion (b) EEM CSA of 8.7 mm^2, giving a remodeling index of 0.52. The minimum lumen CSA measured 5.5 mm^2 – a borderline stenosis by lumen CSA criteria. Note that the pullback continued until the aorta (c) was seen. The guiding catheter has been retracted and is out of view. There is evidence of aortic wall disease (d). Note the minimal reference-segment disease

Can negative remodeling occur early? In two datasets of patients with chronic stable angina and intermediate lesions, negative remodeling was seen in approximately half of the lesions.[30,31] While there is no absolute way to gauge the age of a lesion, these reports suggest that negative remodeling can occur early at some sites within the coronary tree.[12,30,31] An example is shown in Figure 5.12.

Impact of diabetes on remodeling

Insulin use may blunt positive remodeling in diabetic patients. Thus, small vessels in diabetic patients may be the result of inadequate remodeling rather than excessive atherosclerotic plaque accumulation (Figure 5.14); and diabetes – particularly insulin-treated diabetes – may increase the frequency of negative remodeling.[16,32,33] Diabetes also affects remodeling in ACS patients. One study indicated that 48% of non-diabetic ACS patients had positive remodeling compared with only 32% of diabetics.[34] This suggests that unstable lesions in diabetics may be more of the erosive type than actually containing plaque ruptures.

Clinical implications of remodeling

IVUS identification of positive remodeling is not just "academic". Positive remodeling has been shown to be a predictor of (1) CK-MB elevation after percutaneous coronary intervention;[35] (2) no reflow in primary infarction angioplasty;[36,37] (3) recurrent ischemia within one month after thrombolysis for acute myocardial infarction;[38] (4) target-lesion revascularization in patients undergoing non-stent intervention;[9] (5) major adverse coronary events in patients with unstable angina undergoing any form of revascularization;[39] (5) target-vessel revascularization and intimal hyperplasia in patients undergoing bare metal stenting;[40,41] (6) intimal hyperplasia after implantation of drug-eluting stents;[42] and (7) in-hospital complications, major adverse coronary events, restenosis, and new lesion formation in patients with stable angina undergoing single-vessel intervention.[43] A greater degree of positive remodeling has also been associated with multiple plaque ruptures compared with single plaque ruptures, and multiple angiographic complex plaques have been associated with increased adverse coronary events in the first year post-myocardial infarction.[44,45] Thus, the cumulative evidence indicates that positively remodeled lesions are more biologically active than intermediate or negatively remodeled lesions; and positive remodeling occurs (or is a prognostic marker) in patients who are more prone to develop additional unstable lesions or become clinically unstable.

LESION MORPHOLOGY AND PLAQUE RUPTURE

Plaques that are prone to rupture – the so-called thin-cap atheroma – are reported to have the following pathologic features: (1) positive remodeling; (2) a fibrous cap of less than 100 μm (and perhaps less than 65 μm) at it minimum thickness; (3) a large lipid/necrotic core often containing hemorrhage and/or calcification; (4) speckled or diffuse calcification (not enough to increase plaque stability, although the absence of any calcium is also rare in rupture-prone plaques); (5) abundant intra-plaque vasovasorum; and (6) macrophage infiltration of the thin fibrous cap.[18,46,47] Gray-scale IVUS cannot reliably assess the lipid or necrotic core of a plaque, although spectral radiofrequency analysis shows promise in assessing plaque composition. The resolution of IVUS (100 μm, at best) limits its ability to detect and measure a rupture-prone thin fibrous cap – particularly when this fibrous cap is intact and the trailing edge is indistinguishable from the underlying plaque. IVUS cannot detect plaque inflammation.

Nevertheless, although gray-scale IVUS cannot determine plaque composition with histologic accuracy, studies consistently show more hypoechoic (soft) plaque in ACS lesions compared with stable angina.[10,48–50] Conversely, extensive calcification is uncommon in most IVUS studies of unstable lesions. Recently, it has been suggested that spotty calcification – multiple small-sized calcium deposits – is more common in acute myocardial infarction and can be detected within the necrotic core using virtual histology. This is consistent with histopathology in similar patients.

Ruptured plaques

Although there have been no pathologic validation studies, the IVUS features of a ruptured plaque are also consistent with the reported histology – a cavity that communicated with the lumen with an overlying residual fibrous cap fragment.[21,51–54] Once the plaque has ruptured and the fibrous cap remnant is surrounded by blood, it is more easily detectable than pre-rupture – unless the cavity fills with thrombus to recreate the pre-rupture limitations. However, some fibrous cap remnants – particularly very thin fragments – may still be below the resolution of IVUS or lie too close to the transducer where there is a zone of uncertainty. It is hoped that improved transducer design, including higher frequencies, will improve the detection of fibrous cap remnants.

Approximately two-third of fibrous caps rupture at the lateral attachment to the vessel wall, and one-third rupture in the middle (Figures 5.15–5.18).[51] This distribution has important implications in the pathogenesis of plaque rupture since central fibrous cap rupture requires significantly more stress compared with rupture at the lateral attachment.

While the diagnosis of thrombus by IVUS is usually considered presumptive, many studies have also reported more IVUS-evident thrombus in ACS lesions (Figures 5.6, 5.16, 5.18–5.20).[48,51,55] In addition ACS patients are not a homogeneous group. Patients who are troponin-positive have more evidence of thrombus formation than ACS patients who are troponin-negative.[56] IVUS thrombi can also exist without concrete evidence of plaque rupture.

Almost all (90%) angiographic complex lesions – ulceration, intimal flap, lumen irregularity, thrombus, and aneurysm – are associated with IVUS ruptured plaques validating the commonly used Ambrose angiographic identification of ACS lesions.[51,57,58] This is illustrated in the many examples in this chapter. However, the converse is not true; and angiography can miss plaque ruptures, particularly multiple discrete plaque ruptures, in the same artery.

The fibrous cap remnant typically appears to be incomplete relative to the mouth of the ruptured plaque cavity in either its circumferential or axial extent, as is seen in many of the figures in this chapter (Figures 5.17–5.20). It is not clear whether this deficit is because the thinnest portions of the fibrous cap are below the resolution of IVUS, because of geometric changes in the artery post-plaque rupture, or because part of the fibrous cap is lost during plaque rupture.

Frequency of culprit and non-culprit (multiple) ruptured plaques

Various IVUS studies have reported culprit-lesion ruptured plaques in a varying percentage of ACS patients. Overall, the frequency seems to average slightly less than 50%; this is less than has been reported pathologically.[50,54,59]

Rioufol *et al.*[54] reported a series of 24 acute coronary syndrome patients with three-vessel IVUS imaging. In this report, there were 50 ruptured plaques: nine (37.5%) within the culprit lesion and 41 at non-culprit sites, including 16 patients with ruptures in two arteries and three patients with ruptures in all three arteries. Thus, surprisingly, most of the ruptured plaques were at sites remote from the presumed culprit lesion; and 79% of patients had a remote-site plaque rupture. The study by Rioufol *et al.* was hailed with enthusiasm by investigators favoring a "pancoronaritis" concept of ACS; however, these findings have not been confirmed by others (Hong and Sumitsuji, unpublished observations). Hong *et al.* (American Heart Association Scientific Sessions 2003) studied all three arteries in 122 patients undergoing primary infarction intervention: 66% of patients had plaque rupture within the culprit lesion; a remote ruptured plaque was seen in 17% of patients; and multiple ruptures were seen in 20% of patients. Sumitsuju *et al..* (American College of Cardiology Scientific Sessions 2004) reported a similar study in 46 patients with a first ACS event and found culprit-lesion

plaque rupture in 49% of patients and non-culprit ruptured plaques in only 15% of patients. These latter two studies are more in keeping with previous histopathologic reports. An example of multiple plaque ruptures is shown in Figure 5.21.

There are several possible reasons for these findings. (1) Errors may occur in identifying the culprit site. (2) Thrombi may be present and may obscure the ruptured plaque cavity and the fibrous cap remnant. (3) IVUS has a limited sensitivity in detecting plaque rupture, particularly small plaque ruptures. (4) Lesions responsible for symptomatic ACS may not contain ruptured plaques, but merely large, bulky, hypoechoic plaques or erosive morphology. (5) Some fibrous cap remnants may be below the threshold of IVUS resolution or lie too close to the transducer. (6) Some plaque ruptures may have an atypical IVUS appearance. Examples of atypical ruptured-plaque morphologies are shown in Figures 5.22–5.24.

Symptomatic versus asymptomatic ruptured plaques

Not all ruptured plaques are associated with acute events. Thrombotic complications that arise from rupture, fissure (small rupture), or erosion may be clinically silent yet contribute to the natural history of plaque progression and luminal stenosis. In the study by Maehara *et al.*,[51] 20–25% of patients with plaque rupture had stable angina or were asymptomatic. In the unpublished study by Hong *et al.*, 27% of 113 stable angina patients had target-lesion plaque rupture, 5% had a remote plaque rupture, and 6% had multiple plaque ruptures. This supports the hypothesis that plaque rupture may be one of the mechanisms of stenosis progression without causing an acute event.[60–63] Angiographic studies have shown that lesion progression in stable angina is greatest at sites with complex lesion morphology.[64]

Recognizing that some ruptured plaques can be asymptomatic or associated only with stable coronary artery disease, Fujii *et al.*[55] compared the morphology of ruptured plaques that were culprit ACS lesions with "incidental" ruptured plaques. Multivariate analysis identified a smaller minimum lumen area ($p = 0.01$) and the presence of thrombus ($p = 0.01$) as independent predictors of ACS culprit-plaque ruptures. This suggests that plaque rupture, itself, did not lead to symptoms. Instead, it was the association of plaque rupture with a smaller lumen area and/or thrombus formation, causing lumen compromise, that led to symptoms (Figure 5.25). The association of thrombus formation and clinical instability in patients with ruptured plaques was also reported in the study by Maehara *et al.*[51] The location of the IVUS catheter does not necessarily indicate the true lumen versus the evacuated plaque cavity (Figure 5.18).

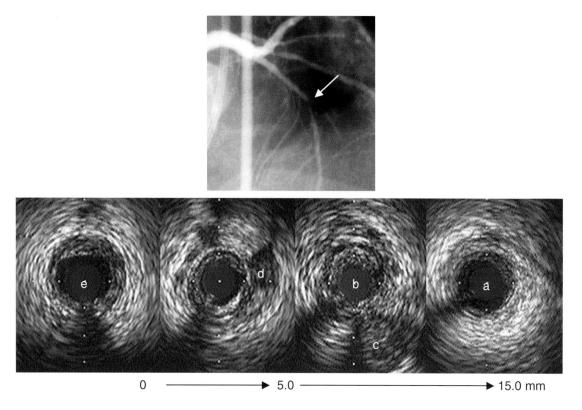

$$0 \longrightarrow 5.0 \longrightarrow 15.0 \text{ mm}$$

Figure 5.14 This woman was a long-standing insulin-treated diabetic patient. She presented with a long stenosis in a small left anterior descending, with almost total occlusion of the small major diagonal (white arrow in the angiogram). The IVUS pullback was performed from the distal reference (a) through the lesion (b) at the level of the diseased diagonal (c) and septal (d) to the proximal reference (e). Note that both references are small and diseased. The distal reference external elastic membrane (EEM) CSA measured 4.7 mm^2 with a plaque burden of 40%, the proximal reference EEM CSA measured 7.3 mm^2 with a plaque burden of 48%, and the lesion EEM CSA measured 4.5 mm^2, giving a remodeling index of 0.75. Small angiographic vessels result from a large amount of atherosclerotic plaque and/or negative remodeling. In this case, the cause is negative remodeling

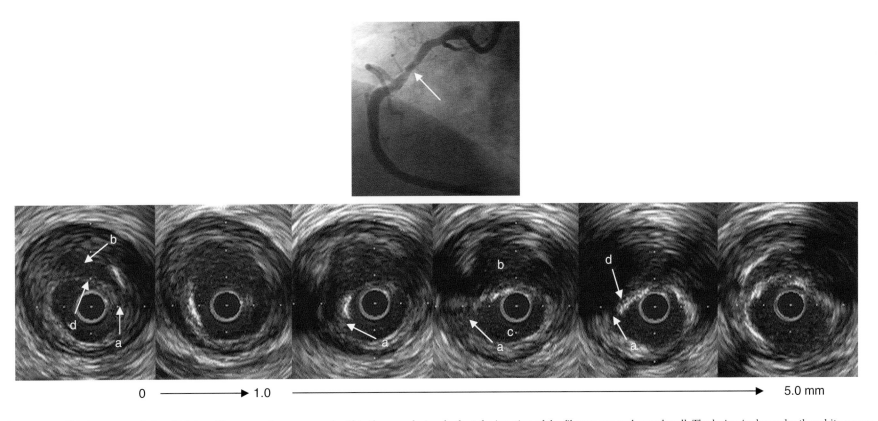

Figure 5.15   This is an example in which two fibrous cap tears occurred within the same lesion, both at the junction of the fibrous cap and vessel wall. The lesion is shown by the white arrow in the angiogram. The IVUS image shows the two lateral tears in the fibrous cap (a), the evacuated cavities (b), the true lumen (c), and the residual fibrous cap fragments (d). The IVUS catheter is in the residual true lumen throughout

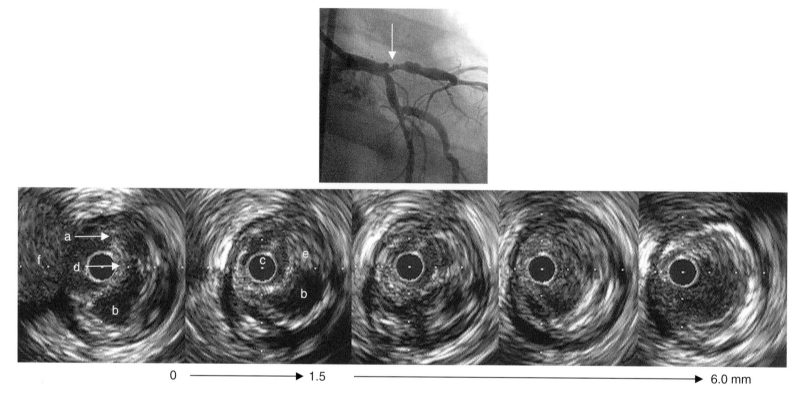

0 ——————→ 1.5 ————————————————————→ 6.0 mm

Figure 5.16   An ostial left anterior descending artery with a complex angiographic lesion is shown (white arrow). The IVUS image shows the lateral plaque rupture (a), the evacuated cavity (b), the true lumen (c), the residual fibrous cap fragments (d), and a probable thrombus (e). Note that the lesion developed opposite the left circumflex (f)

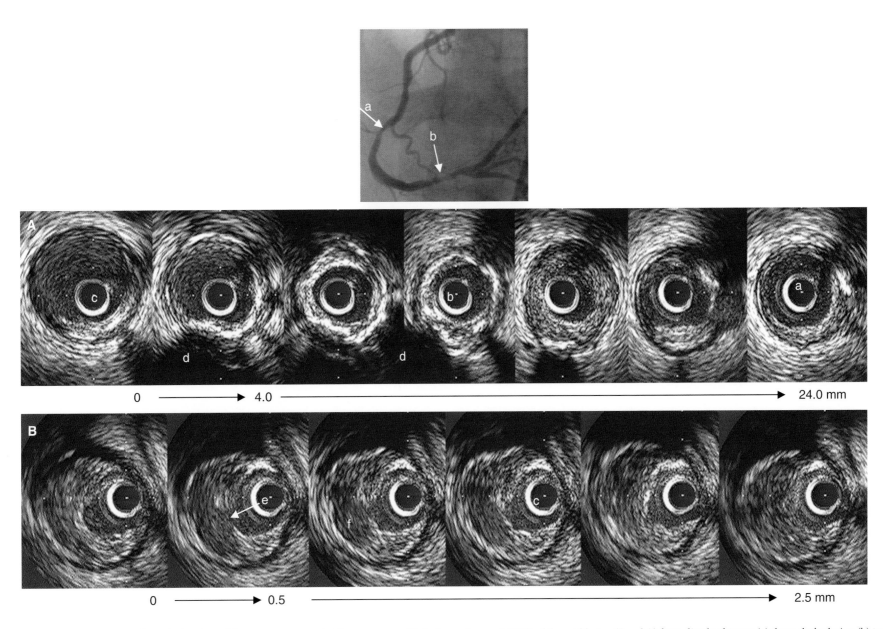

Figure 5.17 This patient had two lesions in a right coronary artery (white arrows a and b in the angiogram). IVUS of the mid lesion (Panel A) from distal reference (a) through the lesion (b) to the proximal reference (c) showed a negatively remodeled lesion. Note the calcific plaque with shadowing (d). The proximal reference external elastic membrane (EEM) CSA measured $14.8\,mm^2$, the lesion EEM CSA measured $11.1\,mm^2$, and the distal reference EEM CSA measured $11.7\,mm^2$. The remodeling index of the mid lesion was 0.84 and the minimum lumen CSA measured $3.0\,mm^2$. IVUS of the distal lesion (Panel B) shows the central plaque rupture (a), the evacuated cavity (b), and the true lumen (c)

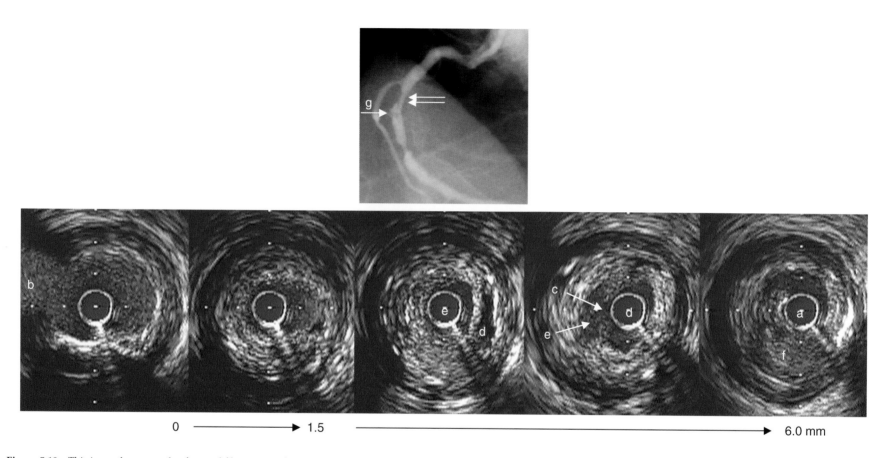

0 ——————→ 1.5 ————————————————————————————→ 6.0 mm

Figure 5.18 This is another example of central fibrous cap plaque rupture. There is a complex right coronary artery lesion just distal to the right ventricular branch (double white arrows in the angiogram). The IVUS study from distal (a) to proximal at the level of the right ventricular branch (b) shows central plaque rupture (white arrow c). Note that the IVUS catheter can be alternatively seen to lie in the false lumen (d) or the true lumen (e) because it can easily enter the false lumen through the central fibrous cap rupture. Therefore, the location of the IVUS catheter cannot be used to identify the true lumen in all cases. There is also suggestion of a thrombus (f) consistent with the filling defect on the angiogram (white arrow g)

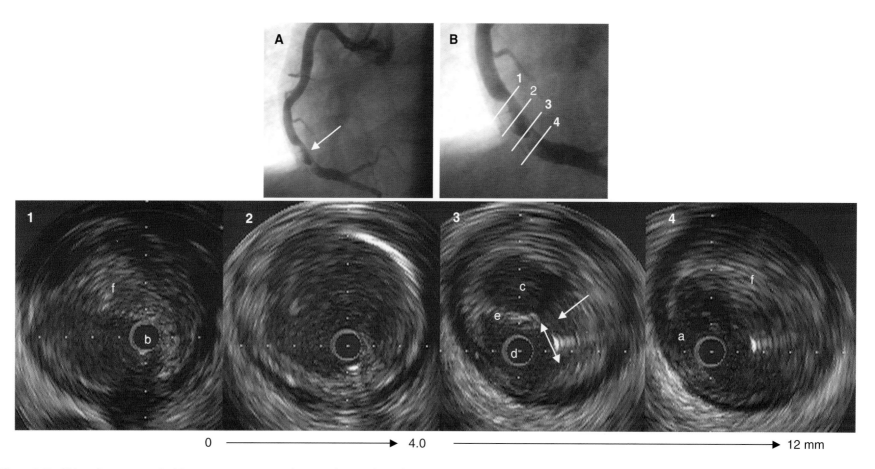

Figure 5.19   This patient presented with an acute coronary syndrome and a complex right coronary lesion (white arrow in Panel A). The IVUS imaging run from distal (a) to proximal (b) shows the evacuated plaque cavity (c), the true lumen (d), the residual fibrous cap (e) and its rupture (white arrow), and evidence of thrombus (f). The IVUS thrombi correspond to the angiographic filling defects; the lines in Panel B correspond to the IVUS image slices 1–4. Note that the fibrous cap remnant does not entirely cover the mouth of the evacuated plaque (double-headed white arrow shows the gap between the fibrous cap remnants)

Figure 5.20 (opposite) This patient presented with an acute coronary syndrome and a complex right coronary lesion (white arrow in the angiogram). The IVUS imaging run from distal (a) to proximal (b) shows the residual fibrous cap (c) and evidence of thrombus (d). Note that the fibrous cap remnant does not entirely cover the mouth of the evacuated plaque (double-headed white arrow)

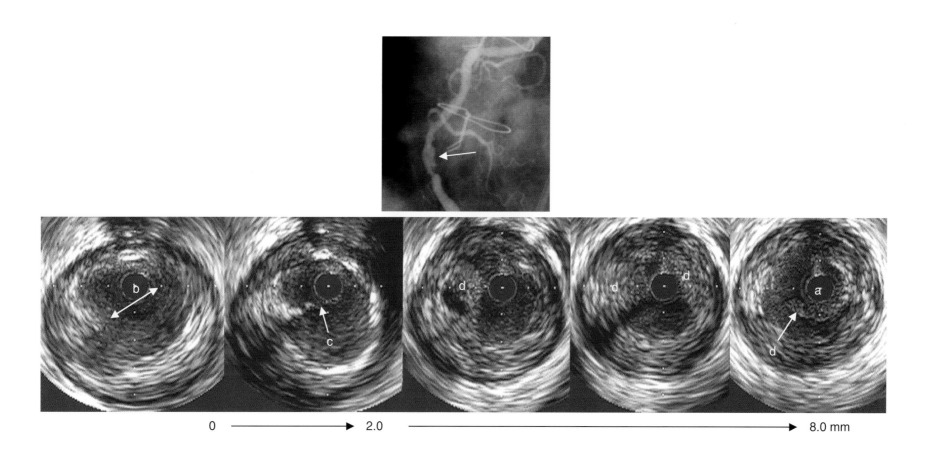

Figure 5.21 (opposite)   This patient presented with an acute coronary syndrome and three complex right coronary lesions (top, middle, and bottom white arrows in Panels A and B). The IVUS studies of these three lesions are shown: Panel C is the proximal lesion, Panel D is the middle lesion, and Panel E is the distal lesion. (The images are shown at 7/8 size compared with the rest of the illustrations.)

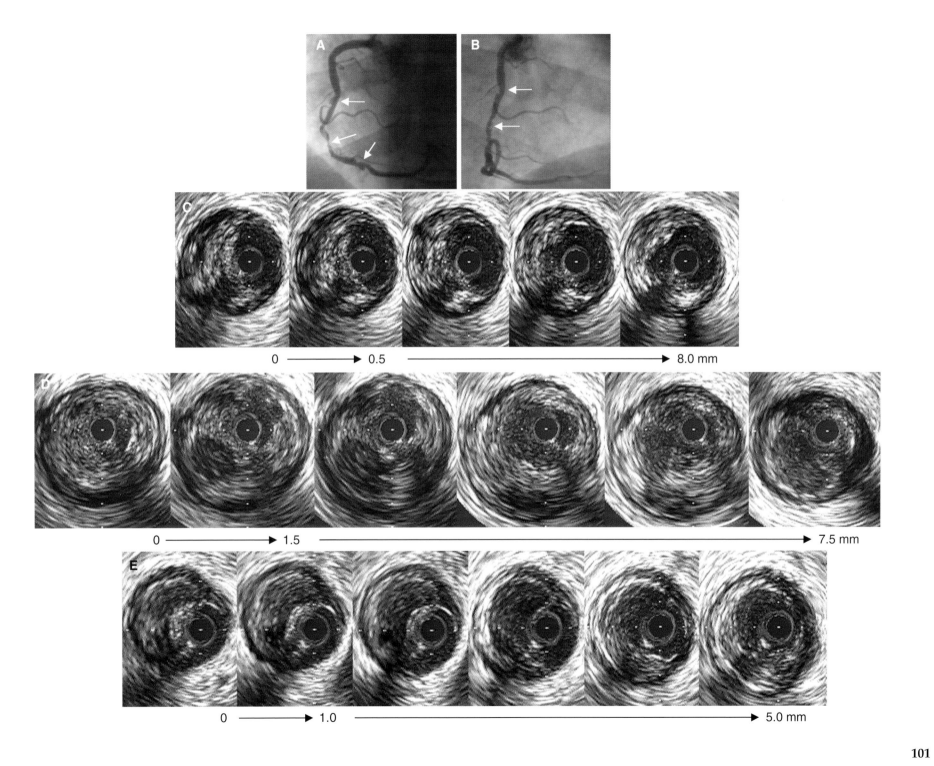

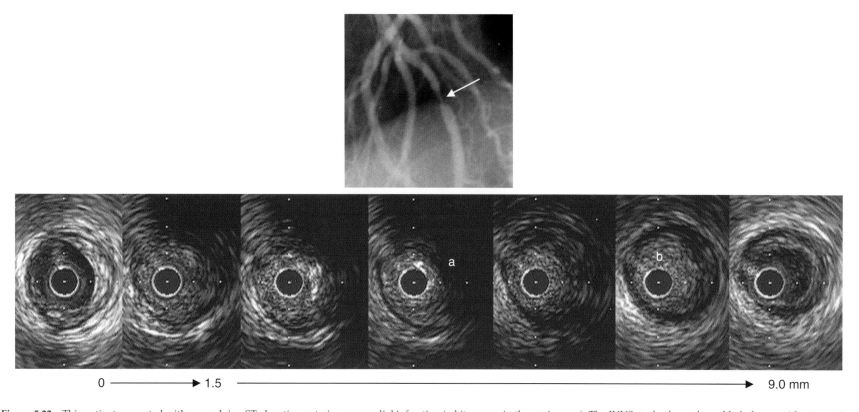

0 ———————➤ 1.5 ————————————————————————➤ 9.0 mm

Figure 5.22 This patient presented with an evolving ST-elevation anterior myocardial infarction (white arrow in the angiogram). The IVUS study showed speckled plaque with attenuation (a) obliterating the lumen, but without the classical features of plaque rupture or thrombus formation. This case suggests that speckled attenuated plaque may represent an unusual appearance of thrombus, in this case either filling the evacuated cavity and lumen or superimposed on an erosive plaque. Note the blood stasis (b) distal to the occlusive lesion

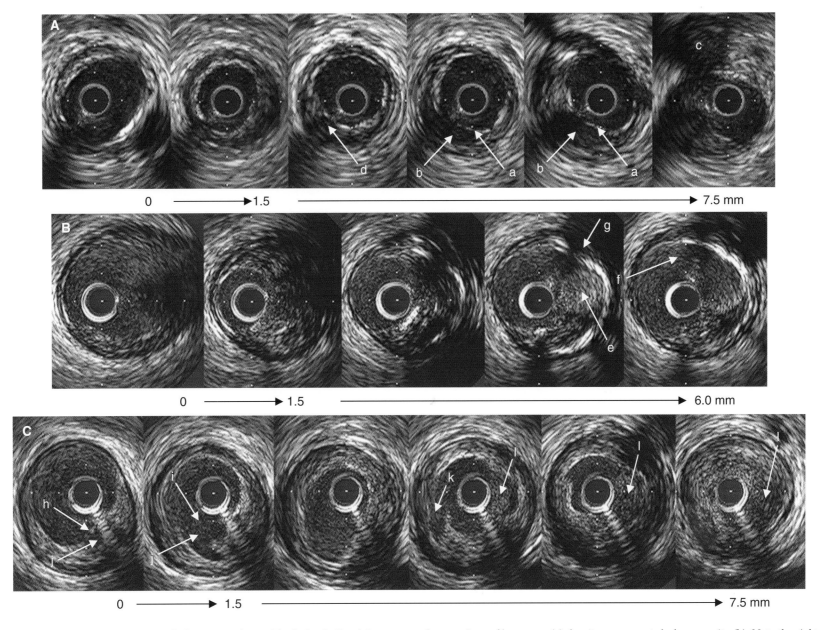

Figure 5.23 Three atypical disrupted plaques are shown. The lesion in Panel A appears to have an intact fibrous cap (a) despite an evacuated plaque cavity (b). Note the right ventricular branch (c) just distal to the plaque cavity. The guidewire artifact (d) suggests a defect in the fibrous cap, but, instead, may actually obscure a defect in the fibrous cap. In Panel B, blood stasis (e) obscures the ruptured plaque cavity. As in Panel A, the lateral disruption of the fibrous cap (f) is also obscured by the guidewire artifact. Note the deep calcium (g) at the base of the ruptured plaque. In Panel C, at the proximal end of the lesion, there is the suggestion of a fibrous cap (h), part of which is particularly thin and almost unnoticeable (i). Note the small cavity (j). There is a secondary site of rupture (k) without a fibrous cap. There is a suggestion of a thrombus (l) that continues proximally

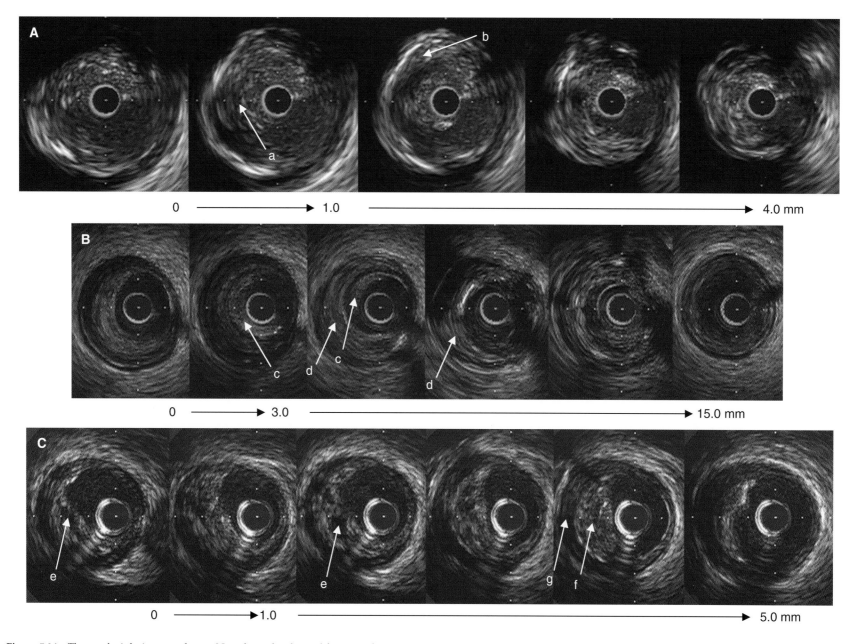

Figure 5.24 Three culprit lesions are shown. None have the classical features of a ruptured plaque. In Panels A and B, there is evidence of a probable thrombus (a and c) that is separate from the underlying plaque (b and d) and that wraps around the IVUS catheter. In Panel C, there are defects in the IVUS plaque (e) that suggest plaque disruption or the presence of thrombus. Note that the possible thrombus becomes more homogeneous distally (f), but is still distinct from the underlying tissue (g)

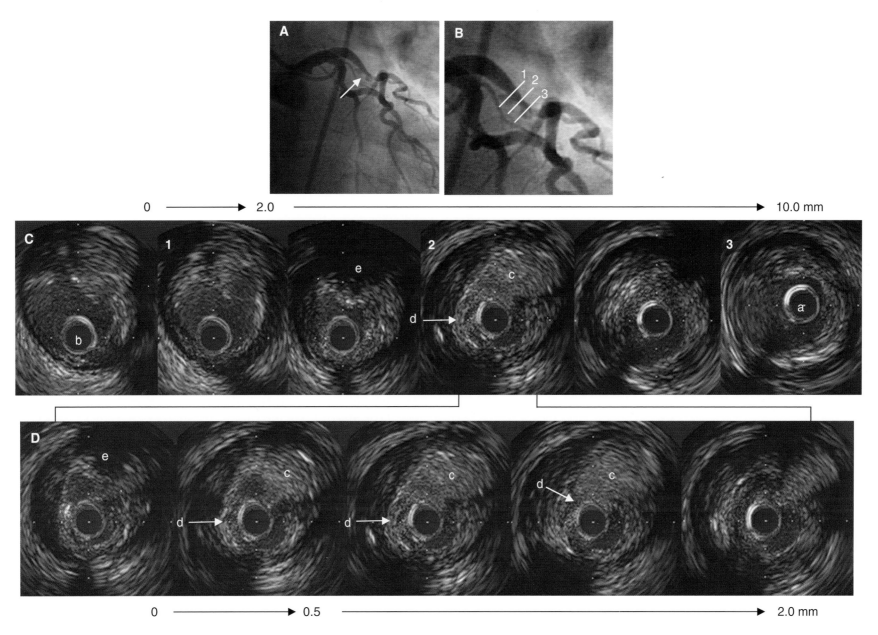

Figure 5.25 This patient presented with a non-Q myocardial infarction and a complex plaque in the left anterior descending artery (white arrow in Panel A). A magnified view is shown in Panel B. Two IVUS imaging runs from distal (a) to proximal (b) are shown; in Panel C, the image slices are 2.0 mm apart, and in Panel D, the slices are 0.5 mm apart, allowing greater detail to be shown. Note the thrombus that originates in the ruptured plaque cavity (c) and that protrudes into the lumen where it wraps around the IVUS catheter to encroach on the lumen (d). In some frames (e), the thrombus is associated with attenuation. The lines in Panel B correspond to the IVUS image slices 1–3. When the angiogram is reviewed with the IVUS information in mind, there is a thrombus (2) within a ruptured plaque cavity (1 and 3)

Other vulnerable plaque morphologies

Erosions are, to an extent, a histopathologic diagnosis of exclusion.[18,46,47] There is no fibrous cap, calcium is less common, positive remodeling is absent, typically the endothelium is absent, and there is minimal inflammation. Erosions are more common in young women and are associated with smoking. Other than the lack of positive remodeling, none of the histopathologic features of erosions can be detected by IVUS.

A more rare type of vulnerable plaque is a superficial calcified nodule within or very close to the fibrous cap of the plaque (Figure 5.26). This structure can protrude through to rupture the cap. It may or may not be associated with a high calcium score.[46]

Finally, some authors have described both fissuring and lipid pools in IVUS images. While these have been seen histologically, there is no current validation of these findings by IVUS. Fissures appear as minor disruptions of the intima and lipid pools as hypoechoic plaque. There are other causes of hypoechoic plaques.

LUMEN COMPROMISE

Despite the fact that most lesions causing an acute event arise from previously insignificant lesions, both angiographic and IVUS studies have shown that the likelihood that any one lesion will lead to an event is related to its baseline stenosis severity.[65–67] This is nicely explained by the following statement from Kern and Meier:[68] "Because the aggregate risk of rupture associated with many nonsignificant lesions (each with an admittedly lower individual risk potential) exceeds that of the fewer significant lesions, a myocardial infarction will more likely originate from a nonsignificant lesion." Thus, lumen dimensions should not be ignored in assessing unstable lesions; and chronically stenotic plaques with severe calcification, old thrombus, and eccentric lumens are included in the list of vulnerable plaque types.[1]

CALCIUM

By IVUS, calcium is seen in most (75%) stenoses in patients with chronic stable angina undergoing intervention.[69–71] The average IVUS arc of calcium in stable stenoses exceeds 100°. Calcium is less common, the amount of calcium is quantitatively less, and the location of calcium is more often deep in ACS lesions.

Calcium and plaque burden

Electron-beam computed tomographic (EBCT) detection of calcium has been shown to be predictive of coronary events.[72–74] If calcium is not related to plaque instability and is less common in plaques associated with ACS, what is the explanation for the predictive value of coronary calcium (as detected and quantified by EBCT) and subsequent events? Both pathologic and IVUS studies have shown that calcium is a marker of plaque burden and that coronary calcium rarely occurs in the absence of coronary atherosclerosis. The overall plaque burden is roughly proportional to an IVUS volumetric measure of calcium.[8,75,76] Total arterial plaque burden is an important determinant of events and patient outcomes;[1] presumably, a greater plaque burden increases the probability that an unstable lesion will develop.

Calcium and plaque instability

Although coronary calcification can be correlated closely with plaque burden, its effect on individual plaque stability is less clear. In one pathologic series of sudden coronary deaths, more than 50% of thin-cap atheromas showed either no calcium or only speckled calcium, while 65% of actual ruptures demonstrated speckled calcium.[47] (The remainder showed showed fragmented or diffuse calcium.) Thus, there is a large variation in the presence and severity of calcium within vulnerable plaques as well as a lack of specificity of the various patterns of calcium. Finally, *in vitro* biomechanical models have shown that, in contrast to lipid pools, which dramatically increase fibrous cap stresses, calcium does not seem to affect the mechanical stability of the atheroma, although it does appear that mildly to moderately calcified plaques are the ones most prone to rupture.[18,77]

PROGRESSION/REGRESSION

Based, in part, on successful studies of restenosis and of transplant vasculopathy, serial IVUS is now being used to study progression and regression as well as strategies to modify the disease process.

In a small study, Takagi *et al.*[78] compared serial IVUS measurements in 36 patients randomized to dietary control versus pravastatin (10 mg daily). At three-year follow-up, IVUS data in 25 of the patients showed a 41% increase in P&M CSA in the diet-only group compared with a 7% decrease in the pravastatin group ($p < 0.0005$).

REVERSAL was a prospective, randomized, double-blind, multicenter study comparing the effects of atorvastatin versus pravastatin on the progression of coronary atherosclerotic lesions.[79] A total of 654 patients were randomized to either 80 mg atorvastatin daily (intensive lipid-lowering strategy) versus 40 mg pravastatin daily (moderate lipid-lowering strategy). The primary endpoint was the percentage change in IVUS P&M volume; the two pre-specified secondary endpoints were the absolute change in P&M volume and the percentage change in plaque burden (defined as P&M volume divided by EEM volume). Paired IVUS data were available in 502 patients. At an 18-month follow-up, low-density lipoprotein (LDL) levels were 110 mg/dl in the pravastatin group versus 79 mg/dl in the atorvastatin group ($p <$ 0.001), while high-density lipoprotein (HDL) levels were not significantly different. There was a 2.7% increase (progression) in the P&M volume in the pravastatin group ($p = 0.01$ compared with baseline) versus a 0.4% decrease (regression) in the atorvastatin group ($p = 1.0$ compared with baseline). The 18-month change was significantly different between the two groups ($p = 0.02$). Secondary endpoints were similarly positive.

Von Birgelen *et al.*[80] analyzed serial IVUS studies of 60 non-stenotic left main coronary arteries obtained 18.3 ± 9.4 months apart to evaluate progression and regression of mild atherosclerotic plaques in relation to serum cholesterol levels. Overall, there was a positive linear relation between the annual changes in P&M CSA and LDL ($r = 0.41$, $p < 0.0001$), with an LDL value of 75 mg/dl as the cut-off where regression analysis predicted, on average, no annual P&M CSA increase. This was remarkably similar to the LDL value in the atorvastatin group of the REVERSAL study. In a subsequent analysis, these same authors showed that annual changes in left main P&M CSA could be correlated with cardiovascular risk factors as reported in the PRO-CAM, SCORE, and Framingham studies.[81–84] In addition, annual changes in non-stenotic left main P&M CSA predicted non-left main cardiovascular events (acute coronary syndromes, including myocardial infarction, or revascularization of new lesions elsewhere in the coronary tree). Patients with events had an annual left main plaque progression significantly greater than patients without events (25.2 ± 19.4% vs. 5.9 ± 15.6%, $p < 0.001$) (Figure 5.27).

Nissen *et al.*[84] used serial volumetric IVUS analysis to study the effect of administering the HDL mimetic ApoA-I Milano – a variant of apolipoprotein A-I, identified in individuals in rural Italy who exhibited very low levels of HDL. In a ratio of 1:2:2, patients received five weekly infusions of placebo or two doses of the drug; 57 patients with ACS were randomized, and 47 patients completed the protocol. IVUS was performed within two weeks after the ACS event and after the five weekly infusions. The primary endpoint was the change in volumetric plaque burden in the combined treatment cohort. Pre-specified secondary endpoints included the absolute change in P&M volume. In the combined treatment group, the volumetric plaque burden decreased by 1.06% ($p = 0.02$ compared with baseline). In the placebo group, volumetric plaque burden increased by

0.14% ($p = 1.0$ compared with baseline). The secondary endpoint results were similar.

Finally, Jensen *et al.*[85] used ECG-gated acquisition volumetric IVUS to study 40 patients at baseline and after 3 and 12 months of simvastatin (40 mg/day). At 12 months, there was a significant reduction in total cholesterol and LDL-cholesterol, a significant reduction in P&M volume of 6.3% and of EEM volume of 3.6%, but no reduction in lumen volume. A correlation could be shown between the percentage change in lumen volume versus the percentage change in P&M volume ($r = 0.74$, $p < 0.001$), but not versus the percentage change in EEM volume; in addition, the percentage change in EEM volume could be correlated with the percentage change in P&M volume ($r = 0.65$, $p < 0.001$), confirming what has long been suspected – that atherosclerosis regression is accompanied by reversal of the positive remodeling process to mask any potential effect on lumen volume. This explains why angiographic findings of progression/regression often lag behind clinical endpoints in progression/regression studies.

These studies indicate that serial IVUS studies have the potential to assess progression and regression in relatively small numbers of patients and over a relatively short time period – certainly compared with angiography, which typically shows no change, and compared with clinical endpoints, which take large numbers of patients followed for long periods of time. The ideal IVUS endpoint – absolute or relative changes in P&M volume or absolute or relative changes in plaque burden – has yet to be determined.

SAPHENOUS VEIN GRAFT DISEASE

Although arterial remodeling and its relationship to lesion formation and plaque rupture in native vessels are well established, the existence of these findings in saphenous vein grafts is the subject of controversy. Some authors have suggested that positive remodeling in vein grafts is an artifact caused by lesion formation at the site of venous valves.[87] This conclusion is disputed by other authors.[88,89] Examples of positive and negative saphenous vein-graft remodeling are shown in Figures 5.27 and 5.28. Similarly, recent observations suggest that vein-graft plaques are also rupture-prone (Figure 5.29). The existence of vein-graft remodeling and plaque rupture is intriguing because it suggests a direct effect of the disease process on the (denervated) vein-graft vessel wall. However, there are no data to indicate that these IVUS findings have the same implications as they do in native arteries, although one recent angiographic study compared patients with single versus multiple complex angiographic plaques and found a worse prognosis in multiple complex plaques similar to native coronary arteries.[45,90]

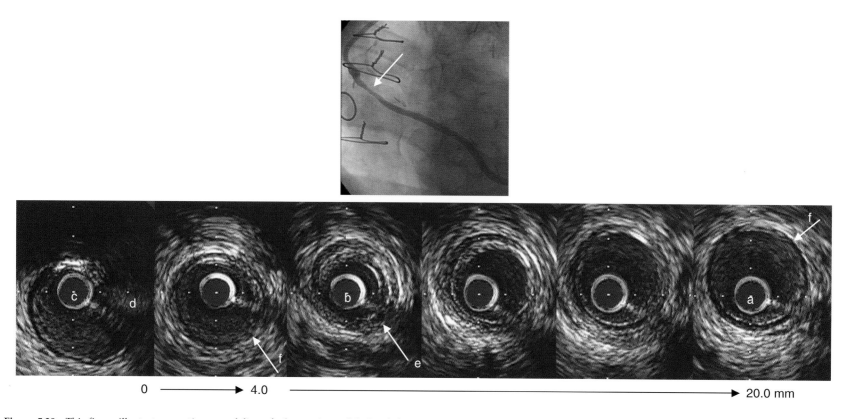

0 ──────▶ 4.0 ───────────────────────────────────────▶ 20.0 mm

Figure 5.28 This figure illustrates negative remodeling of a long vein-graft lesion (white arrow in the angiogram). The IVUS imaging run from distal (a) through the lesion (b) to the proximal reference (c) at the level of the aorta (d) shows a lesion-site vein-graft CSA (e) of 8.4 mm² compared with a mean reference vein-graft CSA (f) of 10.7 mm² for a remodeling index of 0.79

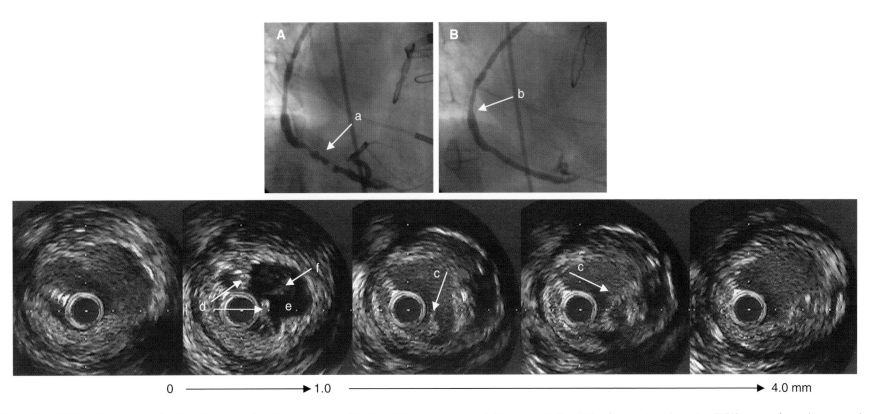

Figure 5.29   This patient presented with a degenerated saphenous vein graft to the right coronary artery (white arrow in Panel A). After stent implantation, IVUS was performed to assess the stent and the proximal vein graft (white arrow in Panel B). IVUS imaging detected mobile plaque elements (c), a residual fibrous cap (d), and an evacuated plaque cavity (e). Contrast was injected during imaging, which explains the absence of blood speckle in the evacuated plaque cavity; note the cloud of echoes (f) that occurred during contrast injection

REFERENCES

1. Naghavi M, Libby P, Falk E, et al. From vulnerable plaque to vulnerable patient: A call for new definitions and risk assessment strategies. Circulation 2003; 108: 1664–72, 1772–8
2. Yamagishi M, Terashima M, Awano K, et al. Morphology of vulnerable coronary plaque: insights from follow-up of patients examined by intravascular ultrasound before an acute coronary syndrome. J Am Coll Cardiol 2000; 35: 106–11
3. Mintz GS, Nissen SE, Anderson WD, et al. Standards for the acquisition, measurement, and reporting of intravascular ultrasound studies: A report of the American College of Cardiology Task Force on Clinical Expert Consensus Documents. J Am Coll Cardiol 2001; 37: 1478–92
4. Shiran A, Mintz GS, Leiboff B, et al. Serial volumetric intravascular ultrasound assessment of arterial remodeling in left main coronary artery disease. Am J Cardiol 1999; 83: 1427–32
5. Von Birgelen C, Hartmann M, Mintz GS, et al. Spectrum of remodeling behavior observed with serial long-term (≥12 months) follow-up intravascular ultrasound studies in left main coronary arteries. Am J Cardiol 2004;93:1107–13
6. Glagov S, Weisenberg E, Zarins CK, et al. Compensatory enlargement of human atherosclerotic coronary arteries. N Engl J Med 1987; 316: 1371–5
7. Mintz GS, Painter JA, Pichard AD, et al. Atherosclerosis in angiographically "normal" coronary artery reference segments: An intravascular ultrasound study with clinical correlations. J Am Coll Cardiol 1995; 25: 1479–85
8. Tinana A, Mintz GS, Weissman NJ. Volumetric intravascular ultrasound quantification of the amount of atherosclerosis and calcium in nonstenotic arterial segments. Am J Cardiol 2002; 89: 757–60
9. Dangas G, Mintz GS, Mehran R, et al. Preintervention arterial remodeling as an independent predictor of target-lesion revascularization after nonstent coronary intervention: an analysis of 777 lesions with intravascular ultrasound imaging. *Circulation* 1999; 99 :3149–54
10. Schoenhagen P, Ziada KM, Kapadia SR, et al. Extent and direction of arterial remodeling in stable versus unstable coronary syndromes: an intravascular ultrasound study. Circulation 2000; 101: 598–603
11. Nishioka T, Luo H, Eigler NL, et al. Contribution of inadequate compensatory enlargement to development of human coronary artery stenosis: An in vivo intravascular ultrasound study. J Am Coll Cardiol 1996; 27: 1571–6
12. Hong MK, Mintz GS, Lee CW, et al. Intravascular ultrasound assessment of patterns of arterial remodeling in the absence of significant reference segment plaque burden in patients with coronary artery disease. J Am Coll Cardiol 2003; 42: 806–10
13. Mintz GS, Kent KM, Pichard AD, et al. The contribution of inadequate arterial remodeling to the development of focal coronary artery stenoses. An intravascular ultrasound study. Circulation 1997; 95: 1791–8
14. Burke AP, Kolodgie FD, Farb A, et al. Morphological predictors of arterial remodeling in coronary atherosclerosis. Circulation 2002; 105: 297–303
15. Iyisoy A, Schoenhagen P, Balghith M, et al. Remodeling pattern within diseased coronary segments as evidenced by intravascular ultrasound. Am J Cardiol 2002; 90: 636–8
16. Kornowski R, Mintz GS, Lansky AJ, et al. Paradoxic decreases in atherosclerotic plaque mass in insulin-treated diabetic patients. Am J Cardiol 1997; 81: 1298–304
17. Schoenhagen P, Ziada KM, Vince DG, et al. Arterial remodeling and coronary artery disease: the concept of "dilated" versus "obstructive" coronary atherosclerosis. J Am Coll Cardiol 2001; 38: 297–306
18. Burke AP, Virmani R, Galis Z, et al. 34th Bethesda Conference: Task Force #2 – What is the pathologic basis for new atherosclerosis imaging techniques? J Am Coll Cardiol 2003; 41: 1874–86
19. Smits PC, Pasterkamp G, de Jaegere PP, et al. Angioscopic complex lesions are predominantly compensatory enlarged: an angioscopy and intracoronary ultrasound study. Cardiovasc Res 1999; 41: 458–64
20. Takano M, Mizuno K, Okamatsu K, et al. Mechanical and structural characteristics of vulnerable plaques: analysis by coronary angioscopy and intravascular ultrasound. J Am Coll Cardiol 2001; 38: 99–104
21. von Birgelen C, Klinkhart W, Mintz GS, et al. Plaque distribution and vascular remodeling of ruptured and nonruptured coronary plaques in the same vessel: an intravascular ultrasound study in vivo. J Am Coll Cardiol 2001; 37: 1864–70
22. Nakamura M, Nishikawa H, Mukai S, et al. Impact of coronary artery remodeling on clinical presentation of coronary artery disease: an intravascular ultrasound study. J Am Coll Cardiol 2001; 37: 63–9
23. Gyongyosi M, Yang P, Hassan A, et al. Arterial remodelling of native human coronary arteries in patients with unstable angina pectoris: a prospective intravascular ultrasound study. Heart 1999; 82: 68–74
24. Schoenhagen P, Vince DG, Ziada KM, et al. Association of arterial expansion (expansive remodeling) of bifurcation lesions determined by intravascular ultrasonography with unstable clinical presentation. Am J Cardiol 2001; 88: 785–7
25. Tauth J, Pinnow E, Sullebarger JT, et al. Predictors of coronary arterial remodeling patterns in patients with myocardial ischemia. Am J Cardiol 1997; 80: 1352–5
26. Weissman NJ, Sheris SJ, Chari R, et al. Intravascular ultrasonic analysis of plaque characteristics associated with coronary artery remodeling. Am J Cardiol 1999; 84: 37–40
27. Hong MK, Park SW, Lee CW, et al. Intravascular ultrasound comparison of chronic recoil among different stent designs. Am J Cardiol 1999; 84: 1247–50
28. Fujii K, Kobayashi Y, Mintz GS, et al. Dominant contribution of negative remodeling to development of significant coronary bifurcation narrowing. Am J Cardiol 2003; 92: 59–61
29. Iyisoy A, Ziada K, Schoenhagen P, et al. Intravascular ultrasound evidence of ostial narrowing in nonatherosclerotic left main arteries. Am J Cardiol 2002; 90: 773–5
30. Hirose M, Kobayashi Y, Mintz GS, et al. Correlation of coronary arterial remodeling determined by intravascular ultrasound with angiographic diameter reduction of 20 to 60%. Am J Cardiol 2003; 92: 141–5
31. von Birgelen C, Mintz GS, Sieling C, et al. Relation between plaque composition and vascular remodeling in coronary lesions with different degrees of lumen narrowing as assessed with three-dimensional intravascular ultrasound in patients with stable angina pectoris. Am J Cardiol 2003; 91: 1103–7
32. Vavuranakis M, Stefanidis C, Toutouzas K, et al. Impaired compensatory coronary artery enlargement in atherosclerosis contributes to the development of coronary artery stenosis in diabetic patients. An in vivo intravascular ultrasound study. Eur Heart J 1997; 18: 1090–4
33. Tsunoda T, Schoenhagen P, Larsen JR, et al. Comparison of coronary plaque volumes and remodeling in Type I diabetes versus matched controls: A quantitative intravascular ultrasound study. Circulation 2003; 108: IV-462
34. Abizaid AS, Mehran R, Mintz GS, et al. Impact of diabetes on coronary remodeling in patients with acute coronary syndromes: an intravascular ultrasound study. J Am Coll Cardiol 2003; 41: 8A
35. Mehran R, Dangas G, Mintz GS, et al. Atherosclerotic plaque burden and CK-MB enzyme elevation after coronary interventions: intravascular ultrasound study of 2256 patients. Circulation 2000; 101: 604–10
36. Tanaka A, Kawarabayashi T, Nishibori Y, et al. No-reflow phenomenon and lesion morphology in patients with acute myocardial infarction. Circulation 2002; 105: 2148–52
37. Kotani J, Mintz GS, Castagna MT, et al. Usefulness of preprocedural coronary lesion morphology as assessed by intravasuclar ultrasound in predicting Thrombolysis In Myocardial Infarction frame count after percutaneous coronary intervention in patients with Q-wave acute myocardial infarction. Am J Cardiol 2003; 91: 870–2
38. Gyongyosi M, Wexberg P, Kiss K, et al. Adaptive remodeling of the infarct-related artery is associated with recurrent ischemic events after thrombolysis in acute myocardial infarction. Coron Artery Dis 2001; 12: 167–72
39. Gyongyosi M, Yang P, Hassan A, et al. Intravascular ultrasound predictors of major adverse cardiac events in patients with unstable angina. Clin Cardiol 2000; 23: 507–15
40. Okura H, Morino Y, Oshima A, et al. Preintervention arterial remodeling affects clinical outcome following stenting: an intravascular ultrasound study. J Am Coll Cardiol 2001; 37: 1031–5

41. Endo A, Hirayama H, Yoshida O, et al. Arterial remodeling influences the development of intimal hyperplasia after stent implantation. J Am Coll Cardiol 2001; 37: 70–5

42. Mintz GS, Tinana A, Hong MK, et al. Impact of preinterventional arterial remodeling on neointimal hyperplasia after implantation of (non-polymer-encapsulated) paclitaxel-coated stents: a serial volumetric intravascular ultrasound analysis from the ASian Paclitaxel-Eluting Stent Clinical Trial (ASPECT). Circulation 2003; 108: 1295–8

43. Wexberg P, Gyongyosi M, Sperker W, et al. Pre-existing arterial remodeling is associated with in-hospital and late adverse cardiac events after coronary interventions in patients with stable angina pectoris. J Am Coll Cardiol 2000; 36: 1860–9

44. Mintz GS, Maehara A, Bui AB, et al. Multiple versus single coronary plaque ruptures detected by intravascular ultrasound in stable and unstable angina and in acute myocardial infarction. Am J Cardiol 2003; 91: 1333–5

45. Goldstein JA, Demetriou D, Grines CL, et al. Multiple complex coronary plaques in patients with acute myocardial infarction. N Engl J Med 2000; 343: 915–22

46. Virmani R, Kolodgie FD, Burke AP, et al. Lessons from sudden coronary death: A comprehensive morphological classification scheme for atherosclerotic lesions. Arterioscler Thromb Vasc Biol 2000; 20: 1262–75

47. Kolodgie FD, Burke AP, Farb A, et al. The thin-cap fibroatheroma: a type of vulnerable plaque. The major precursor lesion to acute coronary syndromes. Curr Opin Cardiol 2001; 16: 285–92

48. Hodgson JM, Reddy KG, Suneja R, et al. Intracoronary ultrasound imaging: Correlation of plaque morphology with angiography, clinical syndrome and procedural results in patients undergoing coronary angioplasty. J Am Coll Cardiol 1993; 21: 35–44

49. Rasheed Q, Nair R, Sheehan H, et al. Correlation of intracoronary ultrasound plaque characteristics in atherosclerotic coronary artery disease patients with clinical variables. Am J Cardiol 1994; 73: 753–8

50. Fukuda D, Kawarabayashi T, Tanaka A, et al. Lesion characteristics of acute myocardial infarction: an investigation with intravascular ultrasound. Heart 2001; 85: 402–6

51. Maehara A, Mintz GS, Bui AB, et al. Morphologic and angiographic features of coronary plaque rupture detected by intravascular ultrasound. J Am Coll Cardiol 2002; 40: 904–10

52. Ge J, Chirillo F, Schwedtmann J, et al. Screening of ruptured plaques in patients with coronary artery disease by intravascular ultrasound. Heart 1999; 81: 621–7

53. Nagai T, Luo H, Atar S, et al. Intravascular ultrasound imaging of ruptured atherosclerotic plaques in coronary arteries. Am J Cardiol 1999; 83: 135–7

54. Rioufol G, Finet G, Ginon I, et al. Multiple atherosclerotic plaque rupture in acute coronary syndrome: a three-vessel intravascular ultrasound study. Circulation 2002; 106: 804–8

55. Fujii K, Kobayashi Y, Mintz GS, et al. Intravascular ultrasound assessment of ulcerated ruptured plaques: a comparison of culprit and non-nulprit lesions of patients with acute coronary syndromes and lesions in patients without acute coronary syndromes. Circulation 2003; 108: 2473–8

56. Fuchs S, Stabile E, Mintz GS, et al. Intravascular ultrasound findings in patients with acute coronary syndromes with and without elevated troponin I level. Am J Cardiol 2002; 89: 1111–13

57. Ambrose JA, Winters SL, Arora RR, et al. Coronary angiographic morphology in myocardial infarction: a link between the pathogenesis of unstable angina and myocardial infarction. J Am Coll Cardiol 1985; 6: 1233–8

58. Ambrose JA, Winters SL, Arora RR, et al. Angiographic evolution of coronary artery morphology in unstable angina. J Am Coll Cardiol 1986; 7: 472–8

59. Sano T, Tanaka A, Namba M, et al. C-reactive protein and lesion morphology in patients with acute myocardial infarction. Circulation 2003; 108: 282–5

60. Burke AP, Kolodgie FD, Farb A, et al. Healed plaque ruptures and sudden coronary death: evidence that subclinical rupture has a role in plaque progression. Circulation 2001; 103: 934–40

61. Kaski JC, Chester MR, Chen L, et al. Rapid angiographic progression of coronary artery disease in patients with angina pectoris. The role of complex stenosis morphology. Circulation 1995; 92: 2058–65

62. Chester MR, Chen LKaski JC. The natural history of unheralded complex coronary plaques. J Am Coll Cardiol 1996; 28: 604–8

63. Yokoya K, Takatsu H, Suzuki T, et al. Process of progression of coronary artery lesions from mild or moderate stenosis to moderate or severe stenosis: A study based on four serial coronary arteriograms per year. Circulation 1999; 100: 903–9

64. Ambrose JA, Winters SL, Stern A, et al. Angiographic morphology and the pathogenesis of unstable angina pectoris. J Am Coll Cardiol 1985; 5: 609–16

65. Little WC, Constantinescu M, Applegate RJ, et al. Can coronary angiography predict the site of a subsequent myocardial infarction in patients with mild-to-moderate coronary artery disease? Circulation 1988; 78: 1157–66

66. Ellis S, Alderman E, Cain K, et al. Prediction of risk of anterior myocardial infarction by lesion severity and measurement method of stenoses in the left anterior descending coronary distribution: a CASS Registry study. J Am Coll Cardiol 1988; 11: 908–16

67. Abizaid AS, Mintz GS, Mehran R, et al. One year follow-up after percutaneous transluminal angioplasty was not performed based on intravascular ultrasound findings. Importance of lumen dimensions. Circulation 1999; 100: 256–61

68. Kern MJ, Meier B. Evaluation of the culprit plaque and the physiological significance of coronary atherosclerotic narrowings. Circulation 2001; 103: 3142–9

69. Mintz GS, Douek P, Pichard AD, et al. Target lesion calcification in coronary artery disease: An intravascular ultrasound study. J Am Coll Cardiol 1992; 20: 1149–55

70. Tuzcu EM, Berkalp B, De Franco AC, et al. The dilemma of diagnosing coronary calcification: angiography versus intravascular ultrasound. J Am Coll Cardiol 1996; 27: 832–8

71. Mintz GS, Popma JJ, Pichard AD, et al. Patterns of calcification in coronary artery disease. A statistical analysis of intravascular ultrasound and coronary angiography in 1155 lesions. Circulation 1995; 91: 1959–65

72. Arad Y, Spadaro LA, Goodman K, et al. Prediction of coronary events with electron beam computed tomography. J Am Coll Cardiol 2000; 36: 1253–60

73. Arad Y, Spadaro LA, Goodman K, et al. Predictive value of electron beam computed tomography of the coronary arteries. 19-month follow-up of 1173 asymptomatic subjects. Circulation 1996; 93: 1951–3

74. Guerci AD, Arad Y. Electron beam computed tomography for the diagnosis and prognosis of coronary artery disease. Circulation 2001; 103: E87

75. Mintz GS, Pichard AD, Popma JJ, et al. Determinants and correlates of target lesion calcium in coronary artery disease: a clinical, angiographic, and intravascular ultrasound study. J Am Coll Cardiol 1997; 29: 268–74

76. Sangiorgi G, Rumberger JA, Severson A, et al. Arterial calcification and not lumen stenosis is highly correlated with atherosclerotic plaque burden in humans: a histologic study of 723 coronary artery segments using nondecalcifying methodology. J Am Coll Cardiol 1998; 31: 126–33

77. Huang H, Virmani R, Younis H, et al. The impact of calcification on the biomechanical stability of atherosclerotic plaques. Circulation 2001; 103: 1051–6

78. Takagi T, Yoshida K, Akasaka T, et al. Intravascular ultrasound analysis of reduction in progression of coronary narrowing by treatment with pravastatin. Am J Cardiol 1997; 79: 1673–6

79. Nissen SE, Tuzcu EM, Schoenhagen P, et al. Effect of intensive compared with moderate lipid-lowering therapy on progression of coronary atherosclerosis. JAMA 2004; 291: 1071–80

80. von Birgelen C, Hartmann M, Mintz GS, et al. Relation between progression and regression of atherosclerotic left main coronary artery disease and serum cholesterol levels as assessed with serial long-term (≥12 months) follow-up intravascular ultrasound. Circulation 2003; 108: 2757–62

81. Anderson KM, Wilson PW, Odell PM, et al. An updated coronary risk profile. A statement for health professionals. Circulation 1991; 83: 356–62

82. Conroy RM, Pyörälä K, Fitzgerald AP, et al. Estimation of ten-year risk of fatal cardiovascular disease in Europe: the SCORE project. Eur Heart J 2003; 24: 987–1003

83. Assmann G, Cullen P, Schulte H. Simple scoring scheme for calculating the risk of acute coronary events based on the 10-year follow-up of the Prospective Cardiovascular Münster (PROCAM) Study. Circulation 2002; 105: 310–5

84. Von Birgelen C, Hartmann C, Mintz G, et al, Relationship between cardiovascular risk as predicted by established risk scores versus plaque progression as measured by serial intravasuclar ultrasound in left main arteries. Circulation 2004; in press

85. Nissen SE, Tsunoda T, Tuzcu EM, et al. Effect of recombinant ApoA-I Milano on coronary atherosclerosis in patients with acute coronary syndromes: a randomized controlled trial. JAMA 2003; 290: 2292–300
86. Jensen LO, Thayssen P, Pedersen KE, et al. Coronary plaque regression by simvastatin is associated with reduction in vessel volume: a three-dimensional intravascular ultrasound study. J Am Coll Cardiol 2004; 42: 12A
87. Nishioka T, Luo H, Berglund H, et al. Absence of focal compensatory enlargement or constriction in diseased human coronary saphenous vein bypass grafts. Circulation 1996; 93: 683–90
88. Ge J, Liu F, Bhate R, et al. Does remodeling occur in the diseased human saphenous vein bypass grafts? An intravascular ultrasound study. Int J Card Imaging 1999; 15: 295–300
89. Hong M-K, Mintz GS, Hong MK, et al. Intravascular ultrasound assessment of the presence of vascular remodeling in diseased human saphenous vein bypass grafts. Am J Cardiol 1999; 84: 992–8
90. Raff GL, Safian RD, Pica MC, et al. Multiple complex plaques in unstable saphenous vein grafts. J Am Coll Cardiol 2004; 42: 261A

6
Pre-intervention and diagnostic imaging, lesion assessment, and device sizing

Despite the many differences between IVUS and angiography (Chapter 4), the concepts involved in the use of IVUS to guide coronary interventions are very similar to angiography. IVUS merely provides a more accurate quantitative and qualitative assessment of the disease.

Pre-intervention, the uses of IVUS are:

- To assess the severity of a coronary artery stenosis, including left main coronary artery disease (i.e. to determine whether revascularization is necessary);
- To assess lesion morphology, including composition, distribution, morphometry, and any unusual features (i.e. to identity any features that would make the procedure more difficult);
- To measure reference vessel size and lesion length (i.e. for device sizing).

In addition, pre-intervention IVUS may be invaluable when attempting to analyze a post-intervention study in order to identify or exclude complications. Again, this is no different from angiography.

As indicated previously (Chapter 3) the following are the basic steps in performing a pre-intervention or diagnostic IVUS study:

- Make sure that the patient is adequately anticoagulated (Most diagnostic angiographic studies are done without anticoagulation);
- Position the guidewire in the distal vessel;
- Administer intracoronary nitroglycerine to avoid coronary spasm
  (If using the solid-state system, perform catheter ring-down subtraction);
- Advance the IVUS catheter distal to the target site;
- Begin imaging and verify that the image is acceptable or, if necessary, tweak the overall gain to compensate for a weak catheter and adjust the zoom (depth) for large vessels;

- If imaging an aorto-ostial lesion, retract the guiding catheter back into the aorta and verify that the path of the IVUS transducer will still be coaxial to the ostium of the vessel;
- Begin recording;
- Withdraw the transducer or catheter to a point proximal to the target site – ideally, back to the aorta, particularly when imaging the left anterior descending or left circumflex, in order to assess left main disease;
- The transducer can be seen fluoroscopically and its position relative to the angiographic anatomy checked using small amounts of contrast injection; contrast or saline injection will also help delineate lumen borders;
- Remove the catheter and review the recorded study to make the necessary measurements and decisions.

The following are the sequence of structures that are viewed (when imaging from distal to proximal) and the basic decisions that must be made:

- *Assessment of distal reference vessel*: (1) amount of disease, (2) selection of the distal reference site, and (3) measurement of the distal reference-site lumen and/or medial and midwall dimensions;
- *Assessment of the target lesion*: (1) measurement of lumen compromise and (2) qualitative analysis of morphology, morphometry, etc;
- *Assessment of the proximal reference vessel*: (1) amount of disease, (2) selection of the proximal reference site, and (3) measurement of the distal reference-site lumen and/or medial and midwall dimensions;
- *Visualization of the rest of the proximal vessel*, checking for occult stenoses and proximal vessel calcification and, particularly if imaging a left coronary artery, assessment of left main disease;
- *Measurement of lesion length* – the distance between distal and proximal reference sites should be measured.

In the stent era, qualitative morphology assessment is less important than quantitative measurements for proper stent sizing (diameter and length).

QUANTITATIVE LESION ASSESSMENT

The IVUS minimum lumen area correlated strongly with Doppler FloWire coronary flow reserve, pressure-wire fractional flow reserve, and exercise thallium. A pre-intervention minimum lumen area $\geq 4.0 \, mm^2$ had a diagnostic accuracy of 92% in predicting a coronary flow reserve ≥ 2.0.[1] Nishioka *et al.*[2] found that this minimum lumen area had a diagnostic accuracy of 93% versus stress myocardial perfusion imaging. Takagi *et al.*[3] found similar results when the IVUS minimum lumen area was compared with fractional flow reserve measured by the pressure wire. These results are shown in Table 1 and Figure 6.1. In two studies – one comparing IVUS with coronary flow reserve and one comparing IVUS with fractional flow reserve – lesion length was also shown to contribute to a lesion's physiologic significance.[1,4]

Outcome

In support of these studies, percutaneous intervention was deferred based on IVUS findings in 300 patients. Events occurred in 24 patients. There was an important difference between lesions with minimum lumen cross-section area (CSA) above and below $4.0 \, mm^2$. In 248 lesions with a minimum lumen CSA $\geq 4.0 \, mm^2$, the event rate was only 4.4%, and the revascularization rate was only 2.8%. These results are shown in Figure 6.2.[5] The predictors for target-lesion revascularization (repeat intervention and bypass surgery) were diabetes mellitus, IVUS lumen CSA, and IVUS area stenosis (minimum lumen area compared to the mean reference lumen area). Examples are shown in Figures 6.3–6.5. When intervention is deferred after IVUS imaging, the long-term event-free survival was similar to previously reported studies of fractional flow reserve > 0.80 (Figure 6.6).[5,6]

Technique and criteria

Thus, based on the above studies, a minimum lumen CSA of less than $4.0 \, mm^2$ correlates with ischemia and indicates worse patient outcomes. However, this cutoff applies only to major epicardial vessels, thereby excluding the left main coronary artery, saphenous vein grafts, and small arteries (branches and distal vessels). There has been no reliable study suggesting a threshold for intervention in saphenous vein grafts. Left mains will be discussed separately. It is interesting to note that even in major native epicardial arteries, the IVUS measure of absolute lumen dimensions correlated better with indices of ischemia compared with the area stenosis (lumen CSA divided by the mean reference-segment lumen CSA). One possible explanation is that these studies included only patients with major epicardial arteries, not small arteries or side branches. An unknown question is the influence of plaque composition on outcomes: should the criteria for treating soft lesions be different from calcific lesions?

This diagnostic use of IVUS depends on image-acquisition technique. Because of the importance of the minimum lumen CSA, it is necessary to interrogate each lesion carefully to identify the image slice with the smallest lumen. Poor technique (too rapid or uneven transducer withdrawal or not interrogating the stenosis carefully) may miss the true minimum lumen CSA.

Once the smallest lumen is identified, careful measurement is required. Intracoronary nitroglycerin should be administered prior to introducing the IVUS catheter to avoid spasm and erroneous measurements and to minimize ischemia. Excessively long imaging runs should be avoided (i.e. it is not necessary to start in the distal left anterior descending when the lesion is in the left main), and the catheter should be removed in the setting of significant angina with ECG changes. Saline or angiographic contrast flush is very useful in delineating intimal borders by clearing the static blood from the lumen (Figures 2.3, 2.4 and 5.29).

In many lesions, the IVUS findings are obvious even without careful measurements – i.e. there is minimal disease or an occlusive lumen. Most importantly, ischemia is determined by lumen size, not by the amount of plaque. Even large plaque burdens (> 70–75%) can exist in the absence of any significant reduction in lumen dimension (Figure 6.4). Therefore, it is important to focus on accurate measurement of lumen dimensions and not to be distracted by the plaque burden. While the plaque burden plays an important role in the natural history of coronary artery disease, it is the identification and correction of lumen compromise that is the focus of an interventional procedure. However, a second unknown question is the influence of plaque burden on outcomes: should the lumen CSA criteria for treating lesions with a large plaque burden be different from lesions with a lesser plaque burden?

Table 6.1 Comparison of IVUS minimum lumen areas with Doppler FloWire coronary flow reserve ($n = 72$) and stress myocardial imaging (^{201}Tl-SPECT, $n = 67$)

	IVUS minimum lumen area $\geq 4.0 \, mm^2$	IVUS minimum lumen area $< 4.0 \, mm^2$
CFR < 2.0	2	27
CFR $\geq$ 2.0	39	4
$+^{201}Tl$-SPECT	4	42
$-^{201}Tl$-SPECT	20	1

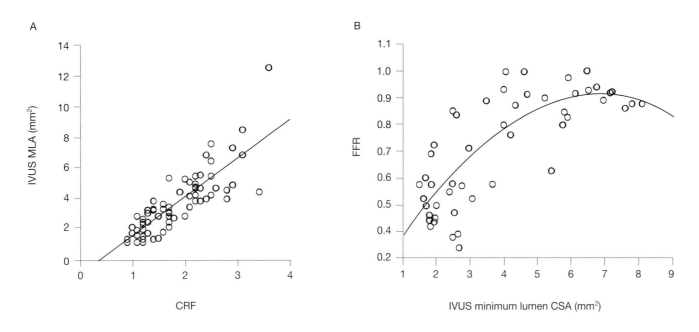

Figure 6.1 IVUS minimum lumen CSA (MLA) correlated with both the coronary flow reserve (CRF) determined by the Doppler FloWire (Panel A, $n = 72$, $r = 0.831$, $p < 0.0001$) and the fractional flow reserve (FFR) determined by the pressure wire (Panel B, $n = 51$, $r = 0.62$, $p < 0.0001$) (Panel A is based on Abizaid et al.[1] and Panel B is based on Takagi et al.[3])

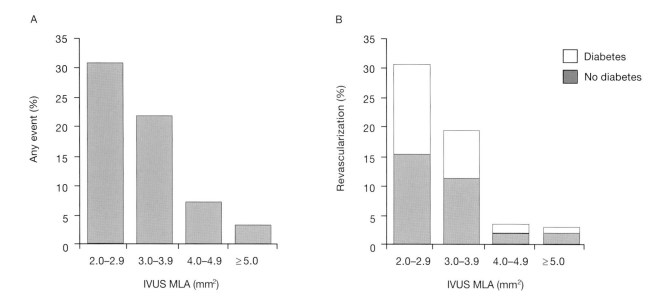

Figure 6.2   After a follow-up period of at least one year after an intervention was deferred, the frequency of cardiac events (death, myocardial infarction, or target-lesion revascularization) depended on the IVUS minimum lumen CSA (MLA) Panel A. Revascularization events were more common in the 20% of patients who were diabetic than in the non-diabetics (Panel B). All events were particularly low in the 83% of patients with a MLA greater than 4.0 mm². (Based on Abizaid *et al.*[5])

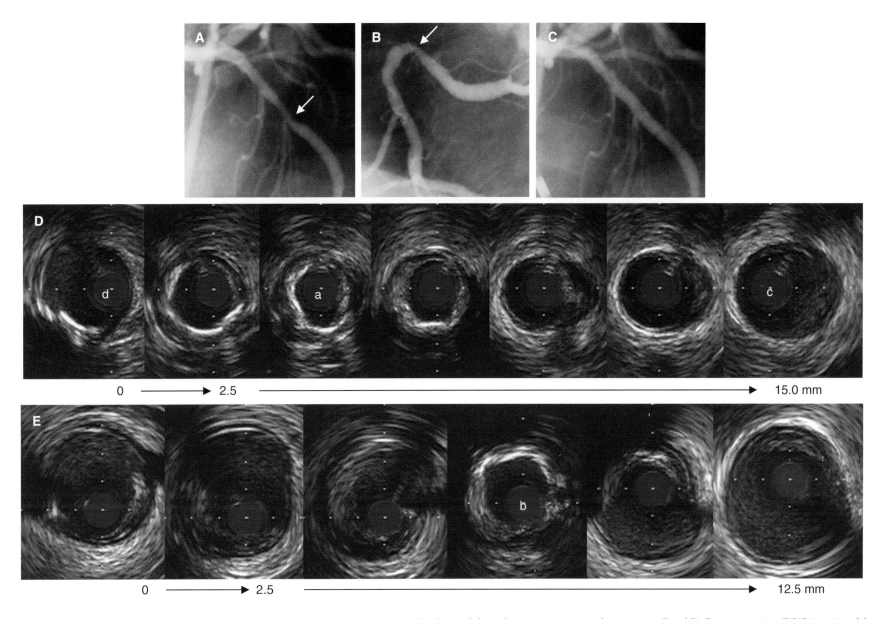

Figure 6.3 This patient had lesions in both the left anterior descending (white arrow in Panel A) and the right coronary artery (white arrow in Panel B). Pre-intervention IVUS imaging of the left anterior descending (Panel D) showed a minimum lumen area of 2.5 mm^2 (a). Diagnostic IVUS imaging of the right coronary artery (Panel E) showed a minimum lumen area of 5.1 mm^2 (b). The quantitative angiographic diameter stenosis measured 41% in the left anterior descending and 46% in the right coronary artery. The coronary flow reserve measured 1.6 in the left anterior descending and 2.6 in the right coronary artery. The left anterior descending lesion was stented. The final angiographic result is shown in Panel C. The angiographic reference measured 2.73 mm. However, the maximum IVUS reference-lumen diameter measured 3.5 mm, and both midwall reference dimensions measured 3.5 mm. Therefore, a 3.5 mm × 15 mm stent was selected. Notice that the distal (c) and proximal (d) reference image slices were the ones with the largest lumens and the smallest plaque burdens (33% and 36%, respectively); the stent length was selected as the distance between the proximal and distal reference image slices

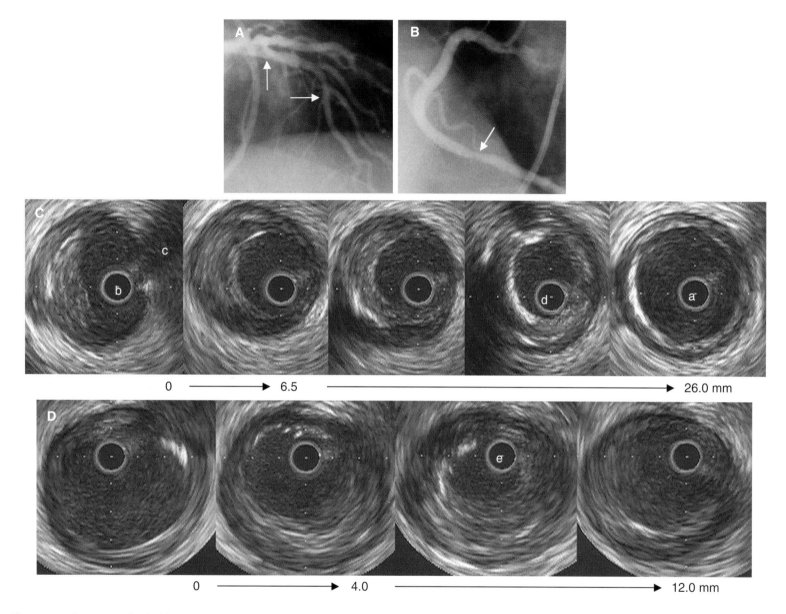

Figure 6.4 This patient also had lesions in both the left anterior descending (between the white arrows in Panel A) and the right coronary artery (white arrow in Panel B). Diagnostic IVUS imaging of the left anterior descending (Panel C) from distal (a) to proximal (b) at the level of the left circumflex (c) showed that the minimum lumen CSA (d) measured 5.1 mm². Diagnostic imaging of the right coronary artery (Panel D) showed that the minimum lumen CSA measured 5.0 mm² (e). Note the large plaque burdens (75% in the left anterior descending and 80% in the right coronary artery) despite an adequate lumen CSA

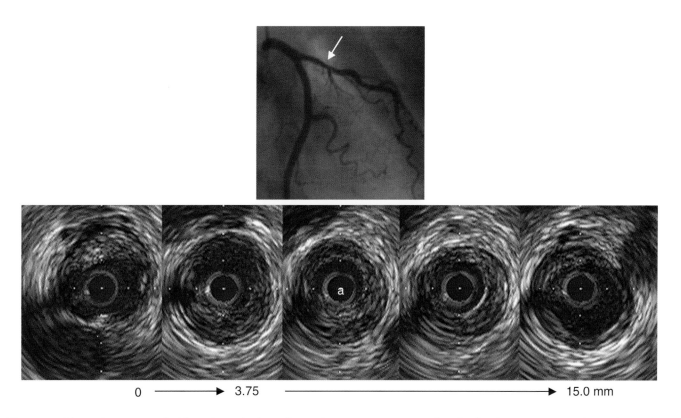

0 ⟶ 3.75 ⟶ 15.0 mm

Figure 6.5   This patient presented with angina and, after a diagnostic angiogram, was treated medically. Her angina persisted, and she then had a marked positive exercise thallium study in the distribution of the left anterior descending. Repeat diagnostic angiography showed this intermediate lesion in the proximal left anterior descending (white arrow). IVUS imaging showed a minimum lumen CSA of 2.2 mm^2 (a). She was treated with a minimally invasive surgical procedure (left internal mammary artery anastamosis)

Ambiguous lesions

Assessment of ambiguous lesions is an important indication for IVUS imaging. Patients frequently present with symptoms, non-invasive tests, and angiographic studies that provide conflicting data. In the USA, most patients undergo coronary angiography without a prior non-invasive study for ischemia. Therefore, every busy catheterization laboratory should have an algorithm for decision-making under these circumstances – either IVUS or invasive physiologic lesion assessment – and its staff should become expert in one of these techniques. Operators who are experienced in physiologic lesion assessment should continue to use physiology to make their decisions. Their results will be more consistent and reliable. The same holds true for IVUS.

Making a decision while the patient is in the catheterization laboratory is always more cost-effective than taking the patient off the table, performing a non-invasive study, and then returning the patient to the catheterization laboratory if a revascularization procedure is necessary. In addition, use of IVUS can reduce radiation exposure and radiographic contrast volume when evaluating difficult-to-assess lesions (bifurcations, aorto-ostial disease, hazy lesions, etc.) or difficult-to-image patients.

Approximately 25% of lesions with a lumen area $< 4.0\,\text{mm}^2$ have an angiographic diameter stenosis $< 50\%$ – that is, they are angiographically not significant. These "silent" lesions tend to be more common in the right coronary artery and in arteries with one angiographically significant stenosis.[7] An example is shown in Figure 6.7. The recent concensus document on vulnerable plaques and patients included the presence of a severe stenosis as a major criteria for detection of a vulnerable plaque; one stenotic plaque may indicate the presence of many non-stenotic or less stenotic plaques.[8]

LEFT MAIN LESIONS

Assessment of left main disease has emerged as an important indication for IVUS imaging. A recently completed left main registry indicated that in half of the patients with an inconclusive angiogram, IVUS detects a significant stenosis.[9]

In general, there are two criteria that have been used to perform revascularization for left main disease: either a minimum lumen CSA below 5.5–6.0 mm^2 or an IVUS diameter stenosis greater than 50% compared with the reference-lumen dimension. The rationale for these two criteria is as follows. In general, when a parent artery bifurcates into two daughter arteries, the sum of the two daughter arteries is approximately 1.5 times the size of the parent. The left main coronary artery provides flow to the left circumflex and left anterior descending, and

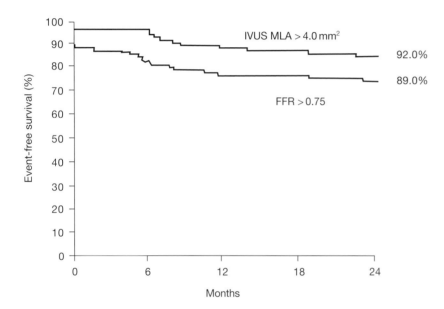

Figure 6.6 When intervention is deferred using the IVUS criteria of a minimum lumen CSA $> 4.0\,\text{mm}^2$, the long-term follow-up is similar to when intervention is deferred using the invasive physiologic assessment criteria of a fractional flow reserve > 0.75. (Based on Abizaid *et al.*[5] and Bech *et al.*[11])

4.0 mm^2 is the minimum lumen CSA necessary for the left circumflex and left anterior descending. The diameter stenosis criterion is based on the standard angiographic definition of a significant left main stenosis (> 50%), but uses the superior measuring power of IVUS to calculate the stenosis. However, the diameter stenosis criterion requires a "normal" reference segment. Because left main disease is frequently diffuse with no true reference segment (producing the so-called "small left main", which is really a diffusely diseased left main), measurement of absolute left main lumen dimensions is preferable. Finally, an IVUS left main lumen minimum lumen diameter of 2.8 mm had a sensitivity of 93% and a specificity of 98%, and an IVUS minimum lumen CSA of 5.9 mm^2 had a sensitivity of 93% and a specificity of 95% compared with a fractional flow reserve of 0.75;[10] previous studies have shown that this fractional flow reserve cut-off is useful for triaging patients with left main disease.[10,11]

Outcome

We reported 122 patients who underwent angiographic and IVUS assessment of left main coronary artery disease severity, who did not have subsequent catheter or surgical intervention, and who were followed for at least 1 year.[12] As with intermediate lesions elsewhere in the coronary tree, there was a poor correlation between quantitative angiographic and IVUS assessment of reference-segment and lesion-site lumen dimensions. The one-year event rate (death, myocardial infarction, or need for revascularization) in these patients was 14% with < 2% having procedure-unrelated deaths. (During follow-up, four patients died, none had a myocardial infarction, three underwent catheter-based intervention of the left main coronary artery, and 11 underwent bypass surgery.) There were three distinct predictors of cardiac events: (1) diabetes, (2) a major epicardial vessel or bypass graft with an angiographic diameter stenosis ≥ 50% that was left untreated, and (3) left main coronary artery lesion-site minimum lumen diameter measured by IVUS (Figure 6.8). The IVUS lumen dimensions were the only independent quantitative predictor of late events. Clinical decisions and events are dichotomous (yes/no), while quantitative parameters are continuous; therefore, there is no absolute lumen dimension cut-off that will guarantee freedom from events. Examples are shown in Figures 6.9–6.14.

Similarly, Wolfhard *et al.*[13] studied 36 patients with significant stenoses of the left circumflex and/or left anterior descending arteries and questionable left main coronary artery morphology. Significant left main luminal reduction was defined as an IVUS area stenosis > 50% or a minimum lumen diameter < 3.0 mm. Additionally, 12 patients showed a ruptured plaque within the left main coronary artery. Of these 36 patients, 30 were originally thought to be candidates for angio-plasty. Based on IVUS findings, 34 of these 36 patients were sent to surgery. No perioperative ischemic complications occurred.

The diagnostic use of IVUS in assessing left main disease depends on technique just like the assessment of a lesion in another part of the coronary tree. In particular, when assessing ostial left main coronary artery disease, it is important to disengage the guiding catheter from the ostium, so that the guiding catheter is not mistaken for a calcific lesion with a lumen dimension equal to the inner lumen of the guiding catheter.

Finally, as with non-left main lesions, sometimes the IVUS findings are obvious even without careful measurements – i.e. there is minimal disease or an occlusive lumen. Plaque burden may be large even in the absence of lumen compromise. While this plaque burden plays an important role in the natural history of coronary artery disease, it is the identification and correction of lumen compromise that is the focus of an interventional procedure. Large left main plaque burdens can coexist with an adequate left main lumen.

LESION MORPHOLOGY

In the stent era, assessment of lesion morphology is less important than it was previously since stent implantation tends to minimize the impact of lesion morphology on the acute and chronic results of percutaneous intervention. Nevertheless, several aspects of morphologic assessments are important. The examples shown here were, with the exception of the patient with a pseudoaneurysm, all acquired before any intervention.

Angiographic filling defects

While most angiographic filling defects are true thrombi, a percentage of filling defects are chronic calcified plaques.[14,15] Others are eruptive, dense calcific nodules that are associated with fibrous cap disruption and thrombosis and are considered a type of vulnerable plaque (Figure 5.26).[16] Clinical clues that angiographic filling defects are calcific lesions include (1) the absence of any decrease in size with prolonged anticoagulation, thrombolytic agents, or glycoprotein IIb/IIIa inhibitors and (2) severe, diffuse coronary calcification. In one analysis of 78 angiographic filling defects, 48 (61.5%) had IVUS evidence of thrombus; and 30 did not (38.5%). Of 30 IVUS non-thrombotic lesions, 13 were calcified plaques, although these lesions were not calcified on angiography. Examples are shown in Figures 6.15 and 6.16. Examples of typical thrombi are shown in Figures 2.30 and 3.7 and in Chapter 5.

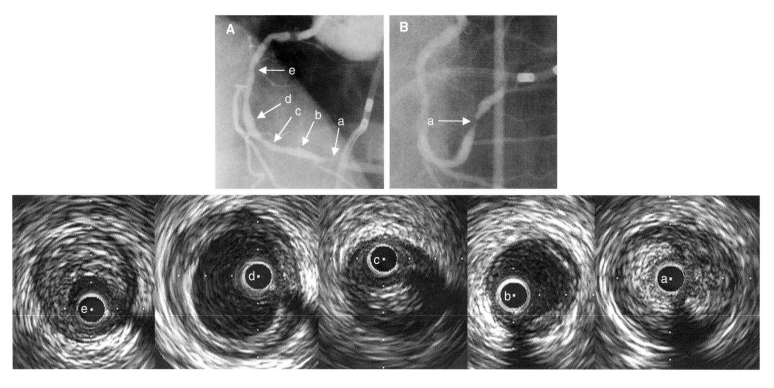

Figure 6.7   This right coronary artery had three IVUS stenoses. The pre-intervention IVUS cross-sections (a–e) correspond to the locations in the angiogram (Panels A and B). Only the distal lesion (a) was severe by angiographic criteria. The two other angiographically silent lesions (c and e) had minimum lumen CSA of 1.8 mm^2 and 2.1 mm^2, respectively. Neither had an angiographic diameter stenosis > 50%. The predictors of an angiographically silent stenosis include one severe stenosis in the artery and right coronary disease

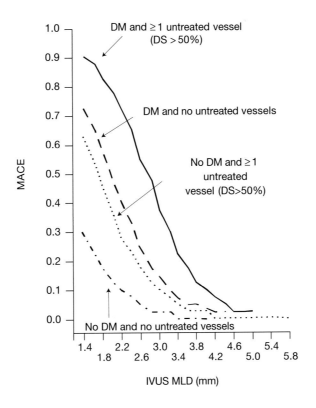

Figure 6.8 The three independent determinants of major adverse cardiac events (MACE) in 122 patients with mostly intermediate left main stenosis who were followed for one year were diabetes mellitus (DM), whether or not there was another stenosis > 50%, and the IVUS minimum lumen diameter (MLD). (Based on Abizaid *et al.*[1])

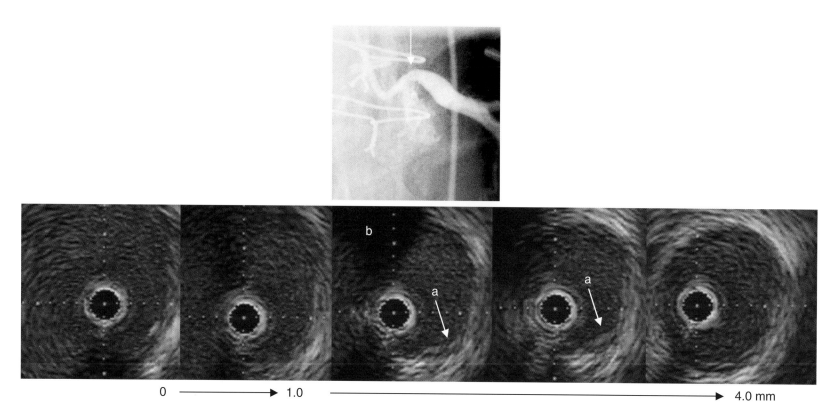

0 ⟶ 1.0 ⟶ 4.0 mm

Figure 6.9 This patient was admitted to a coronary care unit because of chest pain, underwent diagnostic angiography, and then had bypass surgery (left internal mammary artery to the left anterior descending and saphenous vein graft to the left circumflex artery) for an ostial left main stenosis similar to the one shown by the white arrow in this angiogram. He did well for approximately one month, developed recurrent pain, was readmitted to the coronary care unit, underwent repeat angiography that showed closure of both the internal mammary artery and saphenous vein grafts, and had repeat bypass surgery, this time using saphenous vein grafts to both the left anterior descending and left circumflex arteries. He again did well for about a month before developing recurrent chest pain. At this time, he was referred for an IVUS study of the ostial left main stenosis. The pre-IVUS angiogram and its ostial stenosis (white arrow) are shown. The IVUS imaging run shows no left main disease or lumen compromise. There is, at most, mild intimal thickening (a). Note the shadowing caused by the aortic wall (b). The guiding catheter has been retracted and is out of view

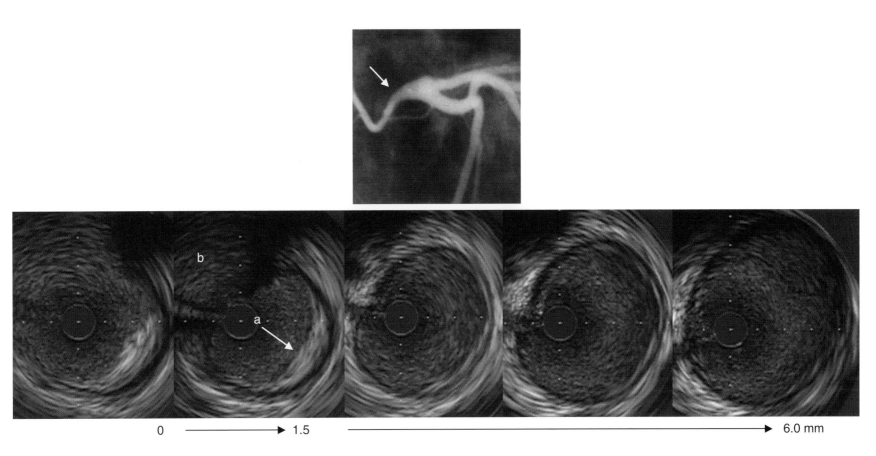

0 ⟶ 1.5 ⟶ 6.0 mm

Figure 6.10 Like the example in Figure 6.9, there is an ostial left main stenosis that, in reality, is an angiographic artifact (white arrow in the angiogram). The diagnostic IVUS study shows, at most, mild plaque (a) just at the junction of the left main with the aorta (b). Although there was a minimum lumen area of 8.8 mm^2 and a plaque burden of 43%, this was an obviously non-stenotic mildly diseased left main ostium

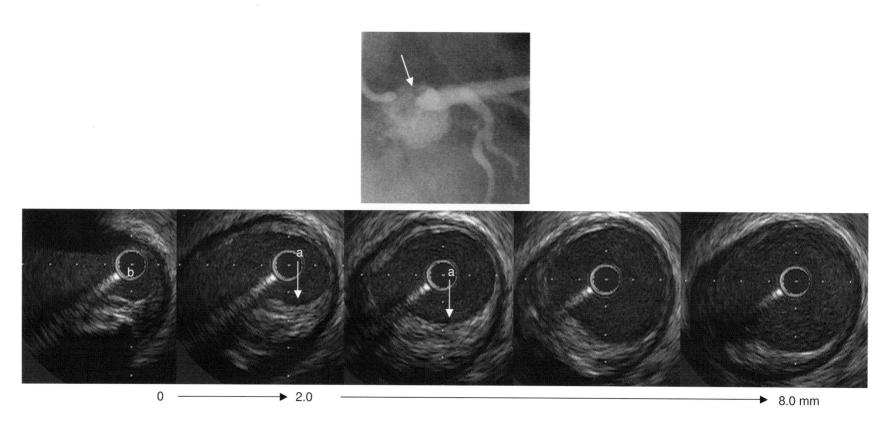

0 ——————▶ 2.0 ————————————————————————▶ 8.0 mm

Figure 6.11   Compared with the examples in Figures 6.9 and 6.10, this shows a significant ostial left main stenosis. It was difficult to engage the angiographic catheter, and non-selective injection shows an ostial stenosis (white arrow in the angiogram). The pre-intervention IVUS imaging run shows a large plaque burden (a), but, more importantly, a minimum lumen CSA of 2.8 mm^2 (b). The patient was referred for bypass surgery

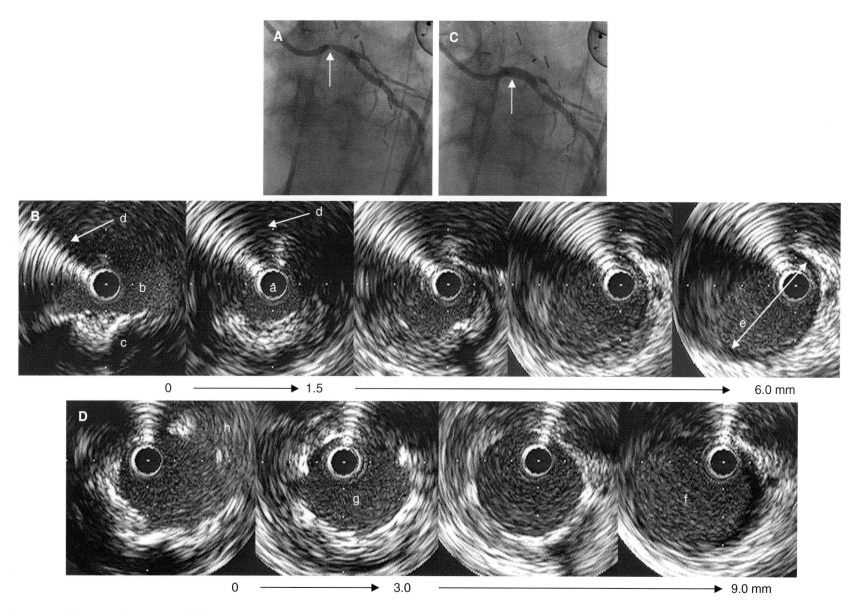

Figure 6.12 This patient has a protected left main stenosis (white arrow in Panel A). The pre-intervention IVUS imaging run showed a minimum lumen CSA of 2.9 mm² (a) just inside the true ostium (b). Note the aortic wall (c) and the very prominent guidewire artifact (d). The distal reference maximum lumen diameter measured 4.1 mm (double-headed white arrow e), and the mean midwall dimension measured 4.2 mm. Therefore, a short 4.0 mm stent was implanted. The final result is shown in the angiogram (white arrow in Panel C) and the IVUS (Panel D). The distal reference-lumen CSA (f) measured 12.4 mm², and the minimum stent CSA (g) measured 10.8 mm². The stent just covers the true ostium, protruding only slightly into the aorta (h)

Figure 6.13 (opposite) This elderly female patient was referred for intervention of a severe proximal left anterior descending artery stenosis (not shown). Pre-intervention IVUS imaging was performed, and, as per routine, transducer pullback was continued until the aorta was seen. This permitted assessment of a hazy distal left main lesion (white arrow on the angiogram). The IVUS imaging run begins at the ostium of the left anterior descending (a, note the left circumflex b), through the distal left main stenosis (c) containing near circumferential calcium (d), to the proximal reference (e). The minimum lumen CSA (c) measured 3.4 mm^2, and the minimum lumen diameter measured 1.3 mm. (The proximal reference-segment lumen CSA measured 16.9 mm^2, with maximum and minimum lumen diameters of 4.8 mm and 4.6 mm, respectively.) Hazy lesions are often more severe than they appear by angiography. When imaging a left anterior descending or left circumflex lesion, it is useful to continue transducer pullback until the aorta is reached. The look at the left main is "free", with the exception of the additional few seconds of imaging time

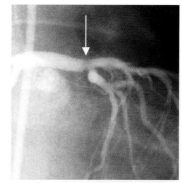

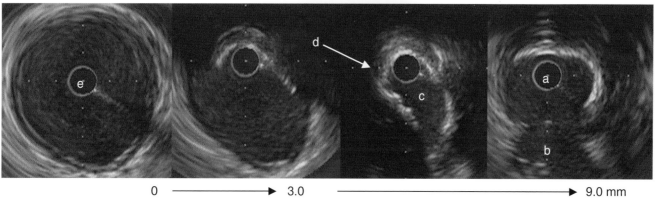

0 ⟶ 3.0 ⟶ 9.0 mm

Figure 6.14 (opposite) This patient has a protected left main stenosis (white arrow in Panels A and B). The pre-intervention IVUS imaging run from distal (a) to proximal reference (b) shows disruption of the intima (c) with intramural blood accumulation (d) that collapsed the internal elastic membrane, intima, and plaque (e). The minimum lumen CSA measured 2.6 mm^2 (f). The maximum reference-segment lumen diameter measured 4.3 mm (double-headed white arrow), as did the distal reference midwall dimension. A 4.5 mm stent was implanted

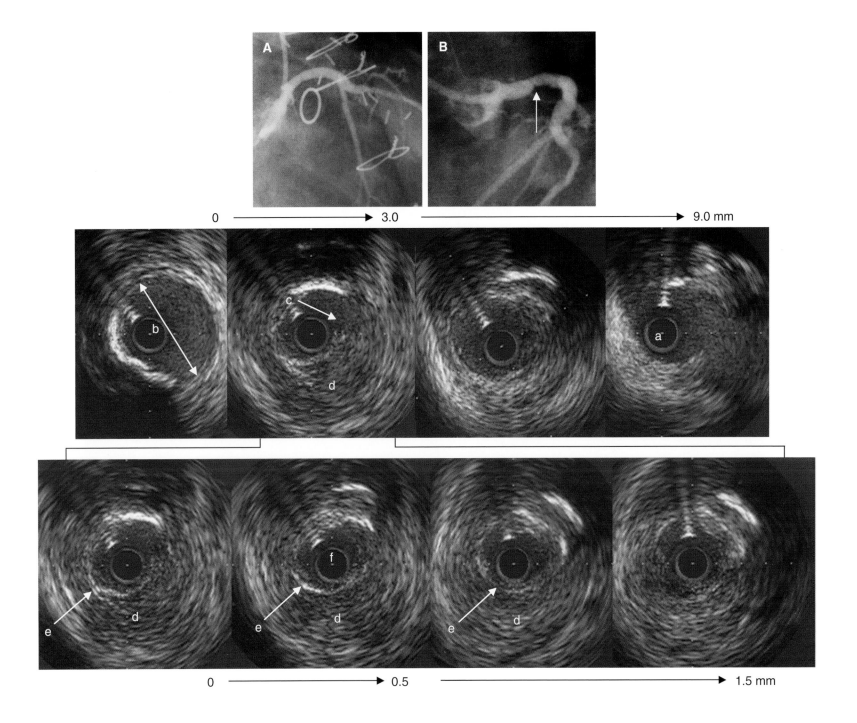

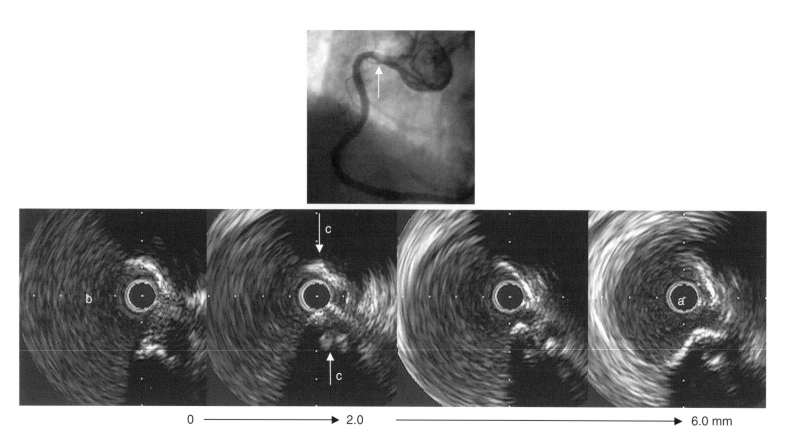

Figure 6.15 Diagnostic IVUS was performed to assess this angiographic filling defect (white arrow in the angiogram). The pullback is from beyond the filling defect (a) to the aorta (b). Note the calcification (c) without any lumen compromise. No intervention was performed

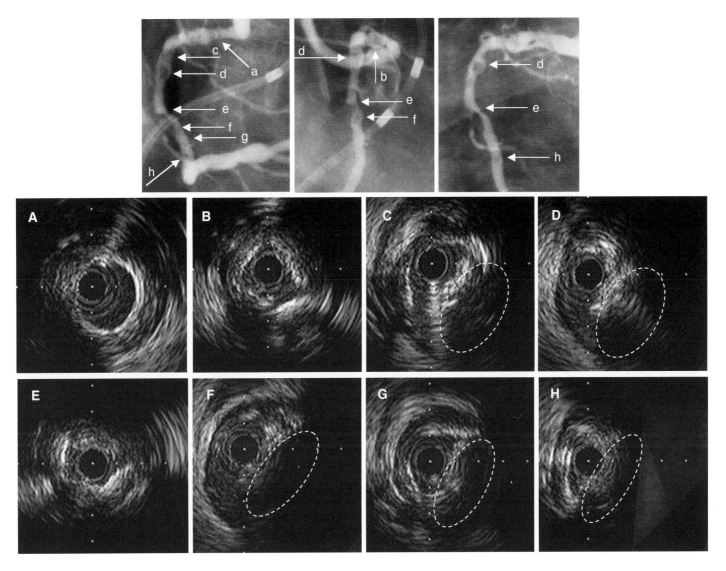

Figure 6.16 This patient presented with an acute coronary syndrome and angiography of the right coronary artery showing multiple filling defects (a–h). The pre-intervention IVUS image slices correspond to the arrows in the angiogram. Note the extensive calcification in each image slice. IVUS shows only the leading edge of a calcified mass or nodule of calcium; the rest of the tissue – regardless of its composition – is shadowed. In several of the IVUS images, a dotted oval is drawn to suggest (speculatively) the potential size and shape of the calcific nodules

Angiographic aneurysms

Maehara *et al.*[17] published an IVUS classification of angiographic coronary artery aneurysms. A true aneurysm was defined as both an external elastic membrane (EEM) and lumen area 50% larger than the proximal reference with an intact vessel wall (Figures 6.17–6.20). As shown in these examples, adjacent to a *very* large aneurysm, there are usually one or more severe stenoses. An unusual type of coronary aneurysm is that associated with Kawasaki's disease (Figure 6.21).[18] A pseudoaneurysm (or false aneurysm) was defined as a maximum lumen area 50% larger than the proximal reference with loss of vessel wall integrity (Figure 6.22). Like pseudoaneurysms elsewhere in the body, coronary pseudoaneurysms are ruptures of the vessel wall that are sealed by an overlying hematoma. This hematoma organizes into thin-walled fibrous tissue that bridges the break in vessel wall integrity. For all practical purposes, pseudoaneurysms are seen only in the setting of a prior intervention, although post-intervention aneurysms can be either true aneurysms or pseudoaneurysms.

One of the difficulties in differentiating true from false aneurysms is the difficulty in determining whether or not the intima, media, and adventitia are intact. In part, this is because the wall of the aneurysm is in the far field, where resolution decreases. Complex plaques were lesions with ruptured or disrupted plaques or spontaneous or unhealed dissections (Figures 6.23 and 6.24). Other examples are shown in Chapter 5. In Maehara's study of 77 angiographic "aneurysmal" lesions, 21 (27%) were classified as true aneurysms; 3 (4%) were classified as pseudoaneurysms (all having had previous intervention), and 12 (16%) were complex plaques.[17] The most common finding – seen in the other 41 patients (53%) – was a normal arterial segment adjacent to one or more stenoses (Figure 6.25).

Coronary ectasia

Coronary ectasia is defined as localized or diffuse dilatation of the coronary arteries more than 150% of the adjacent normal artery; ectasia frequently coexists with atherosclerotic stenoses. There is a standard angiographic classification,[19] and recent Doppler FloWire and quantitative angiographic myocardial blushgrade studies have demonstrated microcirculatory dysfunction – even in the 33% of patients with normal epicardial flow.[19–21] However, there has not been a systematic IVUS study of coronary ectasia. Examples are shown in Figures 6.26 and 6.27.

Ruptured plaques

Ruptured plaques and their variants are discussed in detail in Chapter 5. Most ruptured plaques are associated with acute coronary syndromes and cause angio-graphically complex plaques.[22] However, a minority will be clinically and angiographically silent. Symptomatic ruptured plaques are usually associated with thrombus formation and/or lumen compromise.[23]

Acute coronary syndromes and acute myocardial infarction

Typical features of acute myocardial infarction include (1) plaque rupture, (2) thrombus formation, (3) only either spotty or deep calcium within the minimum lumen site, and (4) positive remodeling (see below). Most authors report a frequency of IVUS-detected plaque rupture in slightly less than half of infarct-related lesions.[24–26] However, in one report, infarct-related plaque rupture was seen in 65% of infarction patients (Hong, American Heart Association Scientific Sessions 2003) and was equally common in Q-wave versus non-Q-wave or ST-elevation versus non-ST-elevation infarct. Pathologic studies have shown that approximately 70% of infarction-related lesions involve plaque rupture; the rest are erosions or other less common morphologies.[8] The IVUS detection of plaque rupture may be influenced by the presence of thrombus (which may obscure the evacuated rupture cavity and the fibrous cap remnant), the thickness of the residual fibrous cap, and the interval from symptom onset to IVUS imaging (which may allow time for healing). Many examples of infarct-related lesions are shown in Chapter 5.

However, not all infarctions result from atherosclerotic coronary disease. Some occur in patients with normal coronary arteries. An example of an infarction in a cocaine addict is shown in Figure 6.28.

Spontaneous dissections

Spontaneous dissections occur in the absence of any history of an intervention; 80% of the cases are in women and 25% occur either post-partum or with oral contraceptive use. Pathologic findings in patients with spontaneous dissection have included (1) medial dissection and intramural hematoma formation, mostly without an intimal tear or evidence of atherosclerosis, (2) eosinophilic infiltration into the adventitia, and (3) cystic medial necrosis. The most commonly reported angiographic finding is the presence of flow in two lumens separated by a radiolucent flap. However, the angiogram may be unimpressive or show diffuse disease.[27,28] On IVUS, medial dissections are often circumferential with an intramural hematoma occupying part of the dissected false lumen. Intimal tears are rare, and there is usually no communication between the true and false lumens.[28] Examples are shown in Figures 6.29 and 6.30.

Spasm

Vasospastic angina can occur in patients with and without angiographic coronary artery disease. Previous IVUS studies have shown that non-calcified atherosclerotic plaque or diffuse intimal thickening is present at the sites of vasospasm, often in association with negative remodeling.[29–31] An example of spontaneous spasm is shown in Figure 5.10.

Catheter-induced spasm is the result of increased vasomotor tone and a myogenic reflex triggered by mechanical stimulation of the catheter tip. IVUS may help to exclude a fixed obstruction. An example of catheter-induced spasm is shown in Figure 6.31.

Myocardial bridges

Normally, EEM and lumen area are largest in mid-systole and smallest in late diastole. In a muscle bridge, the artery (most often the left anterior descending artery) runs under a band of epicardial muscle, causing systolic compression of the artery – i.e. a reversal of the normal pattern. IVUS studies have clarified why ischemia can occur in such patients when the angiogram shows just systolic compression, and coronary flow is minimal during systole. IVUS shows both phasic systolic compression and – importantly – the fact that compression persists into mid-to-late diastole, when most coronary flow occurs. (Doppler FloWire studies show increased flow velocities, retrograde systolic flow, and reduced coronary flow reserve.) Ge *et al.*[32] have described a specific "half moon" phenomenon surrounding myocardial bridges; this is present only over the intramyocardial length of the artery. Visualization of the typical systolic compression depends on the severity of the abnormality, although it can be provoked or exaggerated by nitroglycerin. There is an absence of atherosclerotic changes, both at the level of the intramural coronary artery and in the segment distal to the bridge, although there can be atherosclerotic plaques in proximal segments.[32] An example is shown in Figure 6.32.

Angiographic hazy lesions

Angiography depicts coronary artery cross-sectional geometry as a planar two-dimensional silhouette of the contrast-filled lumen. However, coronary lesions are often complex with markedly distorted lumen shapes.[33] Angiographic hazy lesions can represent the full spectrum of pre-intervention anatomic morphologies, including calcium, spontaneous dissections, thrombus, and a large plaque burden with positive remodeling.

True versus false lumens

A false lumen can be created by a spontaneous dissection or during the wiring of a lesion – particularly a chronic total occlusion. Differentiation of a true from a false lumen is based on (1) recognition of the true three-layered appearance (indicating a true lumen), (2) slower, sluggish, more echogenic blood flow (indicating the false lumen), and (3) identification of side branches (these originating from the true lumen). Examples are shown in Figures 6.27 and 6.30.

Calcified lesions

Using IVUS, calcium can be localized to the lesion versus the reference segment, characterized as superficial (closer to the tissue–lumen interface) versus deep (closer to the media–adventitia junction), and quantified according to its arc and length. IVUS routinely detects target-lesion calcification – even severe calcium – that is angiographically "silent." A detailed discussion of calcium can be found in Chapter 4.

Eccentric lesions

Most lesions appear somewhat eccentric by IVUS in that there is usually more plaque on one side of the lesion than the other. IVUS can assess the degree of eccentricity, whether there is an arc of normal vessel wall within the lesion, and the relationship of the plaque to side branches. Regardless of the angiographic appearance, plaque is deposited preferentially opposite to the major branch, although the exact location of the maximum plaque thickness may be influenced by the angle of the branch relative to the main vessel.[34,35] With conventional IVUS imaging, there is no absolute anterior, posterior, left, or right. If the eccentricity and distribution of the plaque are important to the procedure, it is necessary to identify one or more side branches on both the angiogram and IVUS and to relate the plaque distribution (the maximum and minimum plaque thicknesses and the location of any arcs of normal vessel wall) to these side branches on both studies. This usually requires careful selection of an angiographic projection where the origin and course of the branches are easily identified.[27]

Ostial lesions

IVUS can differentiate between true ostial lesions, in which the minimum lumen CSA and the maximum plaque burden are exactly at the precise ostium, compared with "pseudo-ostial" lesions, in which it is possible to identify a proximal reference segment. True versus pseudo-ostial lesions are shown in Figures 6.33 and 6.34.

Figure 6.17 (opposite) This patient presented with a true saccular aneurysm in the left anterior descending artery (white arrow in Panel A). Pre-intervention IVUS imaging from distal vessel (a) through the aneurysm (b) to the proximal vessel at the level of the diagonal (c) is shown. Note that the intima (d), media (e), and adventitia (f) are intact, making this a true aneurysm. Also note the "septum" (h) that separates the distal end of the aneurysm (g) from the true lumen (i). The white lines in Panel B correspond to the specific image slices (1 and 2) in the IVUS image. The aneurysm external elastic membrane CSA measured 31.7 mm^2, 180% of the proximal reference. This lesion was treated with a standard bare-metal stent (Panel C); by the end of the procedure, the aneurysm had already decreased in size

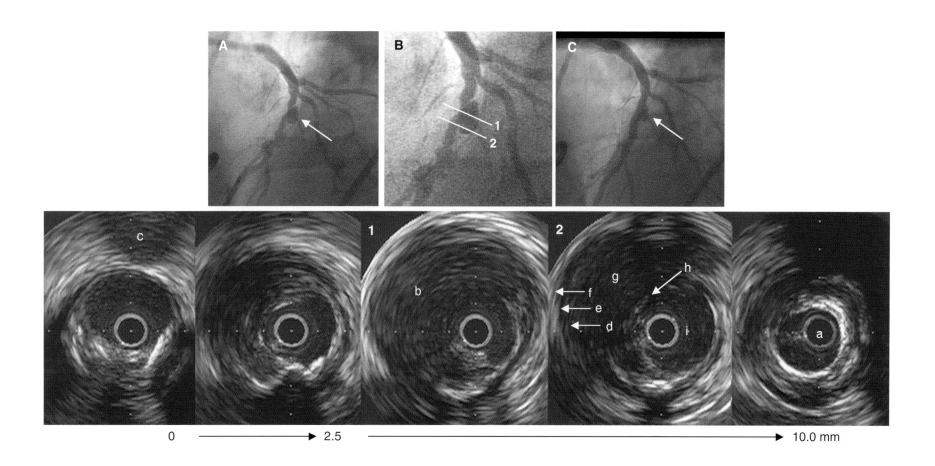

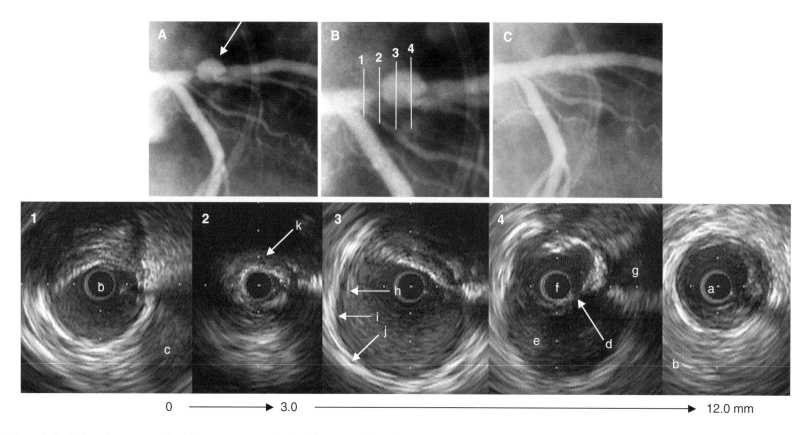

Figure 6.19 This patient presented with a true aneurysm in the left anterior descending (white arrow in Panel A). Pre-intervention IVUS imaging from distal (a), through the aneurysm, to the ostial of the anterior descending (b – note the left circumflex c) is shown. At the level of the aneurysm, note the "septum" (d) separating the aneurysm (e) from the true lumen (f). Also note the diagonal branch (g). The intima (h), media (i), and adventitia (j) are intact. There is a severe stenosis (k) at the inflow to the aneurysm. The white lines in Panel B correspond to the specific image slices (1–4) in the IVUS image. The patient was treated with bare-metal stent implantation, and the post-intervention angiogram is shown (Panel C)

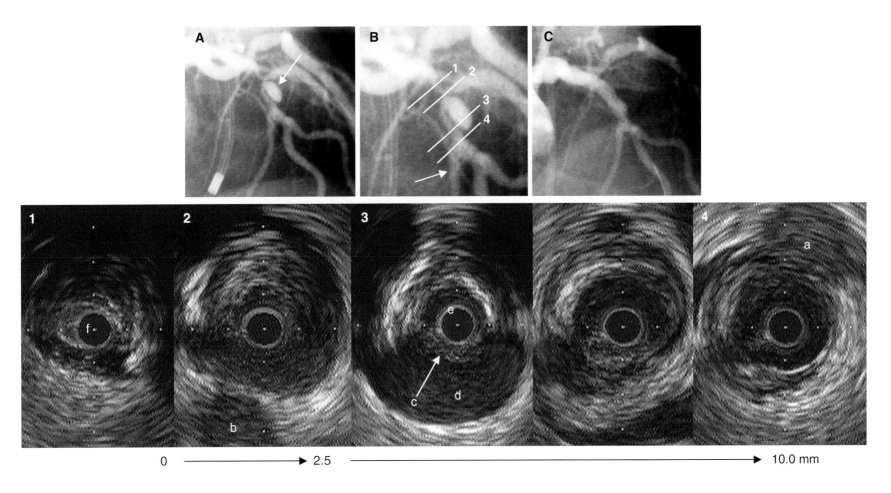

Figure 6.20 This example shows the ability of IVUS to evaluate the relationship between a main vessel aneurysm and side-branches. This patient presented with a true saccular aneurysm in the left anterior descending (white arrow in Panel A). Pre-intervention IVUS imaging is shown from distal at the level of a large, complex septal perforator (a, also shown by the white arrow in Panel B), through the aneurysm and the origin of the major diagonal (b). At the level of the aneurysm, note the "septum" (c) separating the aneurysm (d) from the true lumen (e). There is a severe stenosis (f) at the inflow to the aneurysm. The white lines in Panel B correspond to the specific image slices (1–4) in the IVUS image. The patient was treated with overlapping bare-metal stent implantation, and the post-intervention angiogram is shown (Panel C)

Figure 6.21 (opposite) Kawasaki's disease is the most common acquired heart disease in children. It causes coronary aneurysms in approximately 25% of patients, although half of these will regress. Long-term sequelae of Kawasaki's patients include calcific stenoses, progressive aneurysm enlargement, thrombosis, myocardial infarction, leakage, and rupture.[18] This teenager had known Kawasaki's disease. The coronary angiogram (Panel A) showed a severe right coronary artery stenosis (white arrow, a) followed by marked aneurysmal dilatation (white arrow, b). The IVUS catheter would not cross pre-intervention. Rotational atherectomy was performed using a 1.5 mm burr, and IVUS was then performed. The IVUS study showed the aneurysm (c) with intact intimal, medial, and adventitial layers and the calcific stenosis (d) with reverberations (e). Note the residual layered echolucent contrast (f). (The full size of the aneurysm – more than 9 mm – is not shown because the wall of the aneurysm was off-scale.) The procedure was completed with bare-metal stent implantation (Panel B)

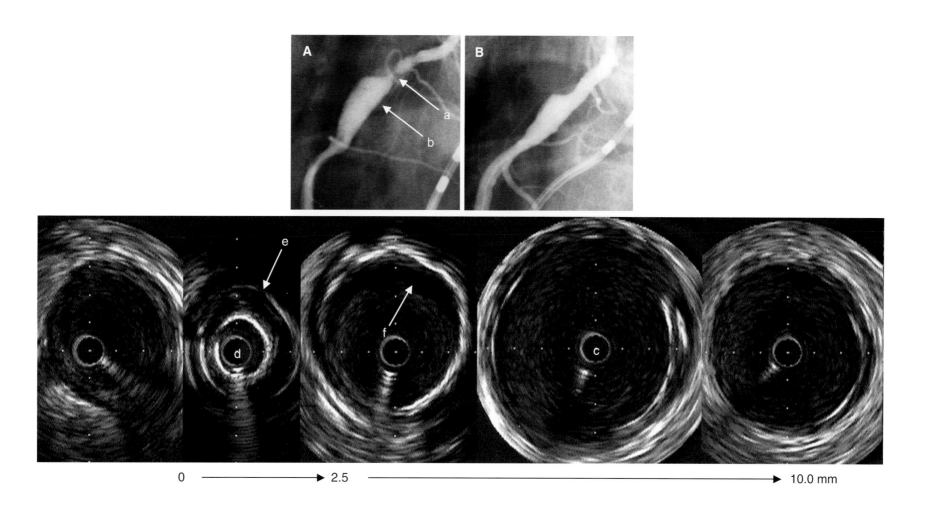

Figure 6.22 (opposite) This patient underwent a previous directional coronary atherectomy of a left anterior descending lesion, during which the artery was perforated, resulting in emergency surgery. Follow-up catheterization (Panel A) showed both restenosis (a) and a large aneurysm (b). Pre-intervention IVUS (Panel C) shows the distal end of the aneurysm (c), the body of the aneurysm (d), the proximal end of the aneurysm (e), and the eccentric restenotic lesion (f). Note that the adventitia stops at the point of transition from the vessel to the aneurysm (g), indicating loss of vessel wall integrity and making this a pseudoaneurysm. The outer extent of the pseudoaneurysm (h) and the wide mouth of the pseudoaneurysm (double-headed white arrow, i) are also shown. The mouth of the pseudoaneurysm measured 4 × 6 mm. It was treated with an autologous vein-covered stent. The final angiogram is shown in Panel B, and the final IVUS is shown in Panel D. Notice the residual contrast (j) and blood (k) in the excluded pseudoaneurysm. Unlike PTFE-covered stents, IVUS can penetrate through the biologic vein (l) to visualize the wall of the excluded pseudoaneurysm (m). The images in Panel D were rotated to correspond to those in Panel C. These images are shown on a 70% scale compared with the other illustrations in this chapter

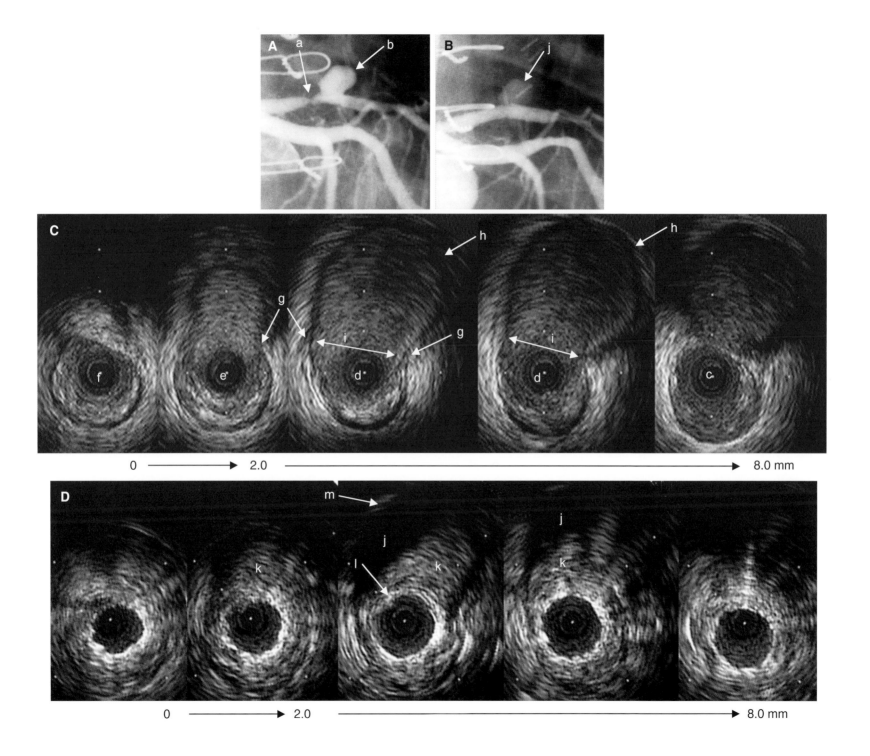

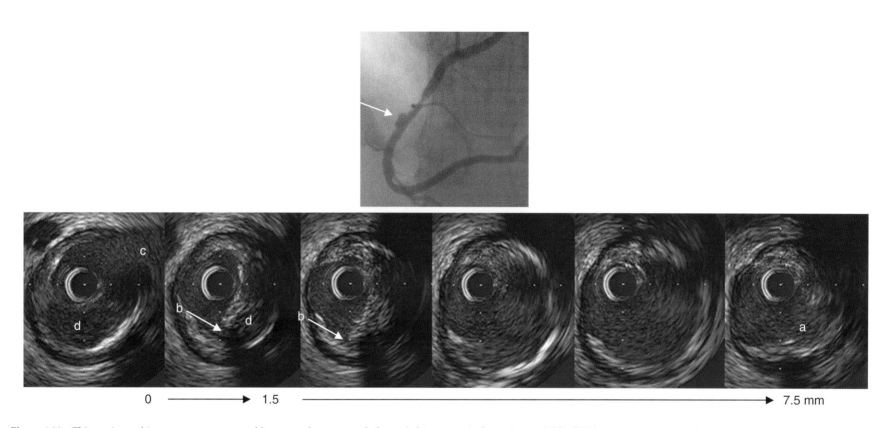

0 ———▶ 1.5 ——————————————————————————▶ 7.5 mm

Figure 6.23 This angiographic aneurysm was caused by a complex, ruptured plaque (white arrow in the angiogram). The IVUS imaging run shows the evacuated plaque cavity (a), evidence of fibrous cap rupture (b), and the right ventricular branch (c) at the proximal end of the lesion. There is a suggestion, but no clear evidence, of a thrombus (d)

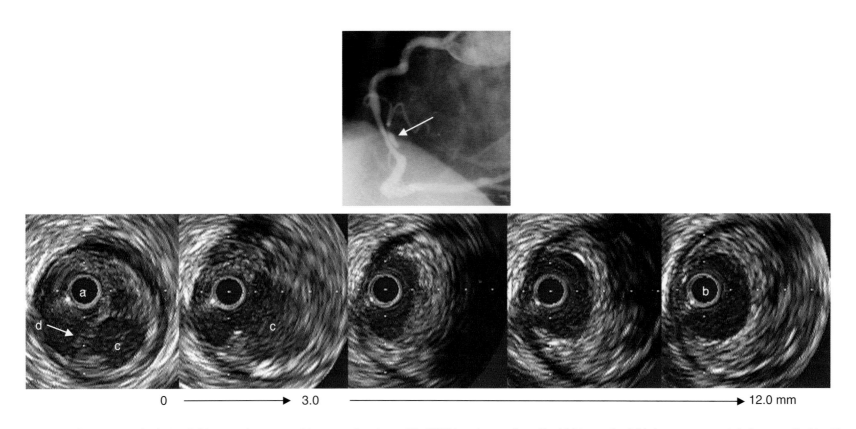

0 ——————————▶ 3.0 ——————————————————————▶ 12.0 mm

Figure 6.24 This angiographic lesion (white arrow) was caused by a complex plaque. The IVUS imaging run from distal (a) to proximal (b) shows an evacuated plaque cavity (c) with a fibrous cap (d)

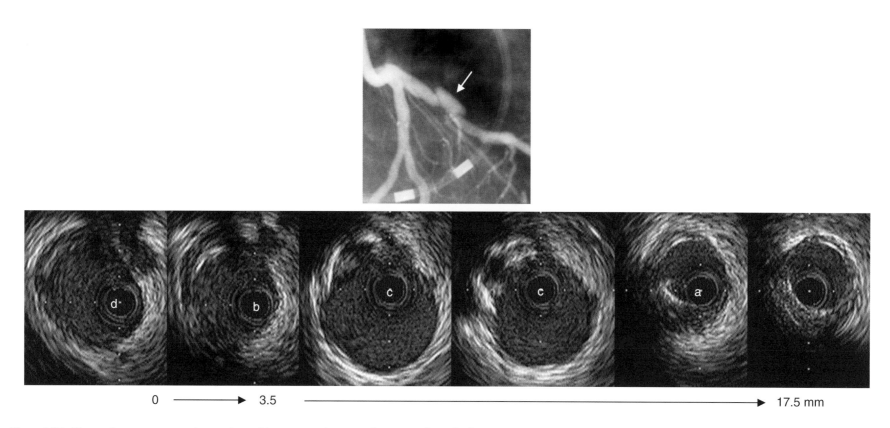

Figure 6.25 The most common cause of an angiographic aneurysm is a normal segment of vessel adjacent to one or more stenoses – the stenoses create the illusion that the normal segment of artery is an aneurysm. This is shown in the angiogram (white arrow) and in the IVUS imaging run. Diagnostic IVUS imaging showed two intermediate stenoses (a and b), in between which was a normal segment of artery (c) whose external elastic membrane measured $19.6\,mm^2$ and whose lumen measured $13.1\,mm^2$, less than 150% of the proximal reference, whose external elastic membrane measured $16.6\,mm^2$ and whose lumen measured $11.0\,mm^2$

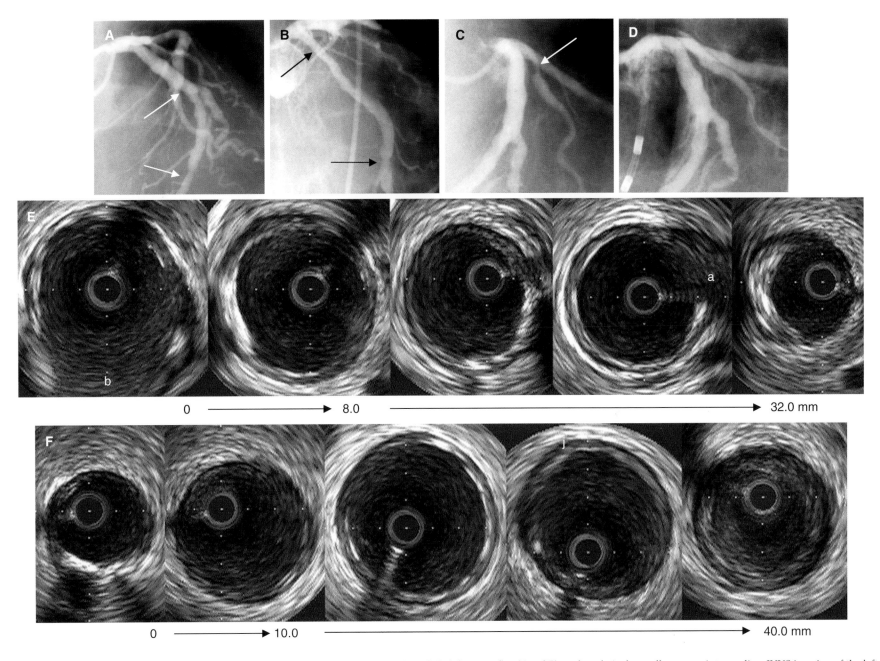

Figure 6.26 This patient presented with ectasia of the left anterior descending artery (Panel A), left circumflex (Panel B), and a relatively smaller ramus intermedius. IVUS imaging of the left anterior descending (Panel E, corresponding to the arrows in Panel A) shows diffuse intimal thickening. Note the location of the septal perforator (a) and ectatic diagonal (b). The proximal LAD (not shown) and the left circumflex (Panel F, corresponding to the arrows in the angiogram, Panel B) showed similar findings. A focal stenosis in the ramus was treated with stent implantation (Panels C and D)

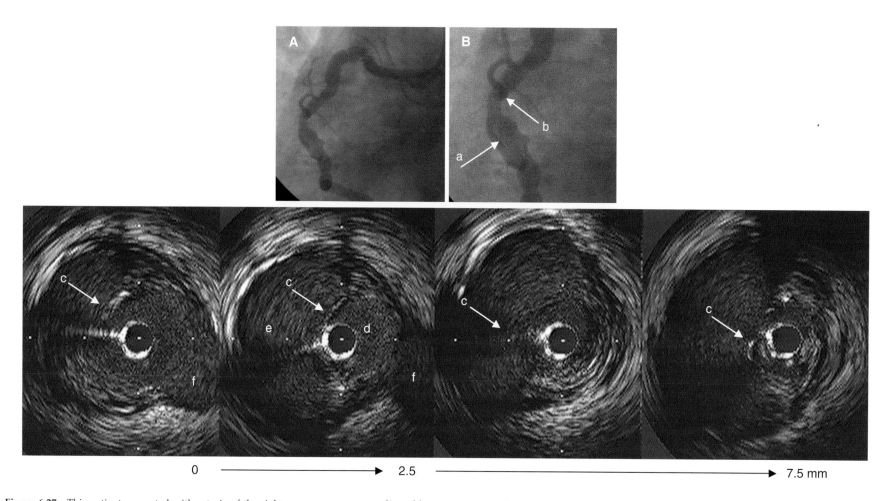

Figure 6.27 This patient presented with ectasia of the right coronary artery complicated by a spontaneous dissection. In the angiograms (Panels A and B) note the faint radiolucency (a) just distal to the right ventricular branch (b), more evident in the close-up (Panel B). In the pre-intervention IVUS imaging run, note the intimal flap (c) that separates the true lumen (d) from the false lumen (e). The flap extends proximally to the level of the right ventricular branch (f), which, by definition, connects with the true lumen. Note that the IVUS catheter is in the true lumen

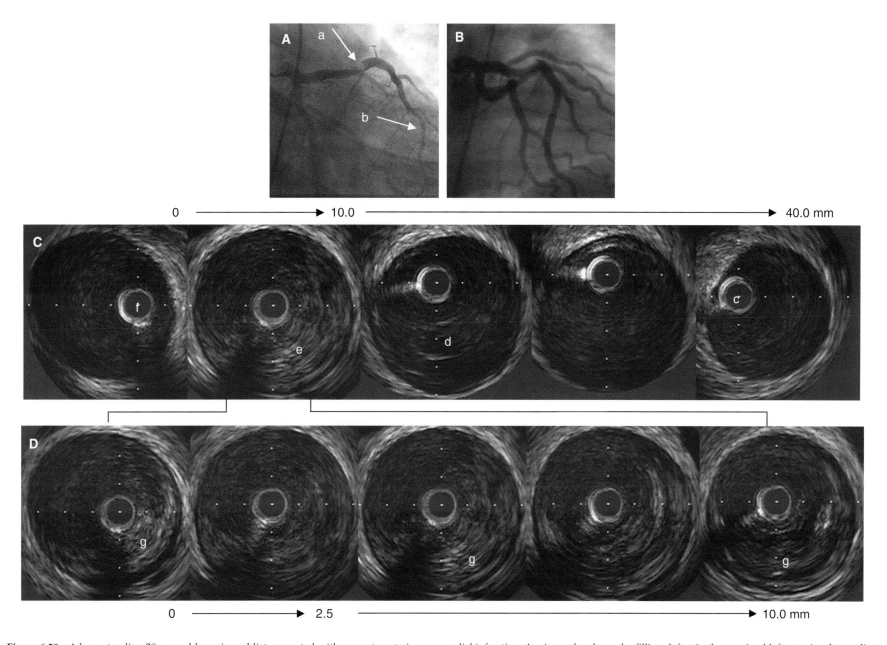

Figure 6.28 A long-standing 28-year-old cocaine addict presented with an acute anterior myocardial infarction. Angiography showed a filling defect in the proximal left anterior descending artery (white arrow a in Panel A) with evidence of decreased distal perfusions (b). Pre-intervention IVUS imaging (Panel C) showed a normal distal vessel (c), a pedunculated (d) and mural (e) thrombus, depending on the image slice, and a normal proximal vessel (f). Panel D shows more closely spaced image slices with a mural, multilayered thrombus (g). Mechanical extraction of the thrombus was performed with Angiojet. Afterwards, the patient was treated with intravenous heparin and eptifibatide for 48 hours. Angiography was then repeated, which showed resolution of the thrombus

Figure 6.29 (opposite)   This is an example of spontaneous dissection. The patient presented with an acute coronary syndrome and only a mild narrowing of the left anterior descending (white arrows in Panels A and B). Pre-intervention IVUS imaging from distal (a) to proximal (b) showed a circumferential medial dissection (c) that was partially occupied by intramural hematoma (d). Note the diffuse intimal thickening and collapse of the vessel (e), but no definitive atherosclerotic changes. The patient underwent stent implantation; the final angiogram is shown (Panel C)

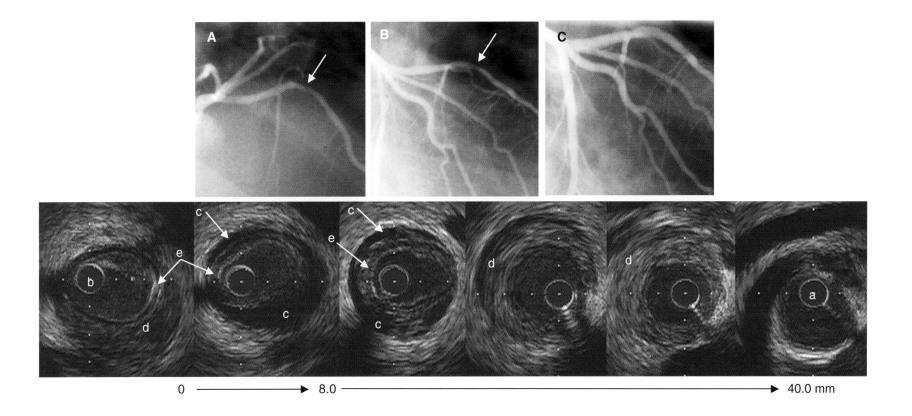

Figure 6.30 (opposite) This is an example of spontaneous coronary artery dissection.The patient presented with an acute anterior-wall ST-elevation myocardial infarction 2 weeks post-partum. The angiogram showed a long severe narrowing in the mid-left anterior descending (white arrows in Panels A and B) and irregular proximal left anterior descending and left main artery. Diagnostic IVUS imaging of the mid-left anterior descending (Panel C) showed a spontaneous dissection. The IVUS catheter is in the false lumen distally (a); note the true lumen (b). There is a skip area that is dissection-free (c). The intimal flap (d) reappears proximally where the false lumen (e) is mostly occupied by hematoma. Note that the artery is free of atherosclerosis. Panel D shows the IVUS imaging of the proximal left anterior descending (f) continuing to the left main. Note the entrance to the left circumflex (g), persistence of the intimal flap (h), the true lumen (i), and the false lumen (j), which is mostly occupied by hematoma. The increased IVUS catheter ring-down in Panel D was probably caused by a small air bubble

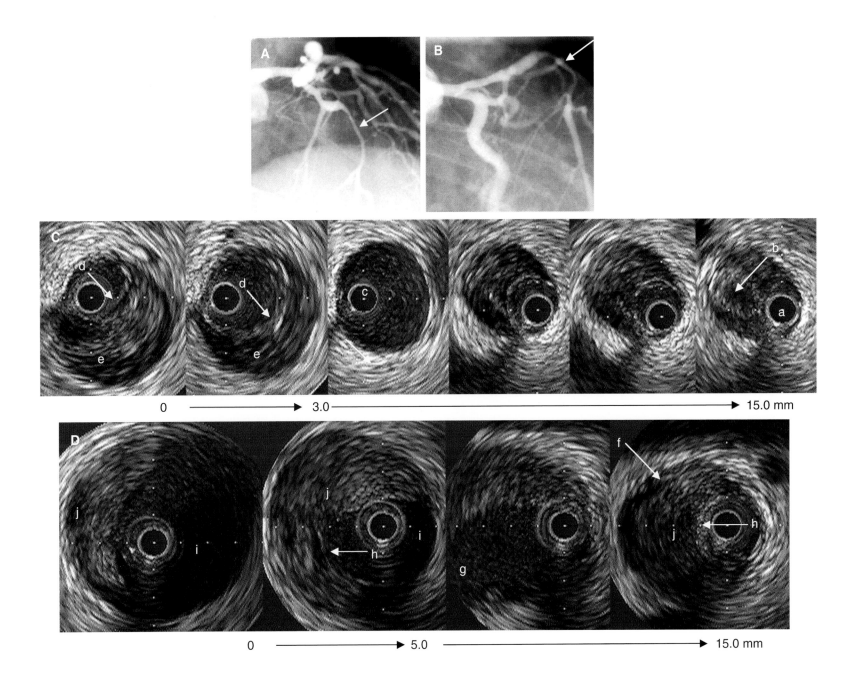

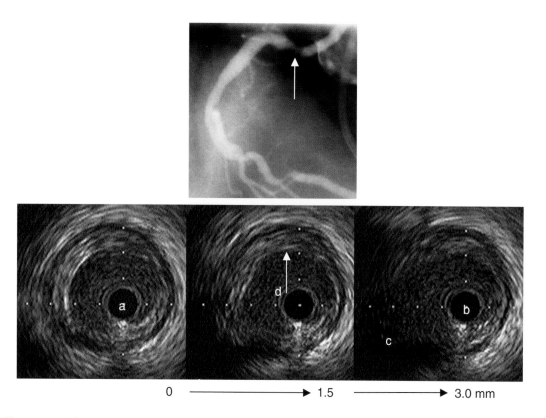

0 ——————→ 1.5 —————→ 3.0 mm

Figure 6.31 Whenever a diagnostic or guiding catheter would engage this right coronary artery, there was a severe ostial narrowing (white arrow on the angiogram). This proved to be catheter-induced spasm. After disengaging the guiding catheters IVUS imaging of the proximal right coronary artery (a) back to the ostium (b, note the transition to the aorta, c) showed a moderate plaque burden of 55% (d), but no stenosis

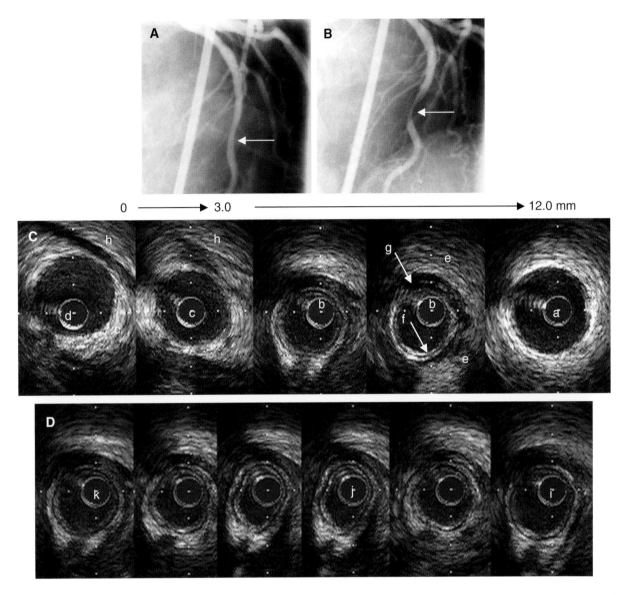

Figure 6.32 This patient presented with a muscle bridge of the left anterior descending artery. Note the systolic compression on the angiograms (white arrows in Panel A, diastole, and in Panel B, systole). The IVUS pullback (Panel C) shows the normal distal epicardial vessel (a), the intramyocardial course of the mid-left anterior descending (b), the point where the left anterior descending first becomes intramyocardial (c), and the normal proximal vessel (d). Note the myocardium (e) surrounding the left anterior descending, the intimal thickening (f) of the intramyocardial vessel, the half-moon appearance that is considered characteristic of this anomaly (g), and the pericardium (h) when the proximal vessel is no longer intramyocardial. Panel D shows one complete cardiac cycle from diastole (i) to systole (j) to diastole (k). Note that the lumen narrows from 4.0 to 2.2 mm², but that there is some deformation of the lumen through most of the cardiac cycle

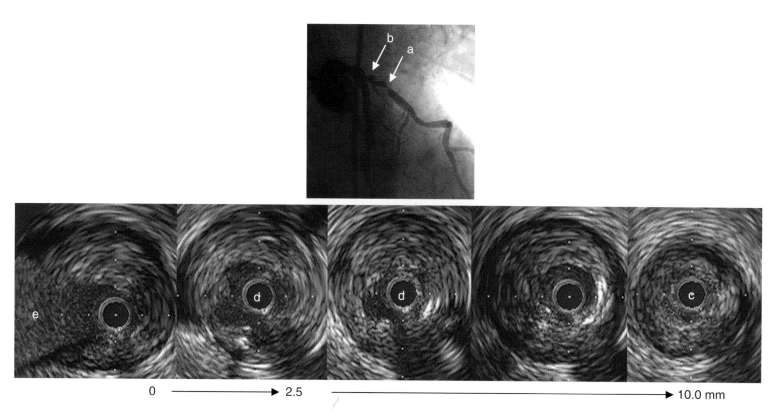

Figure 6.33 This patient presented with a culprit lesion in the left anterior descending artery. Note the proximal stenosis (a) and the ostial complex plaque (b) in the angiogram. The pre-intervention IVUS pullback shows the proximal stenosis (c) and the irregular and disrupted plaque (d) that continued up to and involving the true ostium of the left anterior descending. There was no identifiable proximal reference before the circumflex (e) was seen

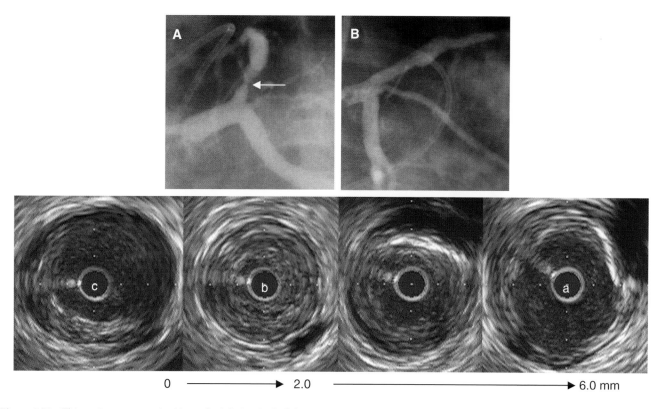

0 ⟶ 2.0 ⟶ 6.0 mm

Figure 6.34   This patient presented with a culprit lesion in the left anterior descending artery (white arrow in Panel A). The pre-intervention IVUS pullback is from the distal reference (a) through the lesion (b) to the proximal reference (c). Note that even though the lesion may be classified as ostial by angiographic criteria, there is a well-defined proximal reference by IVUS. The maximum reference-segment lumen diameter was 4.3 mm proximally and 4.4 mm distally. The midwall dimension was 4.6 mm proximally and 4.9 mm distally. However, because of negative remodeling, the lesion-site external elastic membrane diameter measured 4.0 mm. Therefore, a 4.0 mm stent was implanted. The final result is shown (Panel B)

Side branches

Measurement of side-branch EEM and lumen dimensions and plaque burden requires imaging the branch itself; these measurements cannot be made from the main vessel. Nevertheless, it is possible to assess qualitatively the side branch from the main vessel to determine whether it is normal or diseased and, perhaps, whether or not it is severely diseased (Figure 6.35). This may have implications regarding the likelihood of side-branch compromise during an intervention.

Remodeling

The criteria proposed by Nishioka *et al.*[36] are the easiest for assessing remodeling during real-time image acquisition. Studies have shown that native artery lesions with a large plaque burden, a large EEM CSA, or positive remodeling are at increased risk for acute, subacute, and long-term complications. These lesions can, occasionally, be difficult to dilate even though plaque morphology looks "soft". IVUS identification of positive remodeling is not just "academic". Positive remodeling has been shown to be a predictor of (1) CK-MB elevation after percutaneous coronary intervention;[37] (2) the absence of reflow in primary infarction angioplasty;[38–40] (3) recurrent ischemia within one month following thrombolysis for acute myocardial infarction;[41] (4) major adverse coronary events in patients with unstable angina undergoing any form of revascularization;[42] (5) target-lesion revascularization in patients undergoing non-stent intervention and target-vessel revascularization and intimal hyperplasia in patients undergoing bare-metal or drug-eluting stent implantation;[43–46] and (6) in-hospital complications, major adverse coronary events, restenosis, and new lesion formation in patients with stable angina undergoing single-vessel intervention.[47] Thus, the cumulative evidence indicates that positively remodeled lesions are more biologically active than intermediate or negatively remodeled lesions.

Saphenous vein grafts

There has been little work on the use of IVUS and saphenous vein-graft disease. Saphenous vein bypass grafts that fail early are more likely to (1) be ostial or proximal; (2) have smaller reference vein-graft and plaque CSAs, but a larger plaque burden; and (3) have less calcium and mobile plaque elements compared with vein grafts that fail late.[48] Calcium is found in approximately 40% of saphenous vein grafts, is evenly distributed among the lesion and the proximal and distal reference sites, occurs in older grafts (mean age of 10.5 years), and occurs more often in insulin-treated diabetics and smokers (Figure 6.36).[49] Negatively remodeled vein-graft lesions typically are echodense, contain little plaque, and can have very thick walls without an echolucent zone; they may represent intrinsic vein graft wall or peri-graft fibrosis or occur at anastamotic sites. Negatively remodeled vein-graft lesions can be hard to dilate – even using very high pressures.[50] This may indicate a component of intrinsic or perigraft fibrosis. Examples are shown in Figures 6.37 and 6.38. Finally, vein grafts contain mobile elements, but it is impossible to assess vein-graft thrombus (Figures 6.39 and 6.40). Degenerated vein grafts contain exceptionally large plaque burdens (Figure 6.41). Other unusual IVUS findings are shown in Figures 6.42 and 6.43.

REFERENCE VESSEL IMAGING AND DEVICE SIZING

Proximal reference

The proximal reference is the image slice within the same segment as the target-lesion site that has the largest lumen and smallest plaque burden. At times, it may be necessary to adjust proximal reference-site selection to avoid or deliberately cover a side branch. The typical measurements that are used for device sizing include:

- Maximum and mean lumen diameter
- Mean midwall diameter
- Mean EEM diameter

The entire vessel proximal to the target site should be visualized to determine the extent of the plaque burden and proximal vessel calcification. Calcification causes the proximal vessel to be rigid and non-compliant. This may be important in delivering bulky devices (such as an atherectomy catheter) and direct stent implantation. Occult stenoses may be detected; these appear to be more common in the right coronary artery. Finally, when imaging the left anterior descending or left circumflex arteries, the study should include pullback to the aorta so as to assess the left main artery.

Distal reference

The distal reference is the image slice within the same segment as the target-lesion site that has the largest lumen and smallest plaque burden. At times, it may be necessary to adjust this site selection either to avoid or to deliberately cover a side branch. The typical measurements that are used for device sizing include:

- Maximum and mean lumen diameter

- Mean midwall diameter
- Mean (EEM) diameter

Device sizing

Fundamental to the performance of any intervention is the selection of the size of the balloon, stent, etc. One misconception about device sizing is that the final result begins and ends with correct device-size selection. This is not the case. IVUS device sizing and, then, inflating the stent or balloon according to the manufacturer's package labeling (or until the waist disappears) does not guarantee a good result, or even that the balloon or stent will expand to the diameter on the package. Instead, post-intervention IVUS imaging is important to assure an optimum result. Nevertheless, there are a number of ways to use IVUS to size a device. In general, these strategies will allow safe use of a larger device or balloon when compared to angiographic sizing. It makes sense to adopt one of these strategies, to use a single strategy consistently, and to become familiar with the results.

The only reported work on IVUS device sizing is in relation to balloon angioplasty. IVUS *midwall* measurements can be used to size balloons safely, as was shown in CLOUT (CLinical Outcomes Ultrasound Trial).[51] In essence, the reference-segment plaque burden is a cushion or a sponge that allows safe sizing of a balloon or stent into the vessel wall. The availability of stents to treat severe dissections and glycoprotein IIb/IIIa inhibitors to reduce thrombotic complications has made even more aggressive balloon sizing safe. Therefore, some authorities use lesion-site EEM diameters to select balloon size, recognizing (and accepting) the fact that up to half of the procedures will result in major dissections or other complications necessitating stent implantation.[52–54]

Because there are no data on IVUS-guided stent sizing, the following two suggestions are based on experience – although other authorities may have alternative recommendations. The first suggestion is to identify the maximum lumen diameter – whether proximal or distal to the lesion – and then to use this to select the stent size. This is the simplest and, perhaps, the most reliable approach. In general, this will result in upsizing by (on average) 0.75 mm compared with angiography. The other suggestion is to use mean midwall measurements. In general, this will result in upsizing by 0.85 mm. As shown in Figures 6.44 and 6.45, and in other examples in this chapter, the two measurements are often very similar. Full reference and lesion-site EEM diameters probably should not be used for stent sizing especially with high pressure inflations. Once the stent is implanted, iterative IVUS imaging is important to ensure optimum stent expansion with post-dilation, using larger balloons or higher pressures as necessary. At least with bare-metal stents, restenosis is determined by the final minimum stent cross-sectional area.

Common sense is important to device size selection, and there are certain anatomic situations in which even IVUS imaging will not help – for example, marked vessel tapering (especially if the distal vessel is normal), saphenous vein mismatch compared with the distal native artery, or marked negative lesion-site remodeling (particularly with minimal plaque or an arc of normal vessel wall). In these cases, it may be necessary to temper enthusiasm for aggressive IVUS-guided device sizing and select a balloon or stent appropriately matched to the smaller of the cross-sections. Otherwise, there is a risk of increased complications – particularly rupture and intramural hematoma. Conversely, the distal vessel may be underperfused (and artificially small), particularly with the catheter across the stenosis. For this reason, IVUS-device sizing depends more on proximal reference-vessel measurements.

There are no data on cutting-balloon sizing. However, the cutting balloon should be sized using IVUS reference-segment lumen dimensions.

There are two types of atheroablative devices. Rotational atherectomy and laser angioplasty primarily result in plaque modification rather than definitive plaque removal. The catheter should be larger than the IVUS lesion pre-intervention minimum lumen diameter to have an effect. The maximum catheter diameter is usually determined by the size of the guiding catheter. Both devices typically require adjunct balloon angioplasty or stent implantation. The above recommendation concerning balloon or stent sizing should be followed for adjunctive device or balloon use.

Directional atherectomy devices such as the Atherocath or Silverhawk catheters are designed to perform definitive plaque removal. Limited sizes are available, and the devices are functionally "upsized" when performing the procedure according to the initial results. With the Atherocath, multiple studies have shown that the residual plaque burden determines restenosis as much as the residual lumen CSA. Thus, Atherocath diameters are selected based on the distance to the lesion EEM as well as on plaque distribution. Performance of atherectomy is assisted by knowing the orientation of the maximum plaque thickness to direct the device, and iterative IVUS use with additional atherectomy as necessary helps to minimize the residual plaque burden. If adjunct balloon angioplasty or stent implantation is necessary, the above recommendation concerning balloon or stent sizing should be followed. There are no comparable data for the Silverhawk catheter.

LESION LENGTH AND STENT LENGTH SELECTION

Length measurements are performed using motorized transducer pullback. Unlike angiography, IVUS length measurements are not affected by tortuosity, bend points, or foreshortening. Lengths are more accurate when using motorized transducer pullback through a stationary imaging sheath as compared with pullback of the entire catheter. Lengths are not possible with manual catheter pullback. Length measurements that are useful during an intervention include lesion length and the distance from the lesion to a side branch or the ostium of the artery or between two branches (Figure 6.45).

Precise length measurements are more important in stent implantation than in any other intervention. In general, lesion length – which dictates stent length – is the distance between the proximal and distal reference sites. However, this may need to be adjusted so as to accommodate the planned procedure. For example, the "length" may need to be shortened to avoid jailing a side branch or "lengthened" to cover this branch deliberately. Sometimes the operator may want to select the precise location of one edge (for example, just at the ostium of the left anterior descending) and be less precise about the other edges provided it extends past the reference. At other times, the operator may want to select the proximal and distal ends of the stent based on the anatomy (for example, to sit just between two branches) and will coordinate these points with the IVUS images by looking at the radio-opaque transducer on fluoroscopy.

During bare-metal stenting, there was a tendency to minimize stent length to reduce restenosis – even if some disease was left uncovered. With drug-eluting stents, the trend is to cover as much disease as possible and to end the stent in the segment of artery with the largest lumen and least plaque. Appropriate drug-eluting stent length selection may be very cost-effective compared with ad hoc implantation of additional stents as necessary.

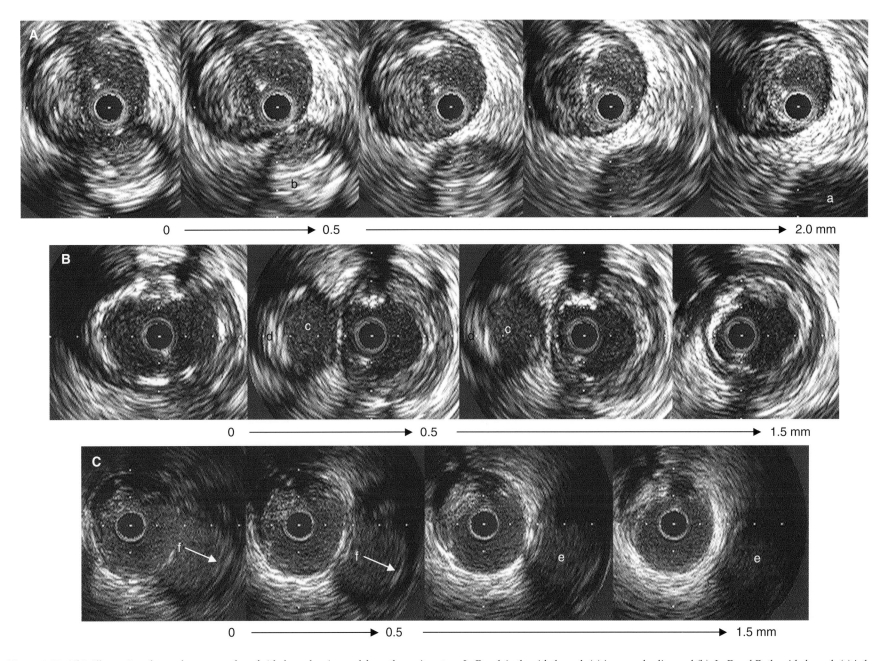

Figure 6.35   This illustration shows three examples of side branches imaged from the main artery. In Panel A, the side branch (a) is severely diseased (b). In Panel B, the side branch (c) is less diseased (d) than in Panel A. In Panel C, the side branch (e) has only mild intimal thickening (f). Nevertheless, it is impossible to assess lumen dimensions and lumen compromise of a side branch from the main artery

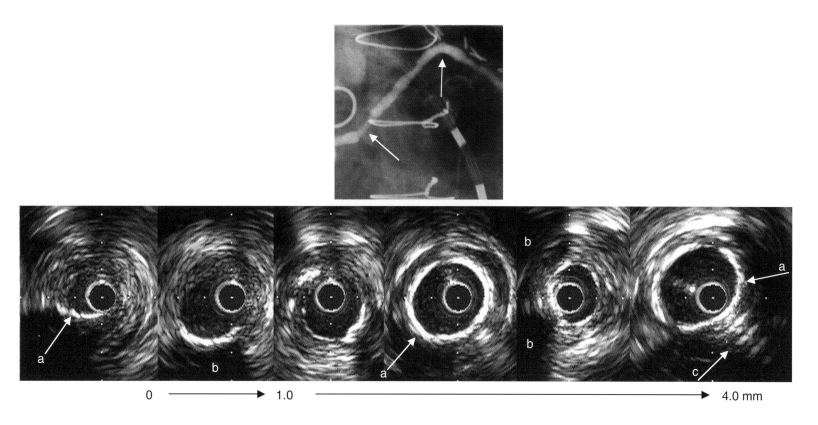

0 ⟶ 1.0 ⟶ 4.0 mm

Figure 6.36 This 12-year-old saphenous vein graft shows multiple areas of calcification. The pre-intervention IVUS image corresponds to the length of graft between the two white arrows in the angiogram. Note the characteristic hyperechoic plaque (a) with shadowing (b) and reverberations (c). Most of the calcium is in the vein-graft wall

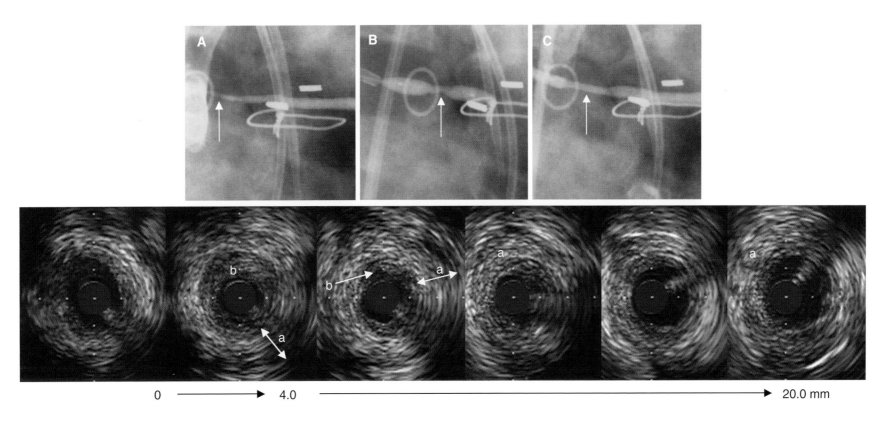

Figure 6.37 This long, ostial saphenous vein-graft stenosis (white arrow in Panel A) proved difficult to dilated despite balloon inflations to 24 atm (white arrow in Panel B). There was a significant residual stenosis (white arrow in Panel C). Pre-intervention IVUS imaging showed a thick vein-graft wall (a, measuring 1.5 mm) and only a modest amount of plaque (b)

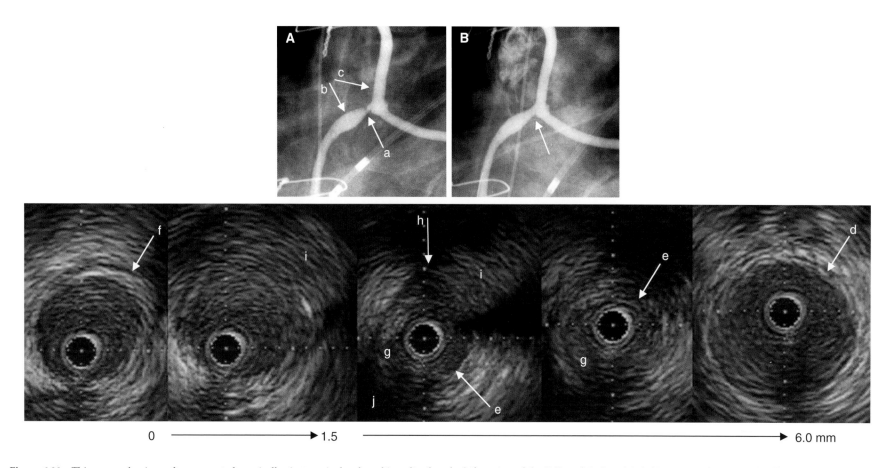

Figure 6.38 This unusual vein graft was created surgically. A stenosis developed just distal to the bifurcation of the "Y" graft in Panel A (white arrow a). It proved difficult to dilate; note the residual stenosis (white arrow in Panel B) despite 24-atm inflations. Pre-intervention IVUS illustrates the length of vein graft between arrows b and c in Panel A. The distal vein graft CSA (d) measured 22.8 mm^2, the lesion-site vein-graft CSA (e) measured 10.1 mm^2, and the proximal vein-graft CSA (f) measured 11.6 mm^2. Note the modest amount of plaque (g), the site of the anastamosis (h), the other limb of the graft (i), and attenuation (j) caused by the fibrotic plaque

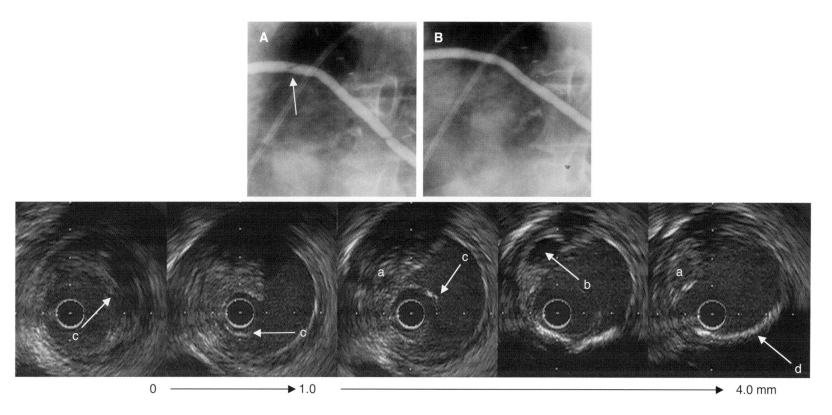

Figure 6.39   The angiogram of this saphenous vein graft showed two linear densities; the proximal linear density is shown by the white arrow in Panel A. The pre-intervention IVUS of the proximal lesion shows eccentric soft plaque (a) with a hypoechoic area (b), mobile elements (c), and deep wall calcium (d). The maximum reference-segment lumen diameter was 4.0 mm distally. Crown stents (4.0 mm) were implanted; the final result is shown in Panel B

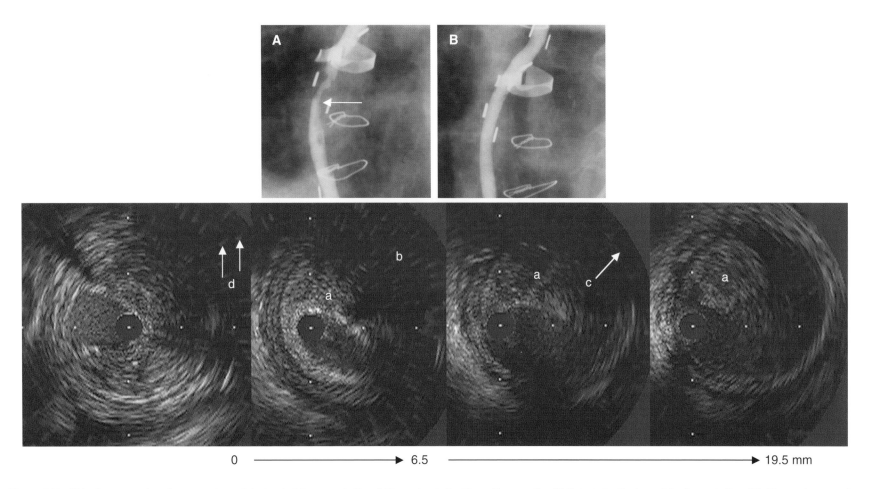

Figure 6.40 This degenerated saphenous vein-graft lesion (white arrow in Panel A) was treated with a self-expanding Wallstent; the final result is shown in Panel B. The pre-intervention IVUS showed a large eccentric plaque burden (a) with attenuation (b). The gain was increased to compensate for the weak transducer in order to penetrate to the vein-graft wall (c); note the appearance of noise (d) when the gain was increased. The scale is 2 mm. The vein-graft CSA measured 30.2 mm^2, and the vein-graft diameter measured 6.0 mm

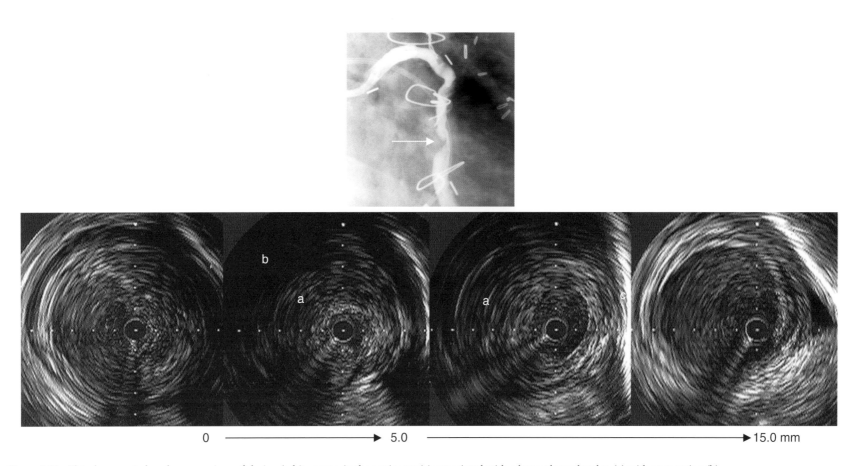

Figure 6.41   This degenerated saphenous vein-graft lesion (white arrow in the angiogram) is associated with a large plaque burden (a) with attenuation (b)

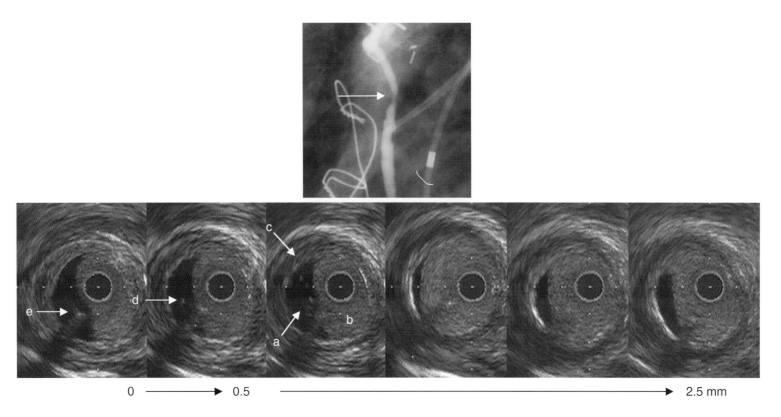

Figure 6.42 IVUS imaging proximal to this saphenous vein-graft stenosis (white arrow in the angiogram) showed a flowing hypoechoic area (a) separating the intense blood speckle (b) from the vein-graft wall (c). Because vein grafts lack side branches, stasis causing blood speckle can be more intense than in native arteries, particularly with an IVUS catheter occlusive across a stenosis. Similarly, contrast injection can layer and stagnate along the vein-graft wall intima, as is the case in this example. Contrast (or saline) is black in appearance; note the small bubbles (d) within the contrast. The position of the guidewire (e) helps to confirm the borders of the lumen

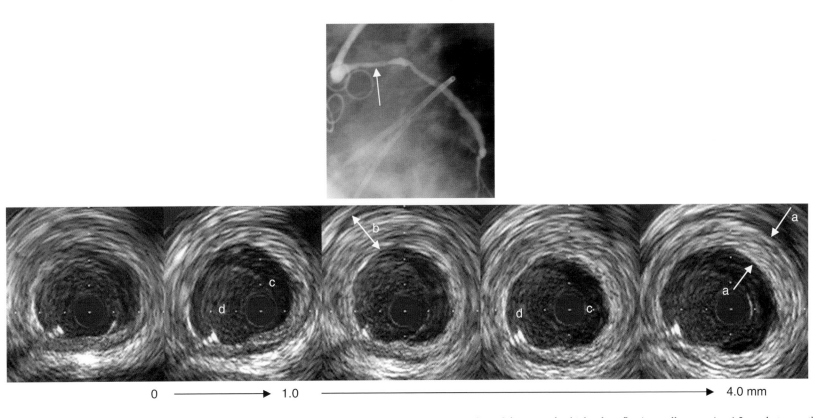

Figure 6.43   This proximal saphenous vein-graft stenosis (white arrow on the angiogram) has the unusual IVUS features of a thick echoreflective wall measuring 1.2 mm between the white arrows (a) and 1.5 mm at the site of the double-headed white arrow (b) and almost completely echolucent plaque (c) when compared with the blood speckle (d). This echolucent plaque has been called a "black hole", which is a misnomer since it is not a hole and is better called a "black wall"

0 ────────► 6.5 ─────────────────────────────────────► 26.0 mm

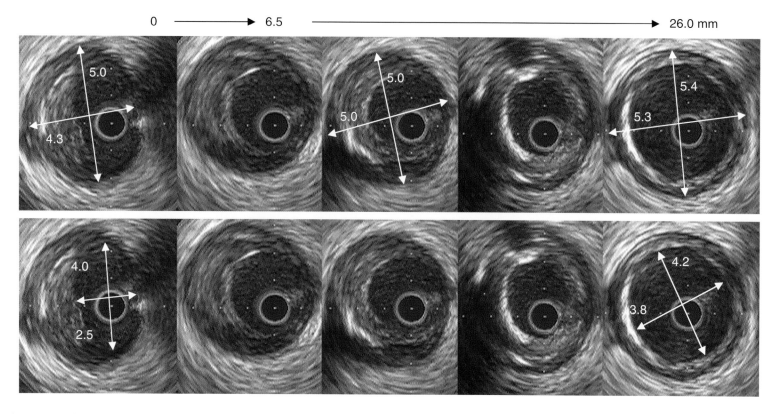

Figure 6.44 This example shows a complete set of measurements used to calculate device size. External elastic membrane (or media-to-media) measurements are shown at the top. Lumen measurements are shown at the bottom. Measurements are in millimeters

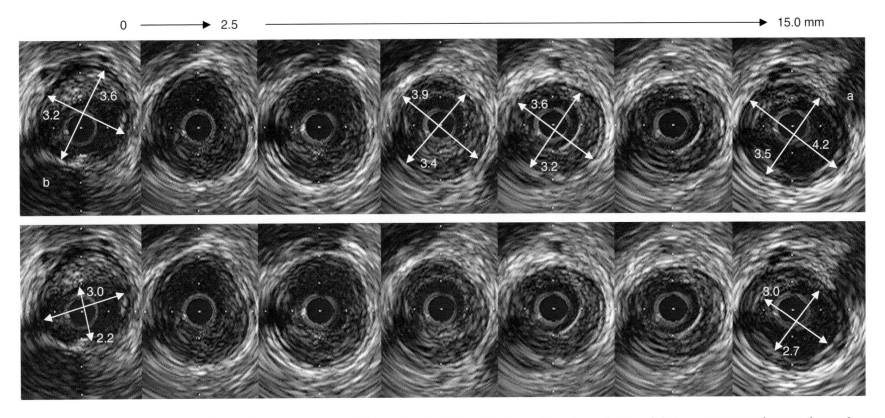

Figure 6.45 This example shows a complete set of measurements to calculate device size. External elastic membrane (or media-to-media) measurements are shown at the top. Lumen measurements are shown at the bottom. Measurements are in millimeters. Note that length measurements can be used to determine the distance between two branches – in this case a septal branch (a) and the left circumflex (b). A 15-mm-long stent will just fit between these two branches without impinging on either of them

REFERENCES

1. Abizaid A, Mintz GS, Pichard AD, et al. Clinical, intravascular ultrasound, and quantitative angiographic determinants of the coronary flow reserve before and after percutaneous transluminal coronary angioplasty. Am J Cardiol 1998; 82: 423–8

2. Nishioka T, Amanullah AM, Luo H, et al. Clinical validation of intravascular ultrasound imaging for assessment of coronary stenosis severity: comparison with stress myocardial perfusion imaging. J Am Coll Cardiol 1999; 33: 1870–8

3. Takagi A, Tsurumi Y, Ishii Y, et al. Clinical potential of intravascular ultrasound for physiological assessment of coronary stenosis: relationship between quantitative ultrasound tomography and pressure-derived fractional flow reserve. Circulation 1999; 100: 250–5.

4. Takayama T, Hodgson JMcB. Prediction of the physiologic severity of coronary lesions using 3D IVUS: validation by direct coronary pressure measurements. Catheter Cardiovasc Interv 2001; 53: 48–55

5. Abizaid AS, Mintz GS, Mehran R, et al. One year follow-up after percutaneous transluminal angioplasty was not performed based on intravascular ultrasound findings. Importance of lumen dimensions. Circulation 1999; 100: 256–61

6. Bech GJW, De Bruyne B, Pijls NHJ, et al. Fractional flow reserve to determine the appropriateness of angioplasty in moderate coronary stenosis: a randomized trial. Circulation 2001; 103: 2928–34

7. Maehara A, Mintz GS, Bui AB, et al. Determinants of angiographically silent stenoses in patients with coronary artery disease. Am J Cardiol 2003; 91: 1335–8

8. Naghavi M, Libby P, Falk E, et al. From vulnerable plaque to vulnerable patient: a call for new definitions and risk assessment strategies. Circulation 2003; 108: 1664–72, 772–8

9. Russo RJ, Wong SC, Marchant D, et al. Intravascular ultrasound-directed clinical decision making in the setting of an inconclusive left main coronary angiogram: final results from the Left Main IVUS Registry. Circulation 2004; 108: IV-462

10. Jasti V, Yalamanchili V, Merrill B, et al. Fractional flow reserve versus intravascular ultrasound for decision making in equivocal left main stenosis. Circulation 2004; 108: IV-462

11. Bech GJW, Droste H, Pijls NHJ, et al. Value of fractional flow reserve in making decisions about bypass surgery for equivocal left main coronary artery disease. Heart 2001; 86: 547–52

12. Abizaid AS, Mintz GS, Abizaid A, et al. One year follow-up after intravascular ultrasound assessment of moderate left main coronary artery disease in patients with ambiguous angiograms. J Am Coll Cardiol 1999; 34: 707–15

13. Wolfhard U, Gorge G, Konorza T, et al. Intravascular ultrasound (IVUS) examination reverses therapeutic decision from percutaneous intervention to a surgical approach in patients with alterations of the left main stem. Thorac Cardiovasc Surg 1998; 46: 281–4

14. Dussaillant GD, Mintz GS, Pichard AD, et al. Intravascular ultrasound identification of calcified intraluminal lesions misdiagnosed as thrombi by coronary angiography. Am Heart J 1996; 132: 687–9

15. Kotani J-I, Mintz GS, Rai PB, et al. IVUS assessment of angiographic filling defects in native coronary arteries: do they always contain thrombi? J Am Coll Cardiol (in press)

16. Virmani R, Kolodgie FD, Burke AP, et al. Lessons from sudden coronary death: a comprehensive morphological classification scheme for atherosclerotic lesions. Arterioscler Thromb Vasc Biol 2000; 20: 1262–75

17. Maehara A, Mintz GS, Ahmed JM, et al. An intravascular ultrasound classification of angiographic coronary artery aneurysms. Am J Cardiol 2001; 88: 365–70

18. Markis JE, Joffe CD, Lohn PF, et al. Clinical significance of coronary arterial ectasia. Am J Cardiol 1976; 37: 217–22

19. Gulec S, Atmaca Y, Kilickap M, et al. Angiographic assessment of myocardial perfusion in patients with isolated coronary ectasia. Am J Cardiol 2003; 91: 996–9

20. Akyurek O, Berkalp B, Sayin T, et al. Altered coronary flow properties in diffuse coronary artery ectasia. Am Heart J 2003; 145: 66–72

21. Maehara A, Mintz GS, Bui AB, et al. Morphologic and angiographic features of coronary plaque rupture detected by intravascular ultrasound. J Am Coll Cardiol 2002; 40: 904–10

22. Fujii K, Kobayashi Y, Mintz GS, et al. Intravascular ultrasound assessment of ulcerated ruptured plaques: a comparison of culprit and non-nulprit lesions of patients with acute coronary syndromes and lesions in patients without acute coronary syndromes. Circulation 2003; 108: 2473–8

23. Rioufol G, Finet G, Ginon I, et al. Multiple atherosclerotic plaque rupture in acute coronary syndrome: a three-vessel intravascular ultrasound study. Circulation 2002; 106: 804–8

24. Fukuda D, Kawarabayashi T, Tanaka A, et al. Lesion characteristics of acute myocardial infarction: an investigation with intravascular ultrasound. Heart 2001; 85: 402–6

25. Sano T, Tanaka A, Namba M, et al. C-reactive protein and lesion morphology in patients with acute myocardial infarction. Circulation 2003; 108: 282–5

26. Oesterle SN, Limpijankit T, Yeung AC, et al. Ultrasoound logic: the value of intracoronary imaging for the interventionalist. Catheter Cardiovasc Interv 1999; 47: 475–90

27. Maehara A, Mintz GS, Castagna MT, et al. Intravascular ultrasound assessment of spontaneous coronary artery dissection. Am J Cardiol 2002; 89: 466–8

28. Yamagishi M, Miyatake K, Tamai J, et al. Intravascular ultrasound detection of atherosclerosis at the site of focal vasospasm in angiographically normal or minimally narrowed coronary segments. J Am Coll Cardiol 1994; 23: 352–7

29. Hong MK, Park SW, Lee CW, et al. Intravascular ultrasound findings of negative arterial remodeling at sites of focal coronary spasm in patients with vasospastic angina. Am Heart J 2000; 140: 395–401

30. Saito S, Yamagishi M, Takayama T, et al. Plaque morphology at coronary sites with focal spasm in variant angina: study using intravascular ultrasound. Circ J 2003; 67: 1041–5

31. Miyao Y, Kugiyama K, Kawano H, et al. Diffuse intimal thickening of coronary arteries in patients with coronary spastic angina. J Am Coll Cardiol 2000; 36: 432–7

32. Ge J, Jeremias A, Rupp A, et al. New signs characteristic of myocardial bridging demonstrated by intracoronary ultrasound and Doppler. Eur Heart J 1999; 20: 1707–16

33. Topol EJ, Nissen SE. Our pre-occupation with coronary lumenology. The dissociation between clinical and angiographic findings in ischemic heart disease. Circulation 1995; 92: 2333–42

34. Kimura BJ, Russo RJ, Bhargava V, et al. Atheroma morphology and distribution in proximal left anterior descending coronary artery: in vivo observations. J Am Coll Cardiol 1996; 27: 825–31

35. Badak O, Schoenhagen P, Tsunoda T, et al. Characteristics of atherosclerotic plaque distribution in coronary artey bifurcations: an intravascular ultrasound analysis. Coron Artery Dis 2003; 14: 309–16

36. Nishioka T, Luo H, Eigler NL, et al. Contribution of inadequate compensatory enlargement to development of human coronary artery stenosis: an in vivo intravascular ultrasound study. J Am Coll Cardiol 1996; 27: 1571–6

37. Mehran R, Dangas G, Mintz GS, et al. Atherosclerotic plaque burden and CK-MB enzyme elevation after coronary interventions: intravascular ultrasound study of 2256 patients. Circulation 2000; 101: 604–10

38. Tanaka A, Kawarabayashi T, Nishibori Y, et al. No-reflow phenomenon and lesion morphology in patients with acute myocardial infarction. Circulation 2002; 105: 2148–52

39. Kotani J, Mintz GS, Castagna MT, et al. Usefulness of preprocedural coronary lesion morphology as assessed by intravasuclar ultrasound in predicting thrombolysis in myocardial infarction frame count after percutaneous coronary intervention in patients with Q-wave acute myocardial infarction. Am J Cardiol 2003; 91: 870–2.

40. Watanabe T, Nanto S, Uematsu M, et al. Prediction of no-reflow phenomenon after successful percutaneous coronary intervention in patients with acute myocardial infarction: intravascular ultrasound findings. Circ J 2003; 67: 667–71.

41. Gyongyosi M, Wexberg P, Kiss K, et al. Adaptive remodeling of the infarct-related artery is associated with recurrent ischemic events after thrombolysis in acute myocardial infarction. Coron Artery Dis 2001; 12: 167–72.

42. Gyongyosi M, Yang P, Hassan A, et al. Intravascular ultrasound predictors of major adverse cardiac events in patients with unstable angina. Clin Cardiol 2000; 23: 507–15

43. Dangas G, Mintz GS, Mehran R, et al. Preintervention arterial remodeling as an independent predictor of target-lesion revascularization after nonstent coronary intervention: an analysis of 777 lesions with intravascular ultrasound imaging. Circulation 1999; 99: 3149–54

44. Okura H, Morino Y, Oshima A, et al. Preintervention arterial remodeling affects clinical outcome following stenting: an intravascular ultrasound study. J Am Coll Cardiol 2001; 37: 1031–5

45. Endo A, Hirayama H, Yoshida O, et al. Arterial remodeling influences the development of intimal hyperplasia after stent implantation. J Am Coll Cardiol 2001; 37: 70–5

46. Mintz GS, Tinana A, Hong MK, et al. Impact of preinterventional arterial remodeling on neointimal hyperplasia after implantation of (non-polymer-encapsulated) paclitaxel-coated stents: a serial volumetric intravascular ultrasound analysis from the ASian Paclitaxel-Eluting Stent Clinical Trial (ASPECT). Circulation 2003; 108: 1295–8

47. Wexberg P, Gyongyosi M, Sperker W, et al. Pre-existing arterial remodeling is associated with in–hospital and late adverse cardiac events after coronary interventions in patients with stable angina pectoris. J Am Coll Cardiol 2000; 36: 1860–9

48. Canos DA, Mintz GA, Berzinge CO, et al. Clinical, angiographic, and intravascular ultrasound characteristics of early vein graft failure. J Am Coll Cardiol 44: 53–6

49. Castagna MT, Mintz GS, Weissman NJ, et al. Calcification in saphenous vein grafts: clinical correlated and intravascular ultrasound findings. J Am Coll Cardiol 2002; 39: 36A

50. Mintz GS, Popma JJ, Pichard AD, et al. The dimorphic pathology of vein graft lesions affects acute procedural and late angiographic outcomes. J Am Coll Cardiol 1995; 25: 79A (abstract).

51. Stone GW, Hodgson JMcB, St Goar FG, et al. Improved procedural results of coronary angioplasty with intravascular ultrasound guided balloon sizing; The CLOUT Pilot Trial. Circulation 1997; 95: 2044–52

52. Abizaid A, Pichard AD, Mintz GS, et al. Acute and long-term results of an IVUS-guided PTCA/provisional stent implantation strategy. Am J Cardiol 1999; 84: 1381–4

53. Schroeder S, Baumbach A, Haase KK, et al. Reduction of restenosis by vessel size adapted percutaneous transluminal coronary angioplasty using intravascular ultrasound. Am J Cardiol 1999; 83: 875–9

54. Schiele F, Meneveau N, Gilard M, et al. Intravascular ultrasound-guided balloon angioplasty compared with stent: immediate and 6-month results of the multicenter, randomized Balloon Equivalent to Stent Study (BEST). Circulation 2003; 107: 545–51

7
Interventional imaging and recognition of complications

Balloon angioplasty was first performed in the late 1970s. Devices were developed in an attempt to improve on the acute and long-term results of balloon angioplasty. Today, most interventional procedures involve routine stent implantation. Provisional stenting – in which aggressive balloon angioplasty is attempted first and stent implantation reserved for inadequate results – has been adopted by a few interventionalists, either for cost reasons or because of the concern for high bare-metal stent restenosis rates. This concern is likely to diminish in the era of drug-eluting stents. The other devices continue to be used by only a small minority of interventionalists. Therefore, the bulk of this chapter will focus on IVUS in stent implantation and, in particular, the recognition of complications that are common to all interventional procedures. The figures in this chapter were collected during a 12-year period in the evolution of interventional cardiology; they are meant to illustrate, not advocate, the approach to lesion morphology and the therapeutic results. All of the IVUS illustrations are at the same scale (magnification). Multiple examples are often included to show the consistency of the IVUS findings.

The goal of an intervention is to eliminate ischemia and optimize lumen dimensions; ideally, the final lumen should be matched to the proximal and distal reference segments. The following chart shows a comparison of the reference-lumen dimensions and the final minimum lumen cross-sectional area (CSA), assuming a final 0% residual stenosis. Even in the setting of a negative angiographic stenosis, a true 0% residual stenosis (assessed by IVUS) is rarely achieved.

Reference	Minimum lumen CSA
2.25 mm	4.0 mm^2
2.5 mm	5.0 mm^2
2.75 mm	6.0 mm^2
3.0 mm	7.5 mm^2
3.25 mm	8.3 mm^2
3.5 mm	9.6 mm^2

In general, IVUS guidance begins with device sizing. Balloon sizing can be more aggressive than stent sizing; lesion-site media-to-media balloon sizing has been successfully used in a number of studies, but lesion-site media-to-media stent sizing is more likely to cause complications such as perforations.[1] However, IVUS-guided sizing does not ensure an ideal result. Post-intervention IVUS followed by additional interventional steps (if necessary) will result in more optimal lumen dimensions in most patients.

IVUS has been fundamental to understanding the mechanisms of all angioplasty procedures. The IVUS findings have often been at odds with *ex vivo* pre-clinical mechanistic studies. Using IVUS, lumen improvement can be attributed to arterial expansion (increase in external elastic membrane (EEM) CSA), plaque & media (P&M) reduction or axial redistribution, and dissection. Ideally, IVUS mechanistic studies should involve volumetric analysis, because planar analysis – regardless of lesion-site selection – cannot easily detect axial plaque redistribution; and the relative contribution of expansion, plaque reduction, and dissection to lumen improvement will be miscalculated. In addition, there is real debate about the mechanism of plaque decrease. Apart from the use of an ablative device, perceived plaque decrease is the result of plaque compression, plaque embolization, unrecognized axial plaque redistribution, or measurement error. Because plaque has solid and liquid (or semisolid), but not gaseous, elements and because only gases are compressible, plaque compression is unlikely. Plaque redistribution and/or prolapse into the lumen of a stent, where it can embolize, appears to depend on plaque composition and pre-intervention remodeling and is more common in soft versus hard plaques.[2,3] A true reduction in plaque volume is IVUS evidence of plaque embolization. Volumetric IVUS analysis requires motorized transducer pullback, careful registration of pre- versus post-intervention images, and a sufficiently long segment of analysis to account for all plaque shifts and edge effects. However, the greater the degree of lesion calcification, the more inaccurate is the pre- versus post-intervention comparison of plaque volume. Similarly, even if post-intervention dissections are small, their size and the decision as to whether to include the dissection plane as part of the plaque or the true lumen will affect plaque volume calculations.

BALLOON ANGIOPLASTY

Mechanism

IVUS studies in stable lesions have shown that balloon angioplasty increases lumen dimensions by a combination of additional vessel expansion, axial plaque redistribution, and dissection.[4–10] As the vessel is dilated, the residual absolute plaque mass is distributed over a larger vessel circumference to reduce the measurable plaque burden (P&M devided by EEM). In unstable lesions, there is also plaque reduction that has been attributed to plaque or thrombus embolization.[11] Experience with distal protection devices supports the fact that plaque embolization is common in unstable lesion subsets. Dissections occur at the junction of plaque components with mismatched compliance – i.e. at the junction of hard and soft plaque or at the junction of plaque and adjacent normal vessel wall.[9,12] It is facilitated by focal calcific deposits.[12] Computer analysis of IVUS images allows investigation of the structural weakness of the plaque and prediction distensibility and post-balloon angioplasty dissections.[13,14] Non-lumen compromising dissections are not associated with adverse events.[15,16] Most heal at follow-up.[17]

In general, the compliance of a lesion decreases as the length and circumference of calcium increases. However, some calcified plaques dilate easily – presumably because the calcium is thin and uniformly distributed. Conversely, some soft-plaque lesions are very "rigid" because the adventitia is maximally remodeled and resistant to further expansion or, perhaps, because of fibrotic adventitial changes. Therefore, IVUS has a limited ability to predict the resistance of an individual lesion although, in general, the more calcium, the harder the lesion, and densely fibrotic lesions can be surprisingly hard to dilate. These issues also apply to stent implantation.

IVUS-guided balloon angioplasty

The exponential increase in stent use, paradoxically, improved the efficacy of stand-alone balloon angioplasty. Stents acted as a safety net to permit more aggressive balloon dilation.

The pilot phase of the Clinical Outcomes Ultrasound Trial (CLOUT) reported that IVUS reference segment midwall dimensions could be used to upsize angioplasty balloons without an increase in complications.[18] Balloon angioplasty was first performed using conventional angiographic sizing. The proximal and distal reference-segment midwall dimensions were then measured, and the smaller of the proximal and distal reference-segment midwall dimensions was used for IVUS-guided balloon sizing. Then angioplasty was repeated using IVUS balloon sizing.

Nominal balloon/artery ratios increased from 1.12 ± 0.15 to 1.30 ± 0.17 ($p < 0.0001$). Acute results were improved; however, this approach did not translate into improved long-term outcomes, perhaps because balloon sizing was only modestly aggressive, with only modest improvements in the final angiographic diameter stenosis ($28 \pm 15\%$ to $18 \pm 14\%$, $p < 0.0001$).[19]

Subsequent reports used even more aggressive balloon sizing strategies. In one study, the pre-intervention lesion-site EEM diameter (often loosely called the "media-to-media" diameter) was used to select the size of the angioplasty balloon (Figure 7.1).[20] Angioplasty balloons were inflated to ≥ 10 atm, and if a persistent waist was present, increased to a maximum of 18 atm. When the operator felt that the best angiographic result had been achieved, IVUS was repeated. Patients were crossed over to stent implantation if angiography showed less than TIMI-3 flow or an NHLBI grade C or greater dissection, or if post-balloon angioplasty IVUS did not show an optimal result (defined as a minimum lumen CSA $\geq 65\%$ of the average of the proximal and distal reference-lumen areas or a minimum lumen CSA ≥ 6.0 mm^2 and no major dissection). A major dissection was defined as a mobile flap, $> 90\%$ of the vessel circumference, or a suboptimal true lumen CSA (excluding the area subtended by the dissection plane).[15]

An example of an optimum balloon angioplasty result is shown in Figure 7.1; examples of inadequate angioplasty results and dissections using this strategy are shown in Figures 7.2 and 7.3. When necessary, stents – at that time either the Palmaz–Schatz or Gianturco–Roubin stents – were implanted followed by high-pressure adjunct inflations. The IVUS criteria for optimum stent implantation were a minimum stent CSA $> 80\%$ of the average reference-lumen CSA (or an absolute minimum stent CSA ≥ 7.5 mm^2) and complete stent-vessel wall apposition. Overall, 206 lesions in 134 patients were treated with balloon angioplasty, while 232 lesions in 150 patients were crossed over to stent implantation because of lumen-compromising dissections (27.9%) or a suboptimal IVUS minimum lumen CSA (72.1%). Of the lesions, 63 (27.2%) were treated with Gianturco–Roubin stents and 169 (72.8 %) with Palmaz–Schatz stents. The one-year target-lesion revascularization (TLR) rate was 8.2% for the balloon angioplasty group and 15.5% for the stent crossover group ($p = 0.016$). However, the TLR rate in the stent group was driven by Gianturco–Roubin-stented lesions (32.2%); The TLR rate was 10.4% in the Palmaz–Schatz group.

A similar study was performed at Tubingen, Germany.[21] The authors reported 252 patients who had 271 lesions treated with IVUS-guided balloon angioplasty. The balloon size was 80–100% of the mean of the proximal and distal reference and lesion EEM diameters. (It actually measured 0.88 ± 0.13 of the EEM diameter.) Dissections were detected by angiography in 157 patients (58%) and by IVUS in 189 patients (70%). The dissections were classified as type B or C in 78% and as type D

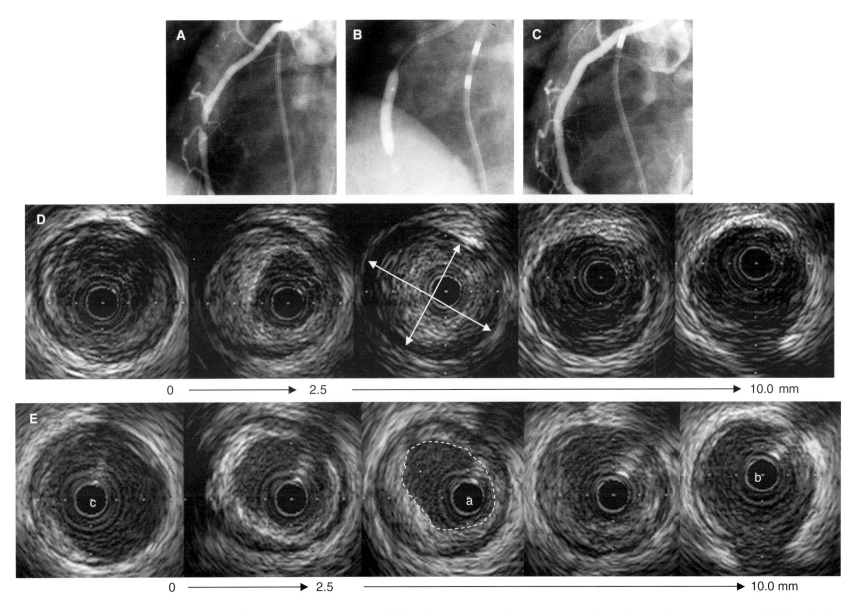

Figure 7.1 This mid right coronary stenosis (Panel A) was treated successfully with IVUS-guided aggressive balloon angioplasty. The pre-intervention lesion-site mean EEM (double-headed white arrows in Panel D) diameter averaged 4.5 mm; therefore, a 4.5 mm balloon was inflated to 12 atm (Panel B). The final result is shown in Panels C and E. The residual lumen CSA (a, dotted white line) measured 8.9 mm^2 – 70% of the mean reference-lumen CSA (b and c); and the residual plaque burden was 58%. The EEM volume increased from 245 mm^3 to 266 mm^3. The P&M volume decreased by 8% (from 147 mm^3 to 135 mm^3), while in the center of the lesion the P&M CSA decreased by 40%. From this, it is possible to infer an axial shift in the plaque from the center of the lesion to its edges. Note that, despite its angiographic appearance, this lesion was concentric, with a maximum/minimum P&M thickness of 1.8:1

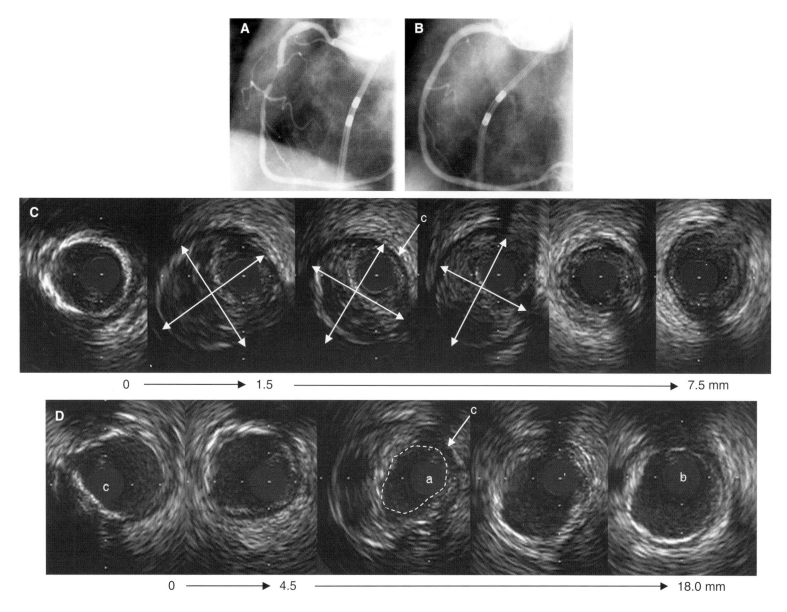

Figure 7.2 This mid right coronary stenosis (Panel A) was treated unsuccessfully with IVUS-guided aggressive balloon angioplasty. The pre-intervention lesion-site EEM diameter (double-headed white arrows in Panel C) averaged 4.5 mm; therefore, a 4.5 mm balloon was inflated to 14 atm. The final result is shown in Panels B and D. The residual lumen CSA (a, dashed white line) measured 4.9 mm^2 – 61% of the mean reference-lumen CSA (b and c), and the residual plaque burden was 76%. The coronary flow reserve was 1.3. A stent was successfully implanted. Note that, despite its angiographic appearance (compared with Figure 7.1), this lesion was highly eccentric, with a maximum/minimum P&M thickness of 5.2:1 and an arc of normal vessel wall (c) within the lesion

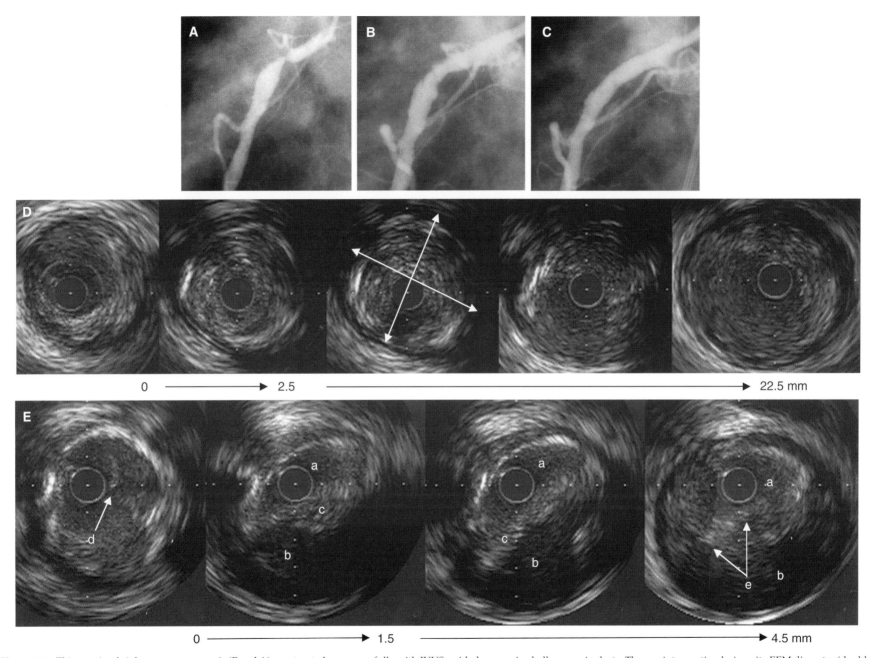

Figure 7.3 This proximal right coronary stenosis (Panel A) was treated unsuccessfully with IVUS-guided aggressive balloon angioplasty. The pre-intervention lesion-site EEM diameter (double-headed white arrows in Panel D) averaged 5.5 mm; therefore, a 5.0 mm balloon was inflated to 12 atm. The angiographic result is shown in Panel B. The post-angioplasty IVUS (Panel E) showed a large dissection. The true lumen (a) was separated from the false lumen (b) by a bulky dissection plane (c); at the proximal and distal ends of the dissection, the flap was thinner and more mobile (d and e, respectively). A stent was successfully implanted (Panel C). Note that this lesion was highly eccentric, with a maximum/minimum P&M thickness of 50:1

or E in 12%, but stent implantation was performed in only 2%. Angiographic restenosis occurred in 19% of the 71% of patients who had angiographic follow-up. The clinical event rate during long-term follow-up was 14%. In fact, in a subsequent publication, the authors reported that the most severe dissections were associated with the best long-term follow-up provided these dissections were not flow-limiting.[16] The UPSIZE Pilot Trial reported similar results.[22]

Most recently, the BEST (Balloon Equivalent to STent) randomized 250 patients to IVUS-guided provisional stenting versus conventional angiographic guidance of deliberate stent implantation.[23] The study was designed to show equivalence between these two strategies, as well as a reduction in the rate of in-stent restenosis in the IVUS-guided provisional stenting group. In the provisional stenting group, balloon angioplasty was first performed using the IVUS lesion-site "media-to-media" dimensions; cross-over to stenting was allowed, and was necessary in 44%. At follow-up, the angiographic restenosis rate was 16.8% in the IVUS-guided provisional stenting group versus 18.1% in the deliberate stenting group; the major adverse event rate was 16% versus 20%. However, even including the cross-overs, the in-stent restenosis rate was only 5% in the IVUS-guided provisional stenting group (versus 15.5% in the deliberate stent group), achieving the investigators' primary objective of limiting the occurrence of in-stent restenosis.

It is difficult to advocate an IVUS-guided provisional-stent strategy in the stent era and, particularly, in the drug-eluting stent era. However, this strategy does make the most use of IVUS information during balloon angioplasty procedures. The aggressiveness of the balloon sizing should depend on operator preference and willingness to deal with angioplasty-induced dissections. IVUS should be repeated post-balloon dilation to assess the result and the need for additional intervention. There has not been a specific study comparing IVUS versus angiography-guided balloon angioplasty; however, half of the patients in the randomized Strategy for Intracoronary Ultrasound-Guided PTCA and Stenting (SIPS) trial underwent balloon angioplasty as the operator-preferred interventional strategy. While the balloon angioplasty group was not analyzed separately, there was an overall reduction in two-year clinically driven TLR in the IVUS group (17% vs. 29%, $p = 0.02$).[24]

CUTTING-BALLOON ANGIOPLASTY

The cutting balloon has three or four microsurgical blades mounted longitudinally on its outer surface. When the balloon is inflated *in vitro*, the blades score into the plaque, after which the shear force of balloon dilation causes widening of these initial cuts to increase lumen dimensions.[25] However, the *in vitro* observations of precise radial cuts are rarely seen using IVUS. Instead, the appearance after imple-

menting the cutting balloon is reasonably similar to post-conventional balloon angioplasty (Figure 7.4).

In one planar IVUS analysis, images in 89 lesions after the use of a cutting balloon (at 8 atm) were compared with 91 lesions after conventional balloon dilation (at standard inflation pressures).[26] Although, overall, the change in EEM CSA did not differ between cutting-balloon versus conventional balloon angioplasty, the mean decrease in P&M CSA was greater ($p < 0.02$), and there was a trend towards a larger increase in lumen CSA ($p = 0.07$) in the cutting-balloon group. These findings were driven primarily by findings in non-calcified lesions, in which plaque reduction accounted for 74% and vessel stretch for 26% of total lumen gain – significantly different from the 56% plaque reduction and 44% vessel stretch in the balloon angioplasty group. In the subgroup of calcified lesions, lumen increase was greater with the cutting balloon, although (1) the changes in EEM and P&M CSA were similar to conventional balloon angioplasty, and (2) the relative contributions of plaque reduction and vessel stretch to lumen increase (62% and 38%, respectively) were also similar to balloon angioplasty. Lesions with cutting-balloon dissections achieved a larger lumen gain than those without dissections, while in the conventional balloon angioplasty group, lumen gain was similar in both those with and without dissections. In another study, plaque compression or plaque shift accounted for 55% and vessel expansion accounted for 45% of lumen enlargement after cutting-balloon angioplasty (compared with 33% and 67%, respectively, after conventional balloon angioplasty, $p < 0.05$).[27] These findings were supported by a separate volumetric IVUS analysis.[28] However, it is notable that none of these studies reported the ex vivo histologic findings of precise plaque scoring after cutting-balloon dilation.

In an IVUS study of cutting-balloon angioplasty followed by stent implantation and increasing inflation pressures, the minimum stent CSA was $7.6 \pm 2.0 \, \text{mm}^2$ at 8 atm, $8.1 \pm 1.5 \, \text{mm}^2$ at 10 atm, and $8.7 \pm 1.6 \, \text{mm}^2$ at 12 atm. The authors felt that these stent CSAs were significantly larger than what would have been achieved with conventional balloon predilation or direct stenting at the same inflation pressures.[29]

Overall, these reports, as well as numerous case examples, suggest that the cutting balloon does facilitate lesion dilation and stent expansion. There are no known IVUS endpoints of optimal cutting-balloon use and no known IVUS predictors of cutting-balloon restenosis.

ATHERECTOMY/THROMBECTOMY DEVICES

These devices were thought to be more efficacious in specific lesion subsets – for example, rotational atherectomy in calcified lesions and directional coronary

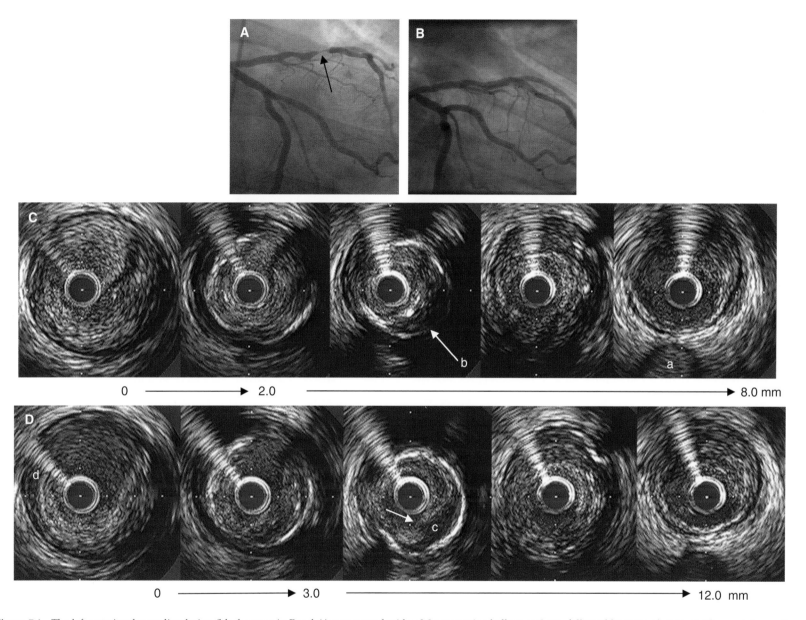

Figure 7.4 The left anterior descending lesion (black arrow in Panel A) was treated with a 3.0 mm cutting balloon at 8 atm followed by stent placement. The pre-intervention IVUS is shown in Panel C. Note the major diagonal (a) distal to the lesion and the deep calcium (b) at the site of the minimum lumen CSA. The post-cutting balloon IVUS is shown in Panel D. There are two dissection planes (c, at the site of the minimum lumen CSA, and d). Note the radial tear in the plaque (white arrow) that leads to the near circumferential dissection plane (c) where the "soft" plaque has separated from the deep calcium. The minimum lumen CSA measured only 2.5 mm². A stent was implanted, with the final angiographic result shown in Panel B

atherectomy in bulky, remodeled, eccentric plaques. IVUS guidance was advocated to match the device to the lesion, since IVUS assessment of calcification and eccentricity was more accurate than angiography.[30] In reality, long-term studies did not support a multi-device lesion-specific approach.

Directional coronary atherectomy (DCA)

Most IVUS studies indicated that tissue removal accounted for more than 75% of the improvement in lumen dimensions after stand-alone DCA.[31,32] Dissections, particularly superficial dissections, were common.[33] Unlike *ex vivo* studies, IVUS showed a consistent and measurable contribution of vessel expansion to lumen improvement – even without the use of adjunct balloon inflations. Adjunct balloon angioplasty or stenting reduced the contribution of tissue removal and increased the contribution of vessel expansion to overall lumen improvement.

The most important factors affecting delivery of the DCA device are vessel size, vessel tortuosity, and vessel compliance. The most consistent factor affecting vessel compliance is calcium. Calcium also affects the ability of DCA to cut and remove tissue. One study indicated that the IVUS arc of target-lesion calcium (even angiographically invisible calcium) is the single most powerful predictor of DCA efficacy regardless of the endpoint measured (Figure 7.5).[34] Superficial calcium limits DCA more than deep calcium; the area subtended by the arc of deep calcium can be used to estimate the post-DCA lumen (Figure 7.6). Interestingly, pre-treatment with rotational atherectomy can modify even a heavily calcified lesion to make it susceptible to tissue removal with the DCA device.[35] This suggests that the most superficial calcified elements are the hardest – a finding that can be supported by histopathology.[36] Plaque composition also affects the mechanism of lumen gain post-DCA; vessel expansion is greater in non-calcified plaques, while dissections are more common (and expansion and tissue removal reduced) in calcium-containing plaques.[37] Lesion characteristics that must be assessed when performing optimal DCA include eccentricity, maximum and minimum plaque thickness, and length. IVUS can also be used to exclude potentially unsafe situations such as when a guidewire has entered into a false lumen.

In order to perform IVUS-guided DCA, the first step is to correlate the IVUS and angiographic images, particularly the relationship of the maximum and minimum plaque thicknesses to major side branches. This requires selecting an angiographic working view in which the lesion and nearby branches are well seen. Side branches are then used to orient the DCA device towards the maximum plaque thickness and away from the minimum plaque thickness (or, more importantly, away from normal vessel wall in a highly eccentric lesion to avoid perforations). In the absence of IVUS imaging when performing DCA of a bifurcation or ostial stenosis, it should be assumed that the maximum plaque thickness is opposite each branch and that the carina is spared – in other words, using a "pair-of-pants" analogy, that the plaque involves the hips and avoids the inseam (Figure 7.7)

If there is no nearby identifiable side branch and if the lesion is eccentric (or if there is uncertainty about plaque distribution on the IVUS image), DCA troughs can be used to direct the device.[38] After pre-intervention IVUS, a single cut is made while carefully noting the fluoroscopic orientation of the device. Comparison of the IVUS images is then used to locate this single trough relative to the maximum and minimum plaque thicknesses and relative to the fluoroscopic appearance of the lesion. The rest of the DCA cuts can then be directed appropriately using this first cut as a reference.

The goal of optimal DCA is not just to maximize lumen dimensions, but also to minimize the residual plaque burden. The residual plaque burden (calculated as P&M divided by EEM CSA) usually occurs at the site of the smallest post-DCA lumen. Minimizing the plaque burden may require iterative IVUS imaging with repeat aggressive atherectomy aimed at the residual plaque – if necessary at higher pressures and/or using larger devices. The residual plaque burden is different from the residual area stenosis (calculated as final lumen CSA compared with the reference-lumen CSA and analogous to the angiographic diameter stenosis); a significant plaque burden can exist in the setting of a 0% or even a negative residual area stenosis (Figure 7.8).

As the residual post-DCA plaque burden decreases, so does the restenosis rate.[39,40] The plaque burden averaged 58% in the Optimal Atherectomy Restenosis Study (OARS, restenosis rate of 28.9%), but 46% in the Adjunct Balloon Angioplasty Coronary Atherectomy Study (ABACAS, restenosis rate of 23.6%).[41,42] (The plaque burden is a predictor of restenosis in non-stent interventions, perhaps by amplifying the constrictive forces that contribute to post-DCA restenosis.[39] More about this appears in Chapter 8.) While it is tempting to "eyeball" or estimate the residual plaque burden, experience has taught that the result always looks better to the naked eye than when it is measured (Figures 7.6 and 7.8). If IVUS guidance is used in an effort to achieve the lowest possible residual plaque burden, careful measurement and calculation are necessary. The goal of DCA should be a residual plaque burden of less than 50% and, ideally, close to 40%. However, from experience as well as from DCA studies, a final residual plaque burden of < 50% is rarely achieved in routine clinical settings.

Adjunct balloon angioplasty did not improve the results of DCA. The randomized ABACAS study showed that adjunct balloon angioplasty did not reduce the restenosis rate beyond what could be achieved with optimal DCA. IVUS analysis showed a lower residual plaque burden in the adjunct balloon angioplasty group compared with the stand-alone group (42.6% vs. 45.6%, $p < 0.001$), but similar restenosis rates (23.6% vs. 19.6%, $p = $ ns) and TLR rates (20.6% vs. 15.2%, $p = $ ns).[42]

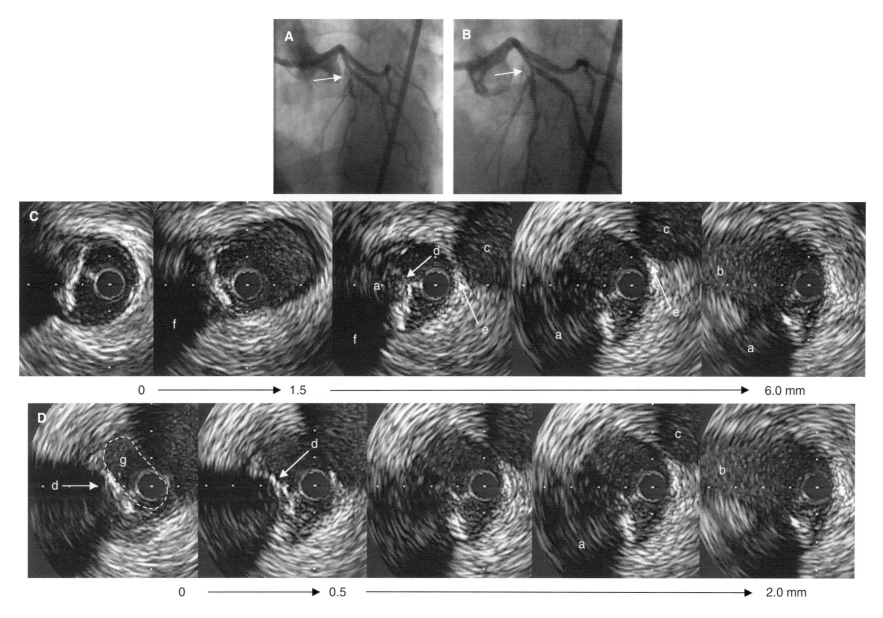

Figure 7.5 This eccentric bifurcation left anterior descending lesion (white arrow in Panel A) was first approached using directional coronary atherectomy. The pre-intervention IVUS (Panel C) showed that the plaque (a) was located adjacent to the major septal perforator (b) and opposite to the major diagonal branch (c). The lesion had the appearance of a filling defect; but the IVUS showed that at least part of its leading edge was calcified (d). Note that the carina (e) was spared; also note the shadowing (f). Post-atherectomy (Panels B and D), there was only minimal lumen improvement; the residual lumen (g, dashed line) measured only 3.6 mm². As this example illustrates, even a modest amount of superficial calcium (d) can limit the effectiveness of directional atherectomy if the calcium is strategically located. The lesion was then stented (the result is not shown)

187

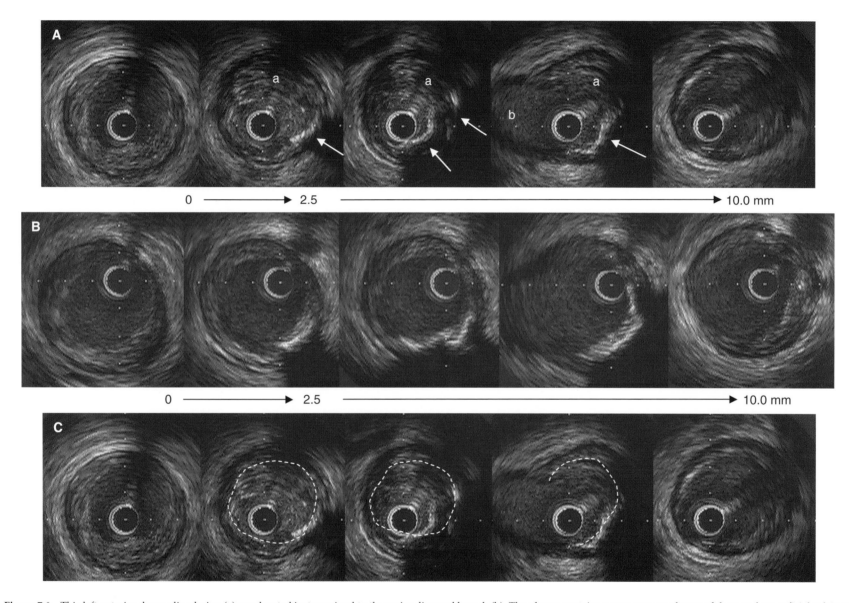

Figure 7.6 This left anterior descending lesion (a) was located just proximal to the major diagonal branch (b). The plaque contains one to two quadrants of deep and superficial calcium (white arrows). Panel B shows the post-directional coronary atherectomy IVUS. The residual lumen measured 7.5 mm², and the residual plaque burden measured 56%. Because directional coronary atherectomy does not cut calcium, the area subtended by the calcium in Panel A can be used to "predict" these final results. To illustrate this, in Panel C, the final lumen from Panel B was traced and superimposed on the pre-intervention IVUS from Panel A; note how this dashed white line closely follows the calcium deposits

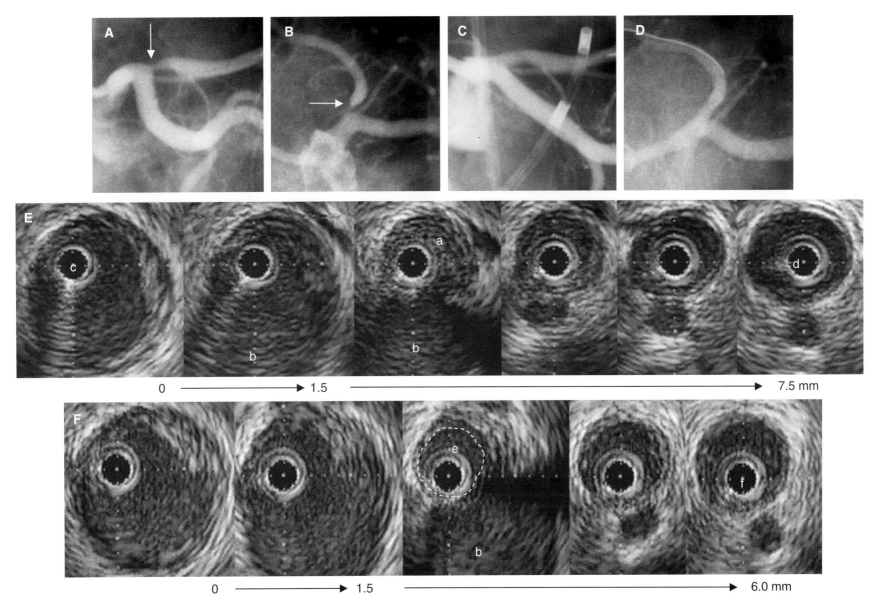

Figure 7.7 This ostial left anterior descending lesion (white arrows in Panels A and B) was treated successfully using directional coronary atherectomy. Despite the angiographic appearance suggesting circumferential plaque, the pre-intervention IVUS (Panel E) showed that the hypoechoic plaque (a) was opposite the left circumflex (b). Note the plaque burden in the left main (c) that measured 38%, but there was virtually no distal reference-segment disease (d). As with most ostial lesions, there was negative remodeling with a remodeling index (compared with the distal reference) of 0.78. The cutter was directed superiorly – away from the circumflex. Post-atherectomy (Panels C and D), there was marked angiographic improvement. The post-atherectomy IVUS (Panel F), showed a final lumen CSA of 6.6 mm^2 (d, dashed line) compared with the distal reference-lumen CSA of 9.5 mm^2, and the residual plaque burden measuring 42%. As shown in this example, when in doubt, assume that ostial or bifurcation plaque is opposite the main side branch. The post-intervention IVUS images have been rotated to correspond to the pre-intervention study

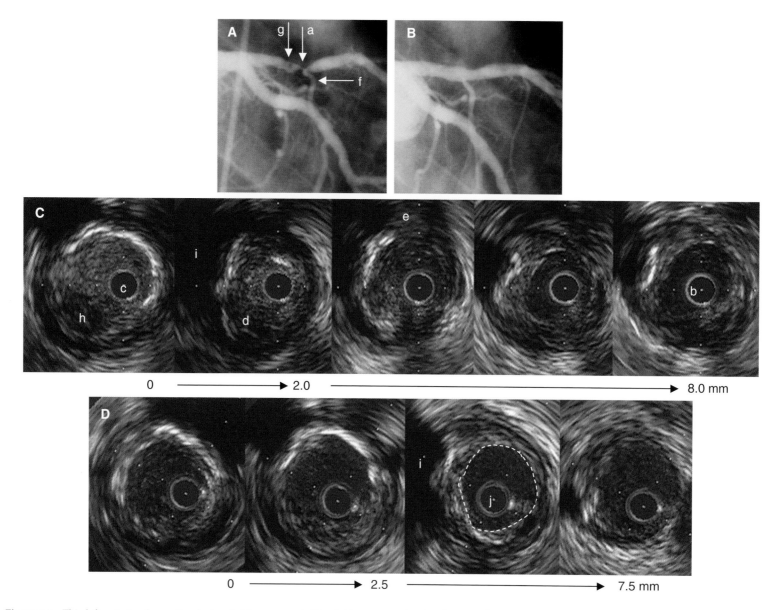

Figure 7.8   This left anterior descending lesion (white arrow a in Panel A) was treated using directional coronary atherectomy. Pre-intervention IVUS (Panel C) from distal (b) to proximal (c) showed the relationship between the plaque (d) and the septal perforator (e) that arose from the lesion and that can also be seen on the pre-intervention angiogram (f). Note the filling defect (g) proximal to the stenosis on the pre-intervention angiogram and the corresponding thrombus (h) on the pre-intervention IVUS study. Also note the deep calcium (i). There was significant angiographic improvement (Panel B). The post-atherectomy IVUS study showed a residual lumen of 6.5 mm² (j, dashed white line). Although the residual lumen was identical to the mean of the proximal and distal reference segments (creating a 0% residual-area stenosis), the residual plaque burden measured 67%. As shown in this example, lumen improvements cannot be used to predict the residual plaque burden. The post-intervention IVUS images have been rotated to correspond to the pre-intervention study

Adjunct bare-metal stent (BMS) implantation post-DCA has theoretical advantages. Stent implantation would counteract the constrictive component of post-DCA restenosis, although pre-stent DCA increases the frequency of late-stent malapposition.[43] In ADAPTS, the restenosis rate of DCA + BMS was 13.3%.[44] The AtheroLink registry reported a restenosis rate of 10.8%. In the SOLD registry, the restenosis rate of DCA + BMS was 13.6%.[45] This led to two randomized trials of DCA + stent versus stent alone: DESIRE (The DEbulking and Stenting In Restenosis Elimination) and AMIGO (Atherectomy before MULTI-LINK Improves lumen Gain and clinical Outcomes) trials. However, in both of these trials, pre-stent DCA did not improve on the results of bare-metal stenting alone, although neither trial achieved the desired objective of optimal atherectomy before stent implantation – a frequent finding in all IVUS-guided DCA studies.

IVUS-guided DCA was used to treat 67 patients with unprotected left main stenosis that involved the distal bifurcation.[46] The residual plaque burden in the left main was 45.6 ± 8.3%, and the residual plaque burden in the major daughter vessel was 46.0 ± 8.8%. Stent implantation, however, was necessary in 25.4%. The restenosis rate was 23.8%. Park *et al.*[47] reported 127 patients with left main disease treated by stenting with or without IVUS guidance, with and without pre-stent DCA. Of the lesions, 59 were located in the ostium, with 19 lesions in the body and 49 lesions in the distal bifurcation. IVUS was performed in 77 lesions. Pre-stent DCA was more frequently performed in the IVUS-guided group (p = 0.019); conversely, DCA was abandoned in four patients after IVUS showed > 90° of calcium. Pre-intervention IVUS of ostial lesions showed negative remodeling in over 50%. A comparison of serial IVUS images before and after DCA showed that the plaque burden decreased from 86% to 55%. Angiographic restenosis was documented in 19%; major adverse cardiac event-free survival was 86.9% at 1 year and 86.9% at 2 years. There was no significant difference in angiographic restenosis between the IVUS-guided versus angiography-guided groups. However, compared with the stenting-only group, the DCA/stenting group had a lower restenosis rate (8.3% vs. 25.0%, p = 0.034) and a lower target-lesion revascularization rate (5.4% vs. 18.8%, p = 0.049). Overall, the reference-artery size was the only independent predictor of angiographic restenosis, while in the IVUS group, the pre-intervention distal reference-lumen dimension was the only independent predictor of restenosis. This suggested to the authors that, in the bare-metal stent era, IVUS guidance and pre-stent DCA were important primarily in smaller left main arteries.

Attempts were made to integrate an IVUS transducer into a DCA device – using both mechanical and electronic-array technologies – with the goal of improving device efficacy and minimizing the residual plaque burden. However, these attempts did not go beyond prototype development.

Rotational atherectomy (RA)

Rotational atherectomy effectively ablates both calcified and non-calcified atherosclerotic plaque relative to the size of the burr tip with little vessel expansion (increase in EEM).[48,49] However, the plaque burden after stand-alone rotational atherectomy is large – much larger than after DCA. This is not surprising. Assuming a pre-intervention EEM diameter of 4.0 mm and a pre-intervention minimum lumen diameter of 0.5 mm, then the pre-intervention P&M CSA would measure approximately 12.0 mm². After the use of a 2.0–2.15 mm burr tip, the lumen CSA typically measures 3.5–4.0 mm²; this results in a residual P&M CSA of 9.0 mm² and a residual plaque burden of 75% or more. IVUS imaging of calcium after rotational atherectomy shows qualitative evidence of calcium removal, evidence of differential ablation, and numerous strong reverberations. Examples are shown in Figures 7.9 and 7.10. While the measured arc of calcium does decrease after rotational atherectomy, this decrease is modest.[48] Full-thickness calcium removal is necessary to decrease the IVUS arc of calcium; and in heavily calcified plaques, full-thickness calcium removal is unusual.

If pre-intervention IVUS is performed, the first burr should be larger than the minimum lumen diameter measured by IVUS. Adjunct balloon dilation or stenting post-rotational atherectomy increases the lumen almost exclusively by vessel expansion and plaque dissection/redistribution.[48] Like primary balloon angioplasty, dissections typically occur at the junction of calcified and non-calcified plaque.

Although rotational atherectomy does not significantly reduce the pre-intervention plaque mass, even modest rotablation renders a lesion more compliant, allowing balloon and/or stent expansion at lower pressures to larger dimensions than would be anticipated from pre-intervention lesion characteristics. For example, in one series, stent expansion was greater in the RA + stent group (91.9 ± 4.4%) compared with the stent-alone group (79.9 ± 3.4%, p < 0.03).[50] In two other series, rotational atherectomy reduced or nullified any impact of severe lesion calcification on stent expansion.[51–53] This has led to the concept that rotational atherectomy results primarily in plaque modification rather than plaque ablation – perhaps by removing the "tougher" superficial plaque elements.[35] In support of this, rotational atherectomy can render even a heavily calcified lesion susceptible to tissue removal with DCA – a device that cuts calcium poorly.[54] The concept of plaque modification is that treatment with an interventional device modifies the lesion so as to improve its compliance and allow dilation (or stent implantation) at lower pressures, resulting in larger lumens. This concept applies also to excimer laser or cutting-balloon angioplasty.

There are no known IVUS endpoints of optimal rotational atherectomy and no known IVUS predictors of rotational atherectomy restenosis. In one non-randomized comparison, stent implantation improved the long-term results of

rotational atherectomy.[55] In another non-randomized comparison, more aggressive rotational atherectomy use (defined as a final burr size ≥ 2.25 mm and/or final burr/vessel ratio ≥ 0.8) was also associated with reduced restenosis.[56]

Excimer laser coronary angioplasty (ELCA)

One IVUS study showed that lumen enlargement was a combination of tissue ablation, vessel expansion, and tissue disruption (Figures 7.11 and 7.12), and there was a large residual plaque burden similar to rotational atherectomy.[57,58] Although variable, the lumen CSA (and the EEM increase) were at times found to be larger than predicted by the size of the laser catheter. This unexpected degree of expansion was attributed to laser-induced shock waves and forced expansion of vapor bubbles into tissue.[59–61] The acoustic trauma from laser angioplasty could be reduced by saline infusion during laser activation and increased by the presence of blood or contrast in the lumen. There was no measurable decrease in calcium; however, superficial calcium developed a fragmented or shattered appearance with newly created sharp-edged gaps in the middle of a previously solid deposit (Figure 7.13) – an effect that was also attributable to acoustic trauma. Adjunct balloon dilation or stenting increased the lumen almost exclusively by vessel expansion and plaque dissection at the junction of calcified and non-calcified plaque. The concept of plaque modification can be applied to excimer laser angioplasty as well as to rotational atherectomy. For example, this device may have resurgent use to facilitate stent delivery when treating chronic total occlusions. There are no known IVUS endpoints of optimal excimer laser angioplasty and no known IVUS predictors of excimer laser angioplasty restenosis.

An attempt was made to integrate an IVUS transducer into a holmium (not excimer) laser catheter, but this attempt did not go beyond prototype development.

Other devices

Other atherothrombectomy devices – transluminal extraction catheter (TEC), x-sizer thromboatherectomy, SilverHawk, and rheolytic thrombectomy (AngioJet) – have been used or are being developed to treat native coronary arteries or saphenous vein grafts. There are few or no IVUS data on these devices, although attempts are being made to integrate an IVUS transducer into the SilverHawk device.

BARE-METAL STENT IMPLANTATION

Mechanisms

The mechanism of lumen enlargement during primary or adjunct stent implantation is similar to balloon angioplasty: a combination of vessel expansion and plaque redistribution/embolization.[2,62,63] Plaque reduction is particularly notable in unstable lesions and has been attributed to plaque or thrombus embolization.[63,64] In one study, the contribution of P&M decrease to lumen increase was 47% in unstable angina compared with only 13% in stable angina.[63] Intrusion or prolapse of plaque through the stent mesh into the lumen – which may then result in plaque embolization – is also more common in acute coronary syndrome and saphenous vein-graft lesions either because of the presence of thrombus or because of the composition of the plaque elements. Findings that are typically associated with acute coronary syndromes such as positive remodeling, thrombus, hypoechoic plaque or lipid-pool-like images, a large plaque burden, and a large lesion-site EEM CSA are associated with CK-MB release and reduced flow during stenting of acute coronary syndrome lesions, in general, and myocardial infarction lesions, in particular (Figure 7.14).[63,65–69] These findings are supported by evidence of embolization obtained using distal protection devices.

Axial plaque redistribution with extrusion of the plaque out of the ends of a stent is the other cause of plaque decrease, particularly if the analysis is limited to the axial length of the stent; it can cause haziness or the appearance of a new lesion at the stent edge.[62,70] One of the limitations of assessing plaque redistribution or embolization is the difficulty of measuring the EEM CSA reproducibly because of the intervening stent metal. Volumetric IVUS analysis is essential.

Practical recommendations

In day-to-day terms, how should IVUS be used during stenting procedures? The following is one suggested algorithm. It begins with pre-intervention IVUS and concludes with iterative IVUS to optimize the final result.

- Perform pre-intervention IVUS to assess stenosis severity, measure reference-vessel size, and measure lesion length.
- Select stent size using maximum reference-lumen diameter, whether proximal or distal to the lesion.
- Select stent length based on the distance between proximal and distal references.
- Determine the optimum stent CSA assuming a 0% residual stenosis.
- Implant a stent according to conventional techniques.

- Repeat IVUS to assess minimum stent CSA. If minimum stent CSA is adequate, stop. If minimum stent CSA is inadequate, perform additional higher-pressure inflations, if necessary using a larger balloon. If there is malapposition, select a balloon sized to the distance between the non-apposed intima and inflate at low pressures. Check to make sure that there are no complications.

As you can see, these steps are, conceptually, little different from angiography-guided stent implantation.

The final stent CSA can be optimized by appropriate stent sizing using pre-intervention IVUS followed by adjunct high-pressure balloon inflations guided by iterative IVUS. Several proposed paradigms exist for stent sizing based on pre-intervention IVUS and appropriate proximal and distal reference-site selection. The simplest is to select the diameter of the stent based on the largest reference-lumen diameter, whether proximal or distal to the lesion. Other authorities advocate reference mid-wall sizing or discounted "media-to-media" sizing. The reference-lumen dimensions will also indicate the size of the balloon that can extend out of the end of the stent without increasing vessel trauma – when performing post-dilations, when tacking up an edge dissection, or when attempting to improve apposition.

The stent length should be based on the distance between the proximal and distal reference sites, although this may be adjusted according to the goals of the intervention – i.e. to deliberately avoid or cover a side branch or to place one end of the stent at a specific point with less concern for the other end.

Combination devices – in which a stent is mounted on a combined balloon dilation/imaging catheter – facilitate post-stent implantation imaging and adjunct balloon inflations, although pre-intervention is not available for stent sizing because the device must be selected prior to IVUS imaging.[24]

Ideally, IVUS guidance should result in a 0% final stenosis; but this is often not achievable. Regardless of stent design, only 1–2 atm are necessary to fully expand stents in air. Inflating a stent according to the package label does not reliably result in the final stent diameter indicated; these measurements were not made *in vivo*. The limitations to stent expansion *in vivo* are plaque composition and plaque burden, not the actual design. Therefore, high-pressure inflations are necessary with all stents. Different operators have different strategies when faced with stent underexpansion. Some increase pressure first while others opt for a larger balloon size; both increase balloon wall tension (Laplace's Law). However, it seems rational to maximize the effect of the first balloon by inflating to higher pressures before upsizing. While it is possible to oversize the stent, it is not possible to achieve a final stent CSA of 9.0 mm^2 in a 2.0 mm vessel. Gross oversizing or overexpansion is associated with increased acute complications such as perforation and rupture. However, there is no evidence that a negative residual stenosis (a stent CSA larger than the reference) increases restenosis.

Angiography does not provide adequate detail for fine-tuning stent dimensions. As seen in the OSTI-I trial, as inflation pressures were raised, IVUS demonstrated increased stent expansion that was not apparent by angiography.[71] A similar study is shown in Figure 7.15. Given the fact that relatively small increases in minimum stent CSA can be associated with significant decreases in restenosis, it is important to actually measure the stent area, not just "eyeball" the result. While increasing stent expansion is associated with more post-procedure CK-MB release, the TLR rates at one year – particularly in stents that are overdilated (minimum stent CSA greater than the reference-lumen CSA) – are reduced, as are overall major cardiac events including mortality.[72]

Importance of the final stent CSA

Statistically, the stent CSA is a stronger predictor of bare-metal stent restenosis compared with stent expansion. Stent expansion is defined as the stent CSA compared with a measure of vessel size (i.e. mean reference-lumen CSA or lesion or reference-EEM CSA).[73,74] However, the stent CSA associated with a 0% residual stenosis is dictated primarily by the size of the vessel (Page 179). The ability to expand a stent to the size that the vessel will accommodate is limited by plaque composition and plaque burden, as is shown in numerous examples in this chapter. As the stent expands, the EEM increases, and the plaque is redistributed axially, prolapses through the stent mesh, or is distributed over the larger EEM circumference. While in some lesions, plaque mass may decrease, there is still a significant residual plaque burden that almost always measures 50–75% at the center of the lesion. Therefore, the stent always looks smaller than the EEM. This does not mean that the stent is underexpanded.

In the CRUISE trial, the 9-month TLR rate was 27% for a final stent CSA $4.0–5.9 \text{ mm}^2$, 19% for a final stent CSA $6.0–6.9 \text{ mm}^2$, 12% for a final stent CSA $7.0–8.9 \text{ mm}^2$, and 4% for a final stent CSA $> 9.0 \text{ mm}^2$. A secondary analysis from the CRUISE trial indicated that the cut-off that separated TLR from non-TLR was a final stent CSA of 6.5 mm^2.[73] An identical cut-off (6.5 mm^2) was found in the overall group of 50 bare-metal stents from the SIRIUS trial.[75] However, these trials excluded many high-restenosis-risk situations. Even so, this single number predicted only 50–60% of bare-metal stent restenosis, indicating that lesion and patient-related variables were responsible for the remaining 40–50%. A minimum stent CSA of 6.5 mm^2 may not be achievable in small arteries, may short-change the anti-restenosis benefit of achieving a larger final stent CSA when possible, and may be inadequate in high-risk subsets where a larger minimum stent CSA may be necessary to accommodate a more aggressive neointimal response. Thus, merely targeting a final stent CSA of 6.5 mm^2 may be too simplistic.

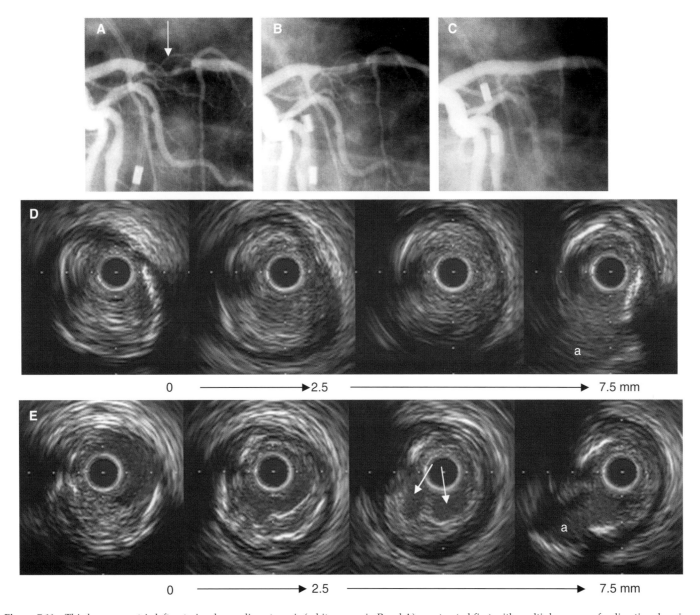

Figure 7.11   This long, eccentric left anterior descending stenosis (white arrow in Panel A) was treated first with multiple passes of a directional excimer laser angioplasty catheter (Panel B) and then with stent implantation (Panel C). A 7.5 mm-long segment of the lesion proximal to the diagonal branch (a) is shown in the pre-intervention and post-laser IVUS studies (Panels C and D). Note the post-intervention troughs (white arrows in Panel E) indicating tissue ablation

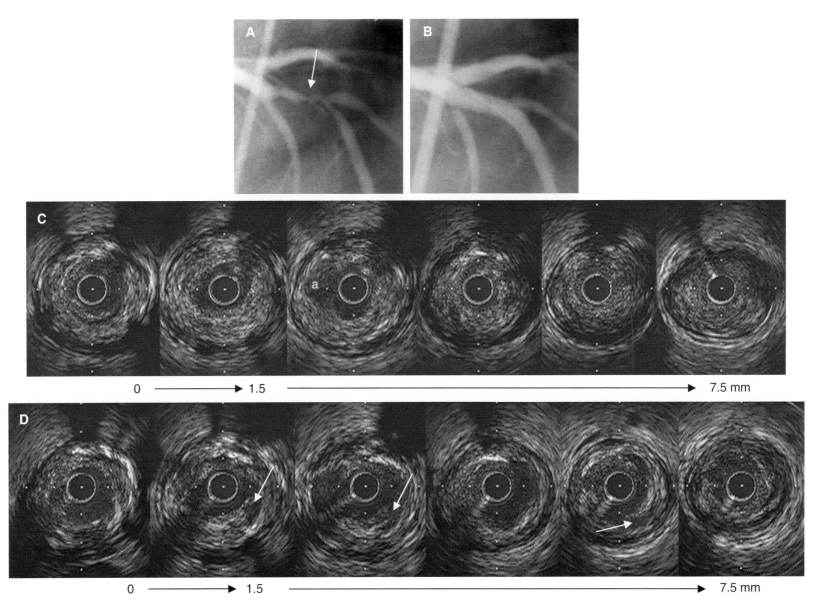

Figure 7.12 This acute coronary syndrome-related left anterior descending stenosis (white arrow in Panel A) was treated first with excimer laser angioplasty and then with stent implantation (Panel B). Note the ruptured plaque cavity (a) on the pre-intervention IVUS study (Panel C) and the superficial tissue disruption (white arrows) on the post-laser IVUS study (Panel D)

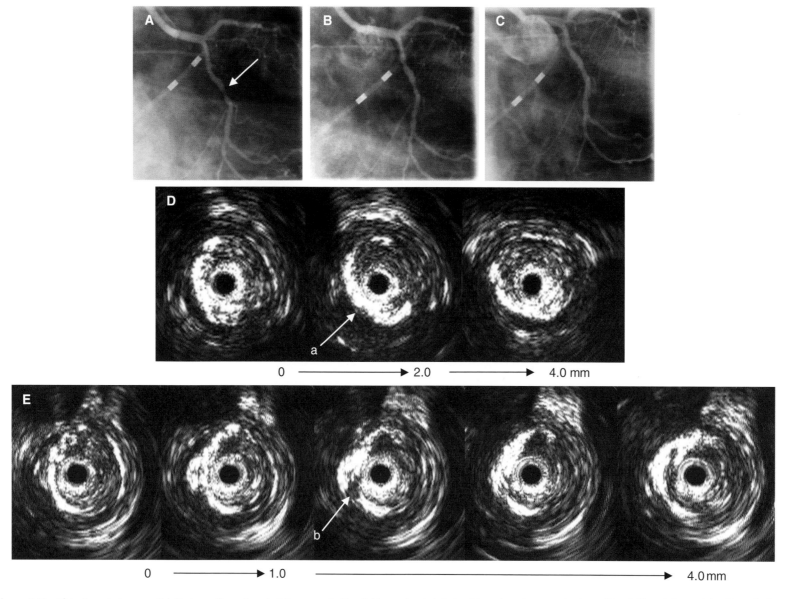

Figure 7.13 This stenosis in a small left circumflex artery (white arrow in Panel A) was treated first with excimer laser angioplasty (Panel B) and then with adjunct balloon inflations (Panel C). The IVUS studies were recorded in 1992 using an InterTherapy instrument that produced a characteristic bistable image (more black and white or contrasty than multiple shades of gray). The pre-intervention study (Panel D) showed a single, two-quadrant, superficial calcific deposit (a) that, on the post-intervention study (Panel E), was broken into two pieces by the excimer laser (b). This fracturing of the calcium was attributed to the intense photoacoustic trauma of excimer laser technology that is exaggerated by blood or contrast in the lumen and reduced by saline in the lumen

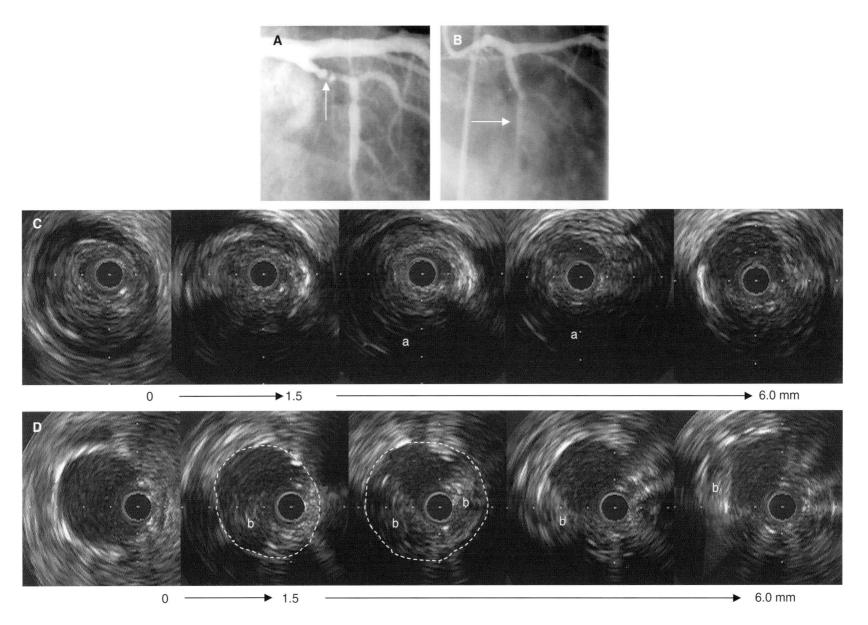

Figure 7.14 This patient presented with an acute coronary syndrome and underwent stent implantation for this culprit lesion in the left circumflex artery (white arrow in Panel A). Post-intervention, there was TIMI grade 1 flow (white arrow in Panel B). The pre-intervention IVUS (Panel C) did not show typical IVUS features of thrombus, but there was a large amount of hypoechoic attenuated plaque (a) that is sometimes seen in unstable lesions and that has been considered to represent a large thrombus burden. The post-stent implantation IVUS (Panel D) showed significant plaque intrusion (b) into the stent (dashed white line)

Between June 1996 and September 1997, 2242 consecutive patients with 2853 unselected native coronary-artery lesions were treated with either tubular-slotted or multicellular bare-metal stents at the Washington Hospital Center. Follow-up was available in 94.7% (2701 lesions in 2123 patients). The overall incidence of major out-of-hospital events (death, non-fatal myocardial infarction, TLR) was 13.7%. The overall one-year TLR rate was 11.0%. Decreasing IVUS final lumen CSA (odds ratio = 0.74; p = 0.0001), ostial-lesion location (odds ratio = 2.8; p = 0.05), and a history of diabetes mellitus (odds ratio = 1.9; p = 0.01) were found to predict late adverse cardiac events. Of note, the difference in TLR comparing non-ostial lesions in diabetics versus non-diabetics was significantly different only for lesions with a final lumen CSA $< 7.5\,mm^2$ (p = 0.0009), not for lesions with a final lumen CSA $\geq 7.5\,mm^2$ (p = 0.4). However, as demonstrated in this and other studies, the final lumen CSA is consistently smaller in diabetics, suggesting that both stent under-expansion and increased intimal hyperplasia contribute to the increased rate of TLR in these patients.[76,77] These data are shown in Figure 7.16.

While the stent CSA is the strongest predictor of clinical restenosis in native arteries, there is no similar consistent evidence that this is true for saphenous vein-graft lesions.[78,79] The possible explanations are that the final stent CSA is almost always large in vein-graft stents and that vein-graft events are usually driven as much by disease progression in the non-stented graft as by in-stent restenosis.

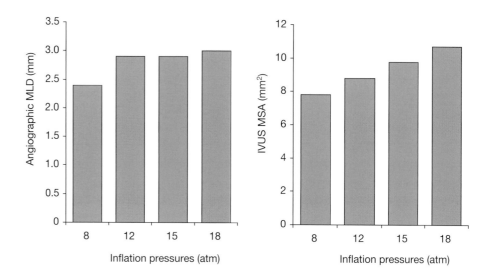

Figure 7.15 Twenty-six lesions with a mean angiographic reference diameter of 3.0 ± 0.5 mm underwent stent implantation using an AVE stent. Quantitative angiography and IVUS were performed after 8, 12, 15, and 18 atm inflation pressures. There was an increase in angiographic minimum lumen diameter (MLD) from 8 atm to 12 atm, but not thereafter. Conversely, there was a stepwise increase in IVUS minimum stent area (MSA) throughout the study. This suggests that angiography is of limited use when fine-tuning stent dimensions

Importance of stent length

Multiple or long coronary stents are frequently implanted in long or tandem lesions. This has been associated with an increased rate of restenosis and, in particular, an increased rate of the difficult-to-treat diffuse type of in-stent restenosis. An alternative strategy to treat long or tandem lesions is spot stenting, in which aggressive balloon angioplasty is followed by IVUS to identify the areas that need to be treated with short stents in order to avoid stenting the entire length of the lesion. In one study by Colombo *et al.*,[80] stents were implanted only if the minimum lumen CSA was less than $5.5\,mm^2$ or the minimum lumen CSA was less than 50% of the lesion EEM CSA. De Feyter *et al.*[81] combined the data from the MUSIC, WEST-II, ERASER, ESSEX, and TRAPIST studies, which included Palmaz–Schatz, Radius, MultiLink, and Wallstents, and calculated restenosis rates over a wide range of stent lengths and areas. They reported that for the same final stent CSA, a longer bare-metal stent was more likely to restenose than a shorter stent. This was particularly true in smaller vessels, while the impact of multiple stents in large vessels was more modest (Figure 7.17). In contrast, in the

analysis from the Washington Hospital Center, stent length and number of stents were not predictive of TLR. TLR was 10.3% for 1 stent, 11.9% for 2 stents, 11.1% for 3 stents, and 10.4% for ≥ 4 stents. One possibility is that more stents and longer stents predispose to focal stent under-expansion somewhere within the longer length of metal. In support of this, the TULIP trial – which specifically addressed longer lesions (> 20 mm) – showed that IVUS guidance can mitigate against this interaction by optimizing the final stent area; in the IVUS-guided group, restenosis was reduced despite the use of more stents and more metal.[82]

Endpoints

The ideal stent implantation results in full and symmetrical expansion, complete stent-vessel wall apposition, no plaque prolapse, and no edge dissections. However, other than the final stent CSA, none of these other "criteria" predict in-stent restenosis.

Apposition is different from expansion; the two terms should not be used interchangeably. Expansion refers to the CSA of the stent relative to a pre-defined

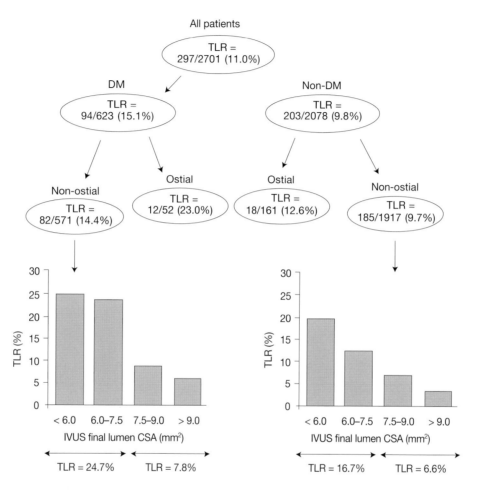

Figure 7.16 In this study of 2701 consecutive lesions (unselected patients) treated with tubular-slotted bare-metal stent implantation with IVUS imaging, the three predictors of target-lesion revascularization (TLR) at 1 year were IVUS final lumen cross-sectional area (CSA), diabetes mellitus (DM), and ostial lesion location. Additional demographics were 41% acute coronary syndrome, 36% left anterior descending, 40% >10 mm long and 12% > 20 mm long, mean reference 3.1 ± 0.5 mm, and multiple stents in 62%. The overall final lumen CSA measured 7.5 ± 2.5 mm^2. The final lumen CSA was larger in ostial lesions compared with non-ostial lesions, but the TLR rate was higher, implying that ostial lesions were associated with more intimal hyperplasia. The final lumen CSA was smaller in diabetics than in non-diabetics; however, in diabetics who achieved a minimum lumen CSA > 7.5 mm^2, the TLR rate was similar to that in non-diabetics with similar final lumen dimensions. Conversely, final lumen CSA < 7.5 mm^2 in diabetics was associated with a significantly higher TLR rate compared with non-diabetics

Figure 7.17 (opposite) de Feyter *et al.*[81] combined the results of five trials to construct four predictive models of restenosis based on the IVUS data: (1) minimum stent CSA, (2) stent volume and stent length, (3) mean stent CSA and stent length, and (4) minimum stent CSA and stent length. (The addition of a third parameter did not improve the predictive model.) They chose the combination of stent length and minimum stent CSA as the most easily obtainable and clinically relevant parameters. Next, the ranges of the two variables were divided into ten groups, and the expected restenosis rate for the median of each range was calculated. The majority of observations were clustered around 15 mm-long stents and a minimum stent CSA of 8 mm^2. In the original manuscript, where there were no actual observations, restenosis rates were interpolated. This figure was adapted from their data; where there was no actual data, the predicted restenosis rates have been deleted

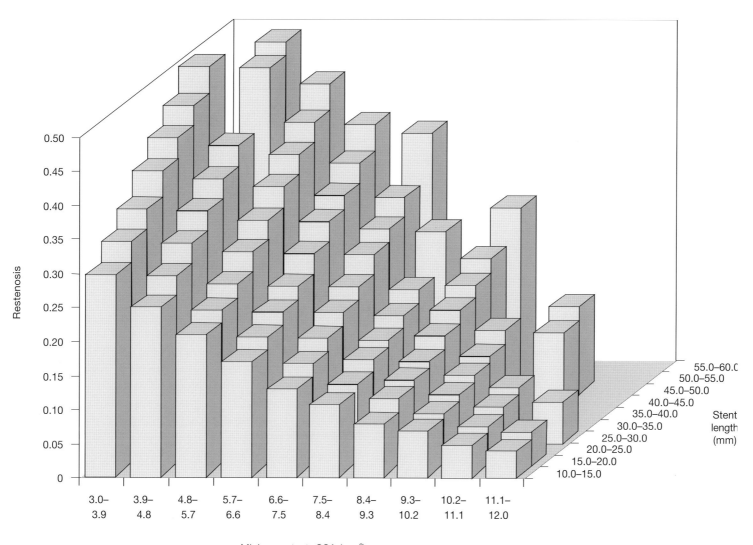

standard such as the reference-lumen CSA. A technical illustration of stent expansion is shown in Figures 7.18 and 7.19. Apposition refers to the contact between the stent and vessel wall. Achieving full apposition is often easier than full expansion. A balloon sized to the intimal diameter is inflated at low pressure. Because there is no plaque limiting full stent apposition (there is only blood flow between the malapposed stent strut and vessel wall), only low pressures are necessary to reduce malapposition (Figure 7.20). Incomplete acute apposition is probably more of a concern in smaller stent CSAs than in larger, more fully expanded stents. Complete apposition may not be possible in large aneurysms or ecstatic segments. Lack of expansion and apposition can occur together or separately, but they have different implications and technical solutions.

Any stent can be associated with tissue prolapse in the right lesion substrate. Tissue prolapse is more common in acute coronary syndromes, degenerated vein grafts, and thrombus-containing lesions. [83,84] Examples are shown in Figures 7.21 and 7.22. Additional balloon inflations, particularly with larger balloons, may not improve and may even worsen tissue prolapse by embedding the stent more deeply into the soft, friable plaque (Figure 7.21). Additional balloon inflations may also promote embolization. The only approach that reduces tissue prolapse is implantation of an additional stent (Figure 7.22). Minor plaque prolapse does not appear to impact on the long-term results of stent implantation.[83] Because tissue prolapse is more common in degenerated saphenous vein grafts, and owing to the limited predictive value of the final stent CSA in vein-graft lesions, high pressures are not routinely recommended when stenting these lesions. The routine use of distal protection devices – which are arguably the standard of care when treating vein-graft lesions [85,86] – can make concomitant IVUS imaging more difficult.

Stent asymmetry, in which the maximum stent diameter is substantially larger than the minimum stent diameter, was one of the original criteria of suboptimum stent implantation.[87] Stent asymmetry is the result of eccentric variations in plaque compliance or an arc of normal vessel wall opposite resistant plaque (Figures 7.23 and 7.24). It is difficult to correct stent asymmetry because additional balloon inflations (or even additional stents) may not improve and may even worsen asymmetry; the compliant parts of the plaque or the arcs or normal vessel wall dilate further, while the non-compliant parts of the plaque continue to resist expansion.

Stent edge dissections are common since the junction between stent metal and reference-segment tissue is a site of compliance mismatch – the typical cause of any dissection. Edge dissections may be more common when the stent ends in a reference segment that contains (1) both plaque and normal vessel wall or (2) distinctly separate hard and soft plaque elements. Minor edge dissections do not

appear to impact on the long-term results of stent implantation.[88] In fact, 75% heal when imaged at follow-up, a frequency similar to balloon angioplasty.[89] Examples are shown in Figures 7.25–7.27,

Does IVUS improve patient outcomes after bare-metal stenting?

Numerous studies have shown that IVUS-guided stent implantation is superior to non-IVUS-guided stenting, and some studies have shown that IVUS use is either cost-neutral or only slightly more expensive. CRUISE was a substudy of STARS in which clinical sites elected to perform IVUS-guided stenting, angiography-guided stenting with documentary IVUS, or no IVUS. The 9-month target-vessel revascularization rate in the IVUS-guided group was 8.5% versus 15.3% in the documentary IVUS group, $p = 0.019$.[90] AVID was a study that randomized patients to IVUS versus angiograph-guided stenting. The IVUS-guided group had a lower clinical restenosis rate: 8.4% versus 12.4% ($p = 0.08$) overall, 4.9% versus 10.8% ($p = 0.02$) in vessels > 2.5 mm, and 5.1% versus 20.8% ($p = 0.03$) in SVGs.[91] TULIP was a randomized comparison of long lesions (≥ 20 mm in a native coronary artery that permitted implantation of ≥ 3 mm stents). Despite more stents and longer stent length (42 ± 11 mm vs. 35 ± 11 mm, $p = 0.001$), the IVUS-guided group had lower angiographic restenosis (23% vs. 45%, $p = 0.008$), TLR (10% vs. 23%, $p = 0.018$), and MACE (major adverse cardiac event) rates (12% vs. 27%, $p = 0.026$).[82]

An earlier study (SIPS) randomized patients to angiographic versus IVUS guidance in which balloon angioplasty or stenting was performed according to operator preference. Half of the patients in each group were treated with stenting. The 2-year clinically driven TLR rate was 17% versus 29% ($p = 0.02$) with a 61% probability that IVUS guidance was both less expensive and more effective.[24,92] In a non-randomized comparison, Choi *et al.*[93] showed that IVUS reduced both in-hospital acute closure ($p = 0.04$) and 6-month TLR ($p = 0.08$) and that the increased costs of IVUS guidance were entirely related to the cost of the IVUS catheter.

CENIC, the Brazilian Society of Interventional Cardiology Registry, reported the acute results of 3375 patients treated with IVUS-guided stenting and 51 151 patients treated with angiography-guided stenting. The IVUS-guided group had lower rates of cardiac death (0.4% vs. 1.1%, $p < 0.001$), Q-wave myocardial infarction (0.06% vs. 0.09%, $p = 0.054$), and the composite of death/Q-wave myocardial infarction (0.08% vs. 1.7%, $p < 0.001$).[94] Gaster *et al.*[95] randomized stent implantation patients to angiography versus IVUS and found a lower frequency of a number of endpoints (including clinical restenosis and recurrent angina) with no increase in short-term costs. A subsequent report showed that accumulated costs at long-term follow-up

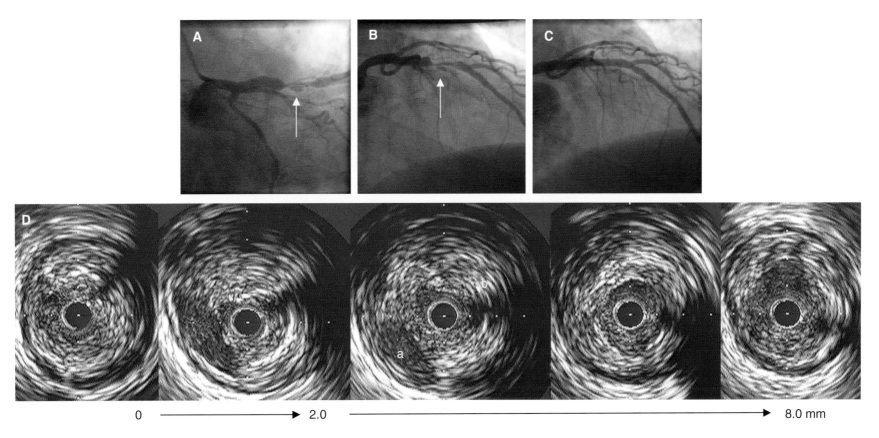

Figure 7.18   This long, complex left anterior descending lesion (white arrows in Panels A and B) in a patient with an acute coronary syndrome was treated with bare-metal stent implantation. The final angiographic result is shown in Panel C. The pre-intervention IVUS (Panel D) showed a ruptured plaque cavity (a) and a large plaque burden with a lesion EEM CSA measuring 37.3 mm^2 and a remodeling index of 1.67. The post-intervention IVUS studies are shown in Figure 7.19

Figure 7.19 (opposite)   Sometimes stents are difficult to expand. These three panels illustrate the initial stent implantation and two successive adjunct balloon inflations during the treatment of the lesion in Figure 7.18. Post-stent implantation (3.5 mm at 16 atm, Panel A), the minimum stent CSA measured 5.6 mm^2 (dashed black line). Note the small amount of tissue prolapse (a) and the proximal incomplete apposition (b). After adjunct balloon inflation (4.0 mm at 10 atm, Panel B), the stent area increased except at the site of the minimum stent CSA (dashed black line) and largest plaque burden; the stent CSA measured only 6.2 mm^2. Note that there is still some tissue prolapse (c) and that there is persistent proximal incomplete apposition. After a second adjunct balloon inflation (4.0 mm at 16 atm, Panel C), the minimum stent CSA increased to 8.2 mm^2 dashed black line). As this example illustrates, it is not always possible to predict stent expansion from gray-scale plaque characteristics, particulary in lesions with a large plaque burden

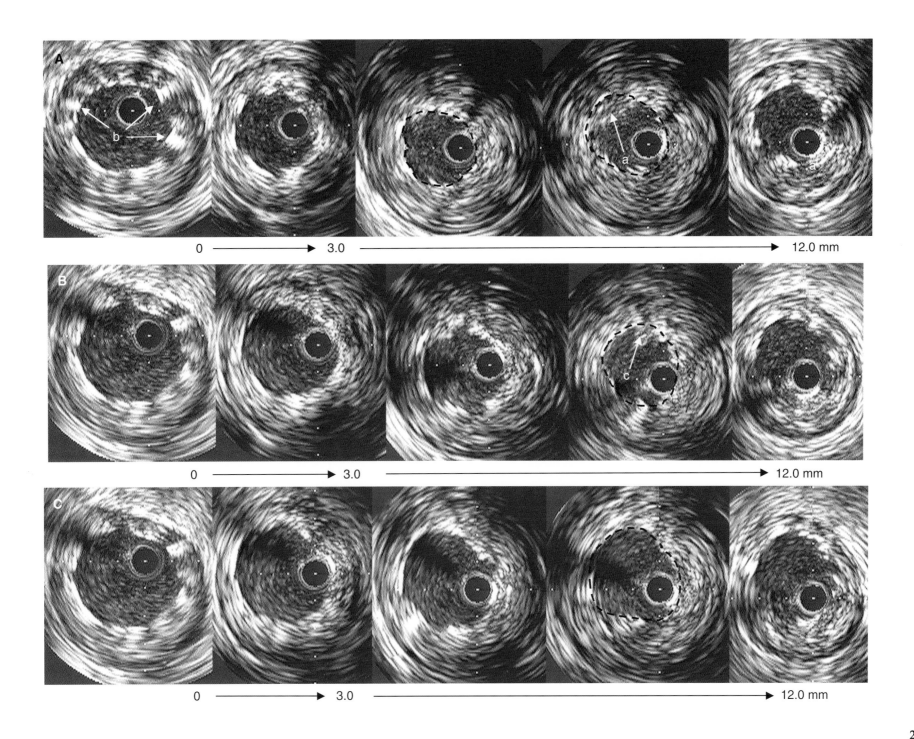

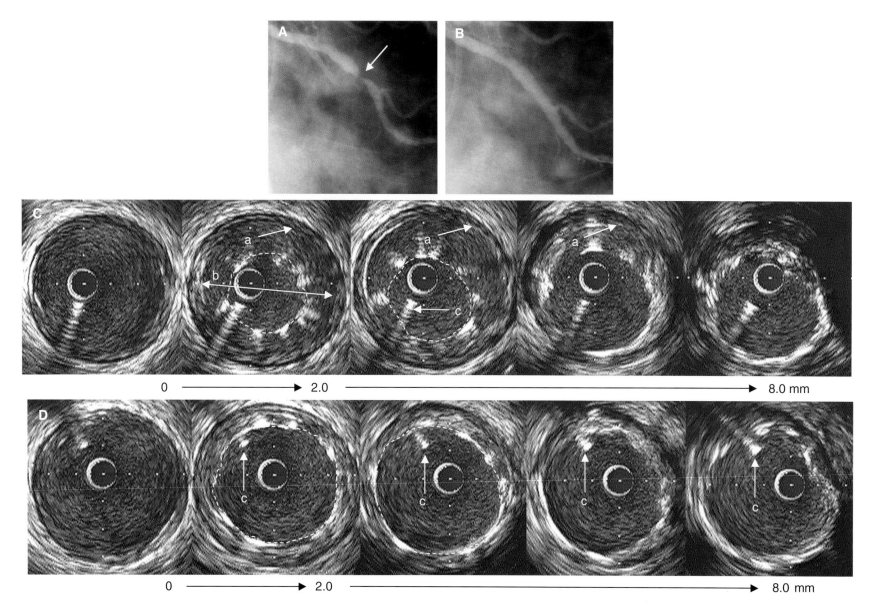

Figure 7.20 Stent malapposition is relatively easy to correct. This left circumflex marginal lesion (white arrow in Panel A) was treated with stent implantation (Panel B). The post-intervention IVUS (Panel C) showed a 6 mm-long segment of proximal stent edge malapposition. Note the space and blood speckle between the stent metal (dashed white line) and the intima of the circumflex (a). The inter-intima distance measured 5.0 mm (double-headed white arrow, b). The stent was post-dilated with a 5.0 mm balloon at low pressures (4 atm). The final IVUS (Panel D) showed marked improvement in the malapposition; the stent (dashed white line) is apposed to the intima throughout most of its circumference (white arrows). The guidewire (c) should not be confused with a malapposed stent strut

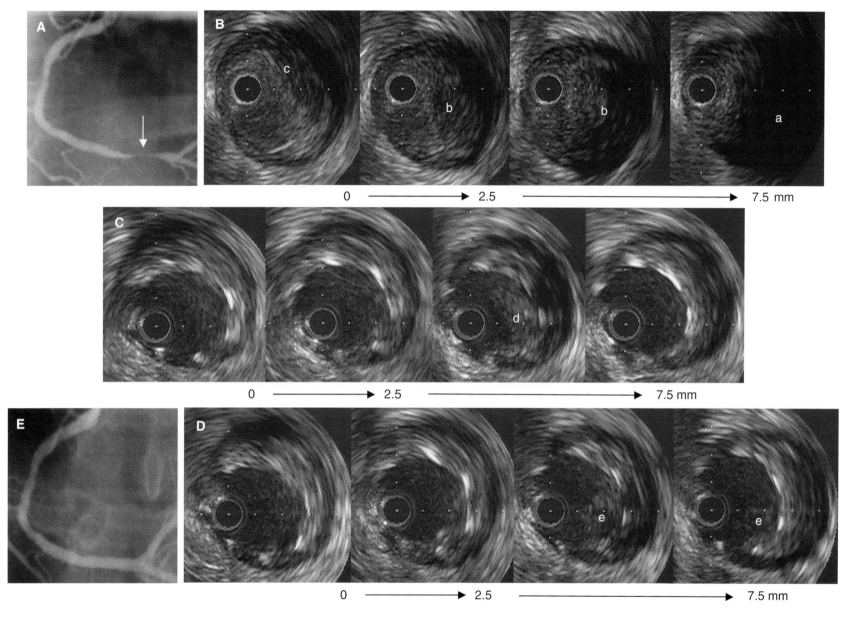

Figure 7.21 This patient presented with an acute coronary syndrome and this culprit lesion in the distal right coronary artery (white arrow in Panel A). The pre-intervention IVUS (Panel B) showed eccentric, hypoechoic, attenuated plaque (a), the suggestion of a thrombus (b), and hypoechoic non-attenuated plaque (c). (As noted elsewhere in this chapter, hypoechoic, attenuated plaque has been considered to represent a large thrombus burden.) After implantation of a 3.5 mm stent at 14 atm (Panel C), there was significant plaque intrusion (d) within the stent. Prolonged adjunct balloon inflation with the same sized balloon at 8 atm did not improve the plaque prolapse and may have made it worse (e in Panel D). The final angiogram is shown in Panel E. After stent implantation, the minimum stent CSA measured 8.8 mm^2, but there was 3.8 mm^2 of plaque prolapse, giving an effective minimum lumen CSA of 5.0 mm^2. These measurements remained essentially unchanged after adjunct balloon inflations

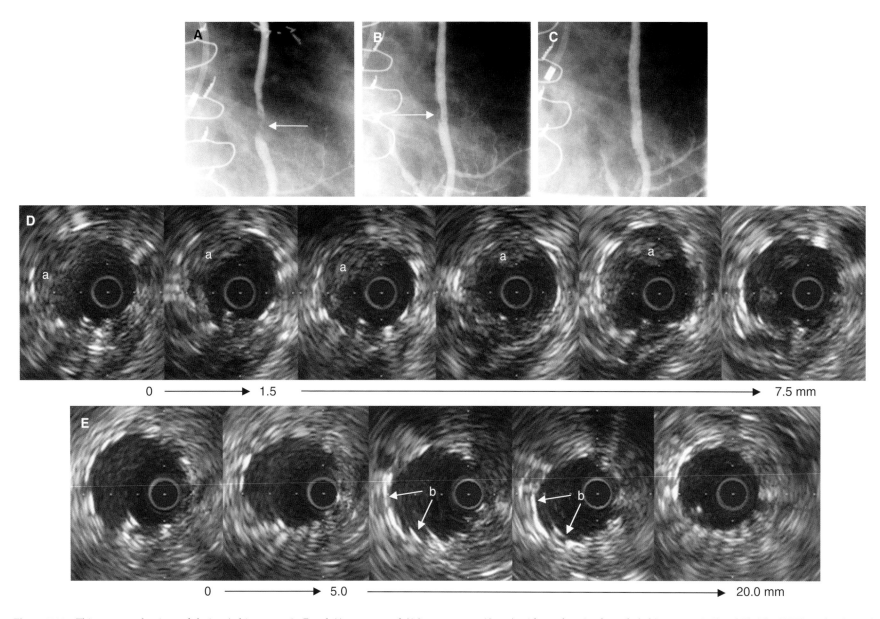

Figure 7.22 This generated vein-graft lesion (white arrow in Panel A) was stented (4.0 mm stent at 12 atm) with a suboptimal result (white arrow in Panel B). The IVUS study showed extensive plaque prolapse (a in Panel D). Implantation of a second stent (3.5 mm) within the first stent eliminated the tissue prolapse (Panels C and E). Note the increased amount of stent metal in Panel E compared with Panel D. After the first stent, the minimum stent CSA measured 10.0 mm^2, but there was 5.3 mm^2 of plaque prolapse, giving an effective lumen CSA of only 4.7 mm^2. After the second stent, the minimum lumen CSA increased to 8.0 mm^2

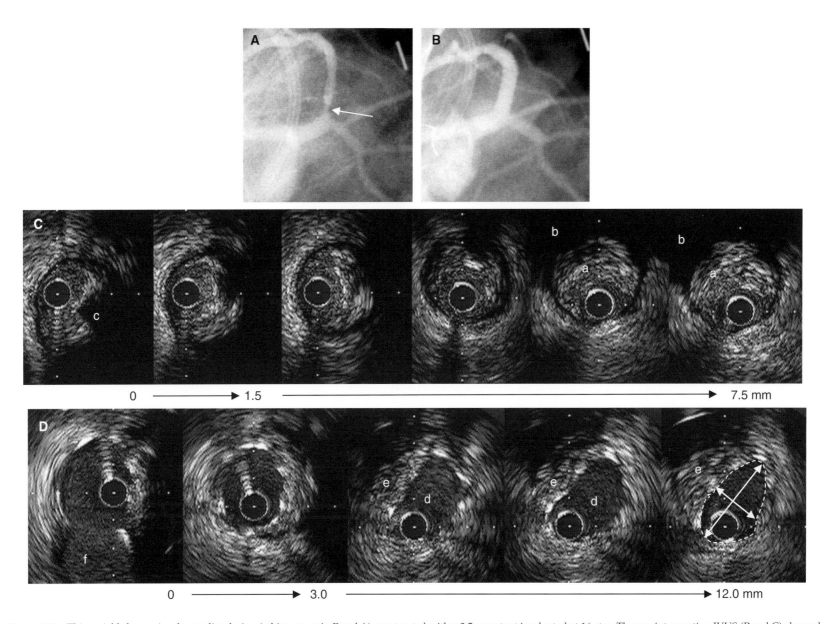

Figure 7.23 This ostial left anterior descending lesion (white arrow in Panel A) was treated with a 3.5 mm stent implanted at 16 atm. The pre-intervention IVUS (Panel C) showed fibrotic plaque (a) with attenuation (b) and, near the ostium, superficial calcium with shadowing (c). The post-intervention angiographic result is shown in Panel B. The post-intervention IVUS (Panel D) showed marked stent asymmetry (d) with a maximum/minimum stent diameter ratio of 3.4/2.0 mm=1.8 (double-headed white arrows). In this example, fibrotic plaque (e) prevented symmetrical stent expansion, which was not evident angiographically and which could not be corrected with additional balloon inflations. The minimum stent CSA (dashed white line) measured 5.0 mm^2. Note that the stent stops just short of the left circumflex (f)

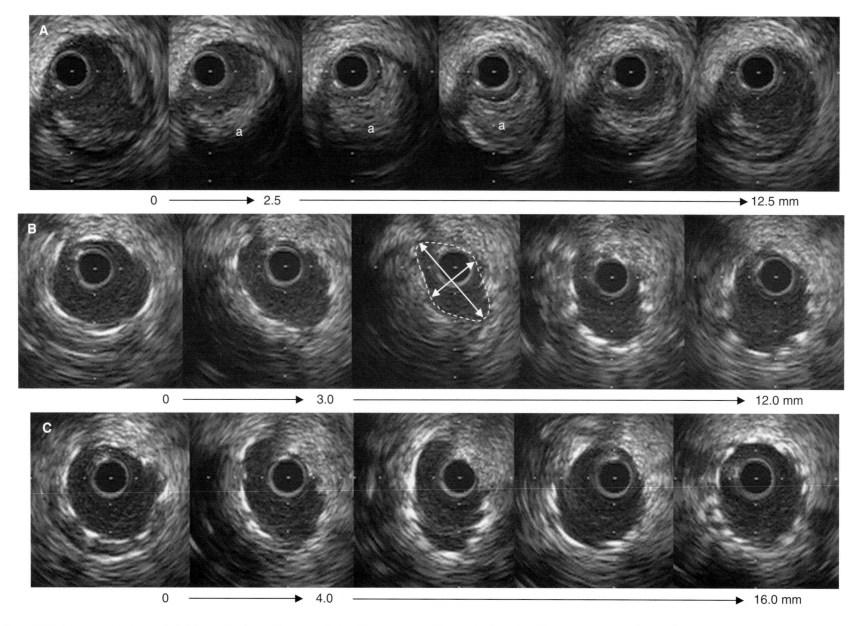

Figure 7.24 This eccentric, hypoechoic left anterior descending artery lesion (a) was treated with stent implantation. The pre-intervention IVUS is shown in Panel A. The remodeling index measured 1.1 and the mean reference-lumen CSA measured 6.9 mm^2. The post-stent implantation IVUS is shown in Panel B. The minimum lumen CSA (dashed white line) measured 6.0 mm^2; and stent symmetry (maximum/minimum stent diameter, double-headed white arrows) measured 1.6. A second stent was implanted (Panel C). The lumen CSA improved to 7.5 mm^2, but stent asymmetry remained. Both stents were 3.5 mm, inflated to 18 atm. As shown in this example, even hypoechoic plaque can resist stent expansion to create stent asymmetry, which is difficult to correct with additional balloon inflations or additional stents

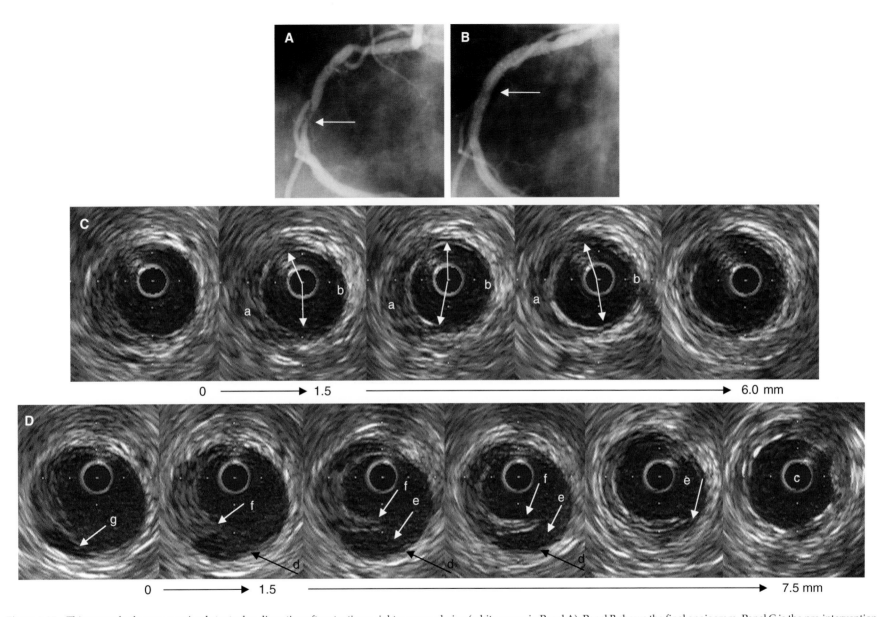

Figure 7.25   This example shows a proximal stent edge dissection after stenting a right coronary lesion (white arrow in Panel A). Panel B shows the final angiogram. Panel C is the pre-intervention IVUS showing only the proximal reference segment. Notice the eccentric, hypoechoic plaque (a); the white arrows indicate the junction between this eccentric plaque and normal vessel wall (b). The proximal reference plaque burden measured 42%. Panel D is the post-stent implantation IVUS; the segment corresponded to the arrow in Panel B, and the frames were selected to be identical to those in the pre-intervention IVUS study. Notice the proximal edge of the stent (c). The stent and/or its delivery balloon caused the adventitia (d) to expand outwards. This, in turn, caused a tear in the intima and media at the junction of the plaque to normal vessel wall (e) to create a dissection flap (f). The dissection propagated proximally for approximately 6 mm (g). The smallest reference lumen CSA measured 7.9 mm^2. Another stent was not implanted

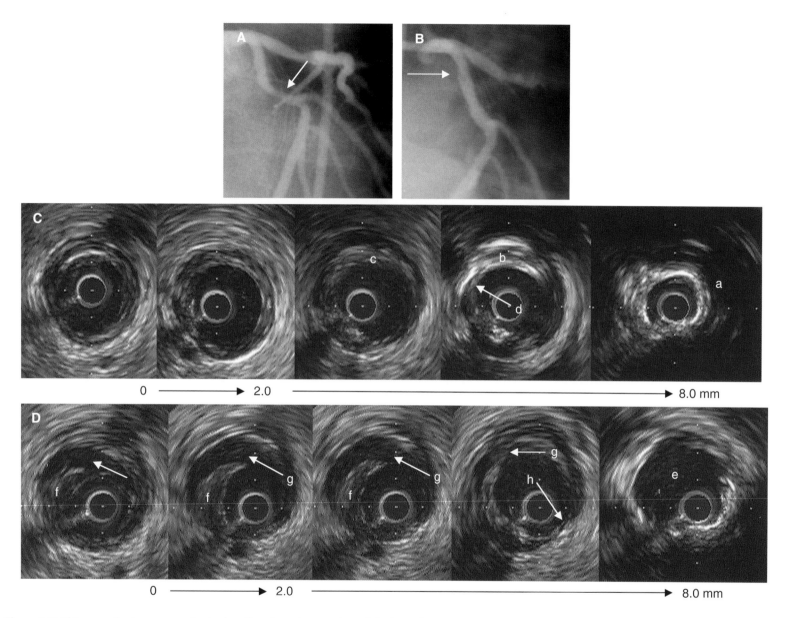

Figure 7.26 This example shows a proximal edge dissection after stenting a left circumflex coronary artery lesion (white arrow in Panel A). Panel B shows the final angiogram. Panel C is the pre-intervention IVUS showing the proximal end of the fibrocalcific lesion and the proximal reference segment. Note the circumferential lesion calcium (a), the fibrotic plaque (b) at the proximal end of the lesion, and the fibrofatty reference-segment plaque (c). The white arrow (d) indicates the transition between hard and soft plaque. Panel D is the post-stent implantation IVUS; the segment corresponds to the arrow in the angiogram in Panel B. Note the proximal edge of the stent (e); the stent ended just at the point of transition between the hard and soft plaque. Note also the tissue flap (f) and the tear (g) down to the media. The dissection occurred at the junction of hard and soft plaque, not at the junction of eccentric plaque to normal vessel wall (h). The smallest reference-lumen CSA measured 7.5 mm². Another stent was not implanted

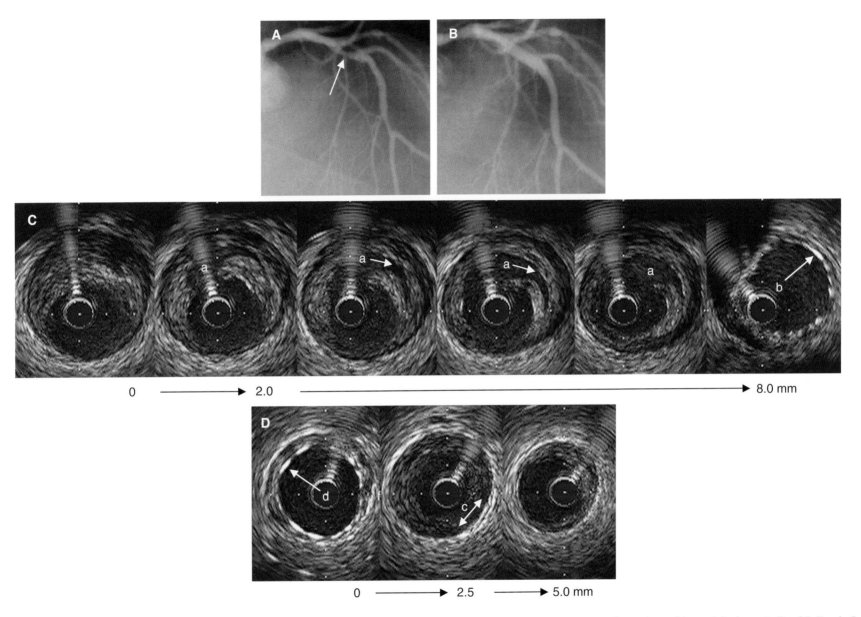

Figure 7.27 This proximal left anterior descending lesion (white arrow in Panel A) was treated with implantation of a 3.5 mm stent. The angiographic result is shown in Panel B. Panels C and D together illustrate the post-stent implantation IVUS. The post-intervention IVUS shows that there is a dissection (a) into the plaque at the proximal end of the stent (b in Panel C) and that there is a dissection between the plaque and the vessel wall (c) at the distal end of the stent (d in Panel D). Additional stents were not implanted

(median of 2.5 years) were lower for the IVUS-guided group ($p = 0.01$); 78% of the IVUS group were MACE-free versus 59% of the coronary angiography group ($p = 0.04$), with an odds ratio of 2.5 in favor of IVUS guidance.[96] Most recently, the BEST (Balloon Equivalent to STent) study showed that IVUS-guided provisional stenting – using lesion site "media-to-media" balloon sizing that necessitated cross-over to stenting in 44% – was equivalent to deliberate stent implantation. At follow-up, the angiographic restenosis rate was 16.8% in the IVUS-guided provisional stenting group versus 18.1% in the deliberate stenting group, and the in-stent restenosis rate was only 5% in the provisional stent group compared with 15.5% in the deliberate stent group.[23]

It is also important to note that there have been two studies (RESIST and OPTICUS) that have reported no benefit from IVUS guidance. In RESIST (REStenosis after IVUS-guided Stenting), patients were randomized after successful stent implantation: no further dilation ($n = 76$) versus IVUS-guided additional balloon dilation to reach optimum stent expansion (minimum stent CSA $\geq$ 80% of the reference-lumen CSA, achieved in 63/79). At 6 months, there was no significant difference in the restenosis rates between the two groups: 28.8% versus 22.5%, respectively. The economic analysis and long-term clinical data of RESIST were reported in a subsequent manuscript.[97] Because of the cost of IVUS catheters and the need for more balloons, acute procedural costs were 18% higher in the IVUS group; however, at 18 months, the cumulative medical costs were nearly equal. The higher acute costs were partially offset by the cost for revascularization procedures (31 in the control group versus 20 in the IVUS group, $p = 0.04$) although sensitivity analysis showed that the additional cost of IVUS remained in the range of 1.0–7.5%. Clinical events (death, myocardial infarction, unstable angina or lesion revascularization) occurred in 37% vs. 25%, respectively. In OPTICUS, 550 patients were randomly assigned to either IVUS-guided or angiography-guided implantation of one or two bare-metal stents. At 6 months, repeat angiography revealed no significant differences between the groups with respect to restenosis rate (24.5% vs. 22.8%), minimal lumen diameter (1.95 ± 0.72 mm vs. 1.91±0.68 mm), and percent diameter stenosis (34.8 ± 20.6% vs. 36.8 ± 19.6%), respectively. At 12 months, neither MACE nor repeat percutaneous interventions were reduced in the ultrasound-guided group.

STENT GRAFTS

Tubular-slotted or self-expanding stent grafts have been developed to seal coronary perforations, treat true and false (pseudo) aneurysms, and prevent distal embolization during degenerated saphenous vein-graft lesion interventions.[98,99]

It has also been hypothesized that the membrane would create a barrier to smooth muscle cell migration and, therefore, reduce intimal hyperplasia and in-stent restenosis. High-pressure dilation (in one series, to 19.3 ± 3.2 atm) is essential for complete expansion; conversely, underexpansion is common with moderate inflation pressures.[98] PTFE (polytetrafluoroethylene, the material most commonly used in these devices) is highly echogenic and, therefore, there is little to no ultrasound penetration into deeper arterial structures. This makes assessment of apposition difficult – except at the edges. Conversely, while autologous vein-covered stents attenuate ultrasound, some penetration is seen. Examples of stent-graft implantation are shown in Figures 6.22, 7.28, and 7.29.

DRUG-ELUTING STENTS

So far, there is only a little practical information about IVUS and drug-eluting stents (DES), although IVUS substudies have been incorporated into most of the clinical trials. It is probable that routine DES implantation will dramatically and irrevocably alter the practice of interventional cardiology. The value of IVUS during interventions will have to be revisited in the DES era. For example, in the various clinical trials and early registries, the event rate after DES implantation is lower than after a deferred intervention in previous studies based on IVUS or physiologic lesion assessment. Therefore, it is possible to argue that all intermediate lesions should be treated with DES without concern as to their true severity. It is no longer clear which approach – appropriate deferred intervention or routine stenting of intermediate lesions – would be associated with the best clinical outcomes.

DES are expensive, and have not been universally adopted in some countries where they are available, for cost reasons. Thus, IVUS could be used to triage lesions into DES versus bare-metal stenting according to the probability of restenosis based on patient characteristics, vessel size, lesion complexity, etc. Diabetes, small vessels, positive remodeling, long lesions, and ostial location all increase the risk of bare-metal stent restenosis; conversely, relatively simple lesions in large vessels in non-diabetics have low restenosis rates if an optimum final stent CSA can be obtained. Even where DES has been generally adopted, misjudging lesion length can be expensive if there is the need to implant a second DES because the first one was too short.

A smaller minimum stent CSA may be acceptable with DES compared to bare-metal stents.[75] Conversely, because DES successfully suppress most of the neointimal response, it is likely that, compared with bare-metal stents, there will be more instances of stent under-expansion or other mechanical complications in patients with DES failure.[100] In the SIRIUS trial, a minimum stent CSA of 5.0 mm^2 predicted 90% of adequate lumen areas at follow-up; thus, in 90% of DES-treated lesions with inadequate follow-up lumen dimensions, the cause was stent under-expansion. However, in a recent report from the RESEARCH registry, the following had higher sirolimus-eluting stent restenosis rates: ostial location (14.7%), diabetics (14.3%), stented length > 26 mm (13.9%), angiographic reference diameter < 2.17 mm, and non-left anterior descending lesions (10.8%).[101] Similarly, in an unpublished series from Lenox Hill Hospital, diabetes mellitus and ostial lesions were more common, stented segments were longer, and final stent CSAs were smaller in sirolimus-eluting stent restenoses. Increased intimal hyperplasia has been noted when DES are implanted into lesions with positive pre-intervention remodeling.[102] In one study, the restenosis rate when treating bifurcations was 26%.[103] Thus, like bare-metal stents, a single minimum stent CSA cut-off may be too simplistic – particularly in higher-risk patient and lesion subsets.

Compared with bare-metal stents, there appears to be less of a restenosis penalty when longer DES are implanted. In fact, the non-IVUS data suggest that "longer is better" and that a DES should cover the lesion from the most normal distal reference to the most normal proximal reference. IVUS may prove useful in identifying these most normal reference segments.

It is commonly assumed that complete (or nearly complete) DES–vessel wall apposition at the time of implantation is necessary for adequate drug delivery. Incomplete apposition at implantation occurs in approximately 10% of bare-metal stents, and there is no reason to assume that this is less common with DES.

DES sizes are currently limited. It is unknown whether stent over-expansion will affect drug delivery. Correct IVUS-guided DES sizing may minimize stent over-expansion.

SPECIAL LESION CONSIDERATIONS

There are some lesions that continue to be problematic despite advances in interventional therapy (including improved stent designs). The issues when treating left main, ostial, and bifurcation lesion location are very similar. In aorto-ostial lesions, correct stent positioning is necessary to cover the lesion adequately without protruding too proximally into the aorta. In ostial left anterior descending lesions, compromise of the left circumflex is a concern. In distal left main lesions, compromise of the left anterior descending and/or left circumflex is also a concern, depending on the technique. In treating bifurcation lesions, side-branch compromise becomes an issue. In all situations, correct device sizing and adequate final stent and/or lumen dimensions are important.

Despite the lack of specific serial IVUS studies, the high restenosis rate of ostial lesions can be attributed to exaggerated intimal hyperplasia because the final stent CSA is larger in ostial lesions compared with non-ostial lesions, and the restenosis rate is higher. Conversely, there has not been a good study of bifurcation lesions to explain their high restenosis rate. It should not be assumed that bifurcation lesions have exaggerated intimal hyperplasia. IVUS studies at implantation in both branches of a bifurcation lesion are necessary to exclude a contribution of chronic stent under-expansion to restenosis. These studies have not yet been done. In particular, the ostium of the side branch – a frequent site of restenosis – must be carefully assessed by IVUS pullback from the side branch to the main branch. It is difficult to assess adequately a side branch from the main vessel, whether pre-intervention, post-intervention, or at follow-up. Furthermore, it should not be assumed that bifurcation stents do not recoil chronically, since previous serial IVUS stent studies did not include bifurcation lesions.[104–106] Examples are shown in Figures 7.30–7.34 (ostial and left main lesions) and Figures 7.35–7.37 (bifurcation lesions). In particular, note the anatomy and final CSA of the ostium of the side branch.

Morphologic assessment, stent sizing, stent lengths, complete stent expansion, final lumen dimensions, and (if possible) complete stent apposition are also important when treating other unusual lesions such as angiographic aneurysms (whether a true aneurysm, normal arterial segment adjacent to a stenosis, or complex plaque – Figures 7.38–7.40), filling defects (Figures 7.41 and 7.42), and acute coronary syndromes (Figures 7.40, 7.42, and 7.43).

Most vein-graft lesions are easy to expand. An exception is a negatively remodeled stenosis with little plaque, which sometimes can be difficult to expand, depending on the degree of fibrosis. Examples are shown in Figure 7.44. Plaque modification may render these lesions easier to expand. Degenerated vein-graft lesions, on the other hand, are friable and are associated with plaque prolapse, plaque disruption if the stent ends in a large plaque burden, or distal embolization (Figure 7.45). IVUS sizing in vein-graft lesions is similar to native arteries (Figure 7.46). Even IVUS sizing does not help when stenting a distal anastamosis stenosis, where there may be a marked mismatch between the vein graft and distal native-artery dimensions. However, the use of distal protection devices makes IVUS imaging – particularly pre-intervention IVUS imaging – difficult.

Chronic total occlusions

There has been no consistent IVUS study of chronic total occlusions. Prototype forward-looking IVUS systems were developed to assist in recanalization, but they were never commercialized.[107]

Figure 7.28 (opposite)   This proximal saphenous vein-graft lesion (white arrow in Panel A) was treated with a Symbiot stent (Panel B). This device has a fully encased self-expanding stent (the Radius stent design) that is sandwiched between two 0.000 63 inch ePTFE layers. The pre-intervention IVUS is shown in Panel C, and the post-intervention IVUS is shown in Panel D. The two layers of ePTFE are strong ultrasound reflectors and have the appearance of a single bright membrane (a) with acoustic shadowing (b). (Compare the appearance of this PTFE stent graft with an autologous vein-covered stent in Figure 6.22.)

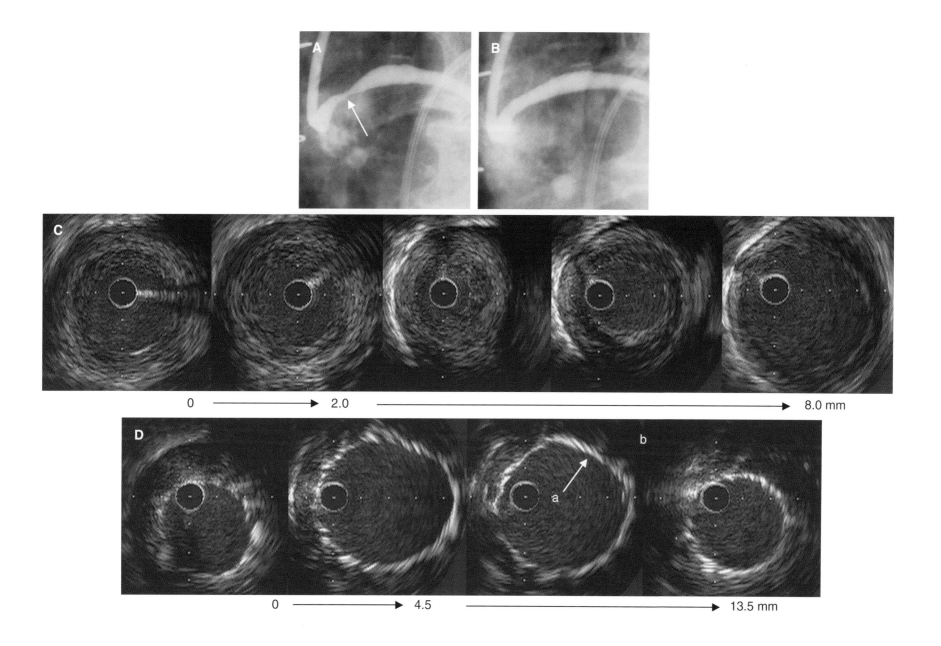

Figure 7.30 (opposite) This ostial right coronary stenosis (white arrow in Panel A) was treated with rotational atherectomy followed by implantation of a 3.0 mm stent (Panel B). The post-rotational atherectomy IVUS is shown in Panel C. The IVUS study is oriented to correspond to the angiographic image with distal on the left and proximal on the right. Note the circumferential calcium (a) and the transition from the right coronary at its ostial (b) to the aorta (c). The guiding catheter has been retracted so as not to be confused with the lesion. The image slices in the post-stent implantation IVUS (Panel D) were selected to correspond to the pre-intervention IVUS. Despite pre-stent rotablation and high-pressure (18 atm) inflations, the minimum stent CSA measures 4.6 mm^2 (d), compared with the distal reference lumen CSA of 7.2 mm^2 (e). However, this minimum stent CSA was not at the site of circumferential calcium (6.8 mm^2, f), but at the transition between the right coronary artery to the aorta. Note that the guiding catheter has been retracted so as to visualize the true aorto-ostial junction, with the proximal end of the stent (white arrows) protruding into the aorta (g). As shown in this example, when a stent is implanted in a lesion with superficial calcium, it can be difficult to distinguish the stent metal from the calcium. IVUS can be used to document ostial stent expansion, whether an ostial lesion is completely covered by a stent, and how much of the stent protrudes into the aorta

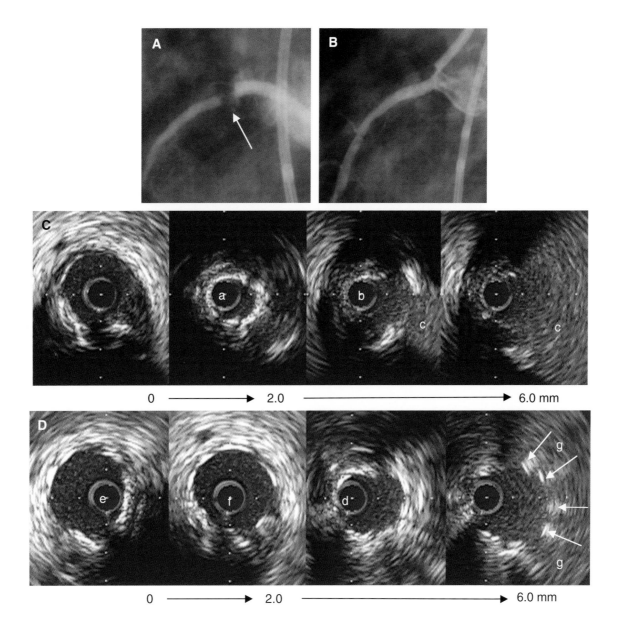

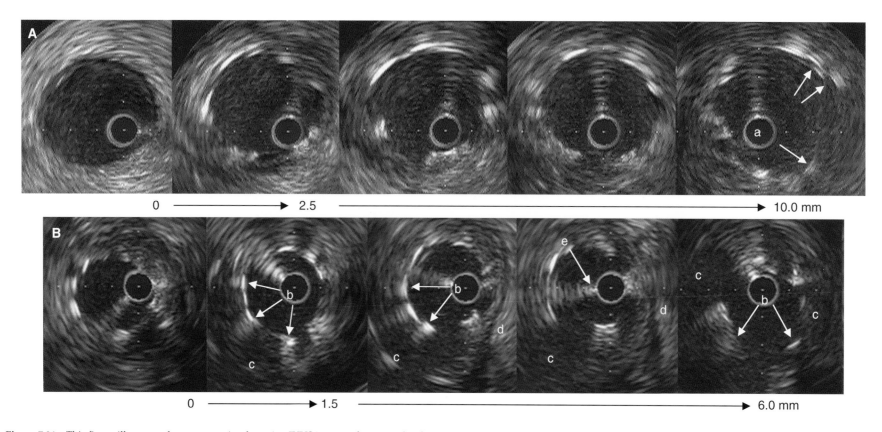

Figure 7.31 This figure illustrates the post-stent implantation IVUS images of two ostial right coronary artery stenoses with proximal on the right and distal on the left. In Panel A, the stent ends almost exactly at the junction of the right coronary artery with the aortic ostium (a). In Panel B, there is protrusion of the stent (b) into the aorta (c) over a length of several millimeters. Note the aortic wall (d) and the guidewire (e) which should not be mistaken for a stent strut. As also shown in Figure 7.30, IVUS can be used to document than an ostial lesion is completely covered by a stent as well as how much of the stent protrudes into the aorta

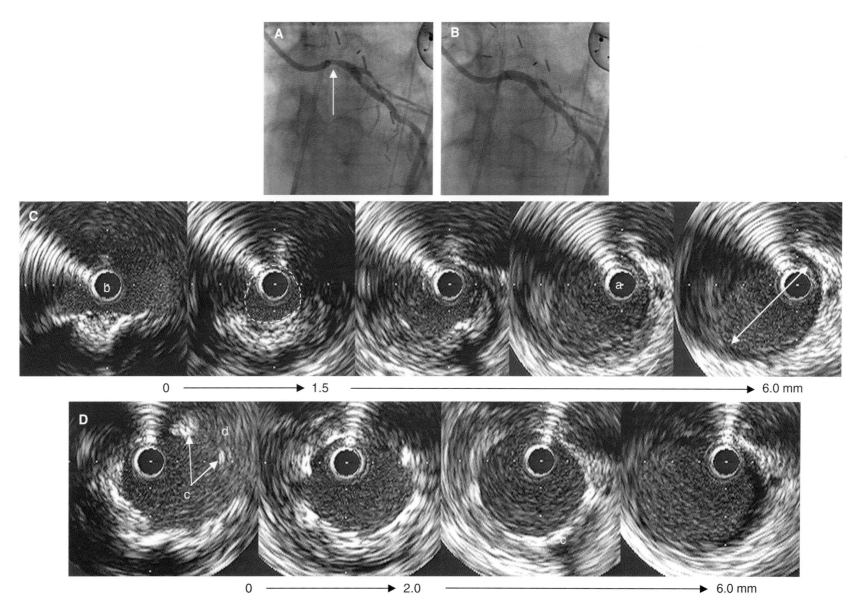

Figure 7.32   This ostial protected left main stenosis (white arrow in Panel A) was treated with stent implantation. The final angiographic result is shown in Panel B. Pre-intervention IVUS imaging (Panel C) from the left main (a) to the aorta (b) shows mostly fibrotic plaque and a minimum lumen CSA (dashed white line) of 3.0 mm^2. Based on the maximum distal reference-lumen diameter (double-headed white arrow), a 4.0 mm stent was implanted at 16 atm. The post-intervention IVUS (Panel D) shows a minimum stent CSA of 11.3 mm^2. Note that the ostium of the left main is fully covered with just a few stent struts (c) protruding into the aorta (d)

Figure 7.33 (opposite)   This distal protected left main stenosis (white arrow in Panel A) was treated with a 4.0 mm stent from the left circumflex across the bypassed left anterior descending to the aorta; the stent was implanted at 16 atm and post-dilated with a 4.5 mm balloon at 12 atm. The final angiographic result is shown in Panel B. The pre-intervention IVUS is shown in Panel C. Note the hyperechoic (fibrotic) plaque (a) with attenuation (b) and the elliptical left main ostium (c) with its transition to the aorta (d). The post-intervention IVUS is shown in Panel D. The minimum stent CSA measured 11.5 mm^2. Note that the left anterior descending (e) is covered (jailed) by the stent and that the stent continues to the left main ostium (f) at its transition to the aorta (g)

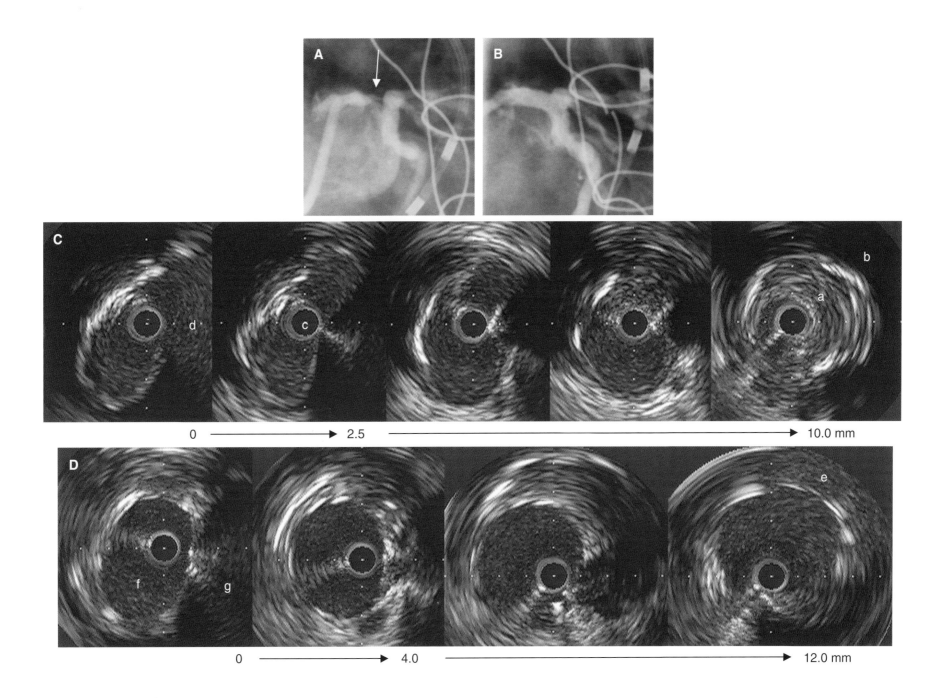

Figure 7.35 (opposite)   Both the left anterior descending and its major (second) diagonal branch were imaged pre-intervention and then stented, but only the left anterior descending was imaged after stent implantation. The pre-intervention IVUS of the left anterior descending is shown in Panel A. Note the distal reference (a), the eccentric hypoechoic plaque (b) that is located opposite the major diagonal branch (c), the proximal left anterior descending (d), a large septal perforator (e), and a proximal (first) diagonal branch (f). The minimum lumen CSA (dashed white line) was just distal to the diagonal (c); it measured 2.2 mm^2. The pre-intervention IVUS of the major diagonal branch is shown in Panel B. Note the distal reference (g), the eccentric plaque (h) that was located adjacent to a small branch (i) in the diagonal and just distal to the left anterior descending (j), the proximal left anterior descending (k), and the proximal (first) diagonal branch (l) that is also seen in Panel A. At the site of the minimum lumen CSA in the diagonal (dashed white line), the IVUS catheter was occlusive. The post-intervention IVUS of the left anterior descending is shown in Panel C. Note the stent in the left anterior descending (m), the second stent in the diagonal (n), the ostium of the diagonal (o), and the proximal septal perforator (p) that was not covered by the stent. The stent stopped just short of the proximal (first) diagonal branch (q). The adequacy of major diagonal branch stent expansion cannot be assessed from the left anterior descending

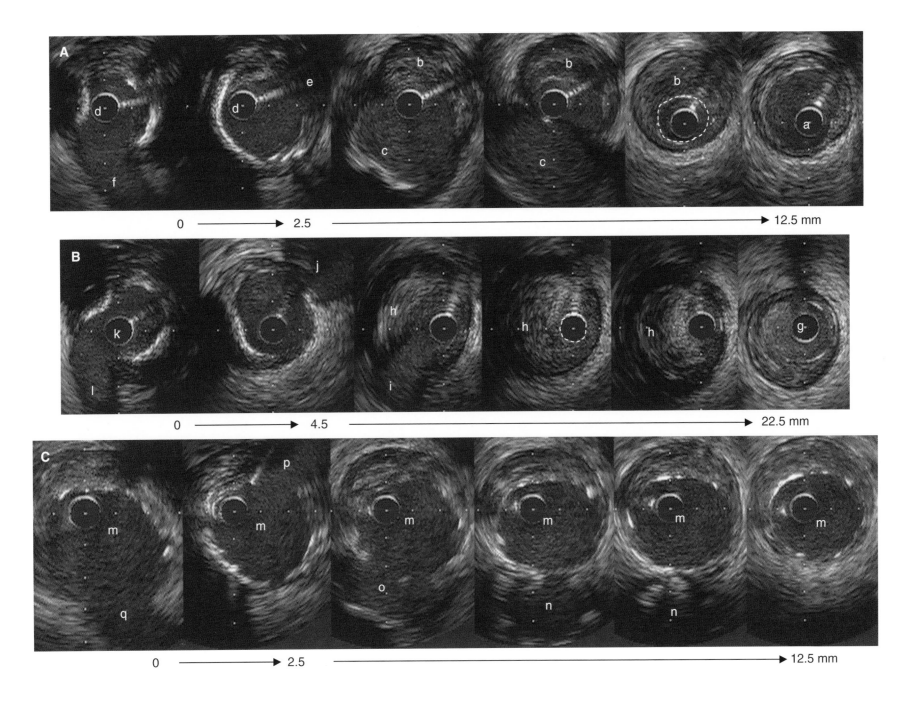

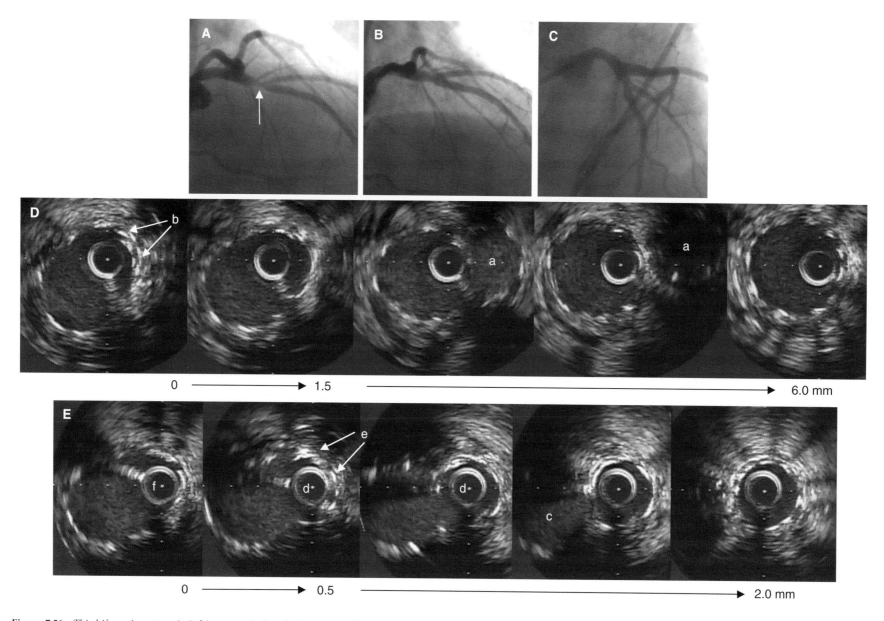

Figure 7.36 This bifurcation stenosis (white arrow in Panel A) was treated with bifurcation stenting using the "crush" technique. A 3.5 mm stent was implanted at 16 atm into the left anterior descending, and a 2.5 mm stent was implanted at 16 atm into the diagonal. The final angiogram is shown in Panels B and C. The final IVUS of the left anterior descending is shown in Panel D; note the diagonal stent (a) as viewed from the left anterior descending and the multiple proximal layers of stent metal (b) proximally. The final IVUS of the diagonal is shown in Panel E; note the left anterior descending stent (c) as viewed from the diagonal, the transition from the diagonal to the left anterior descending (d), and the multiple proximal layers of stent metal (e). The left anterior descending stent appears elliptical (f) in Panel E because of the oblique angle of the transducer in its transition from the diagonal to the left anterior descending. The left anterior descending stent CSA measured 8.7 mm^2, and the diagonal stent CSA measured 3.8 mm^2, with a minimum stent diameter of 2.0 mm

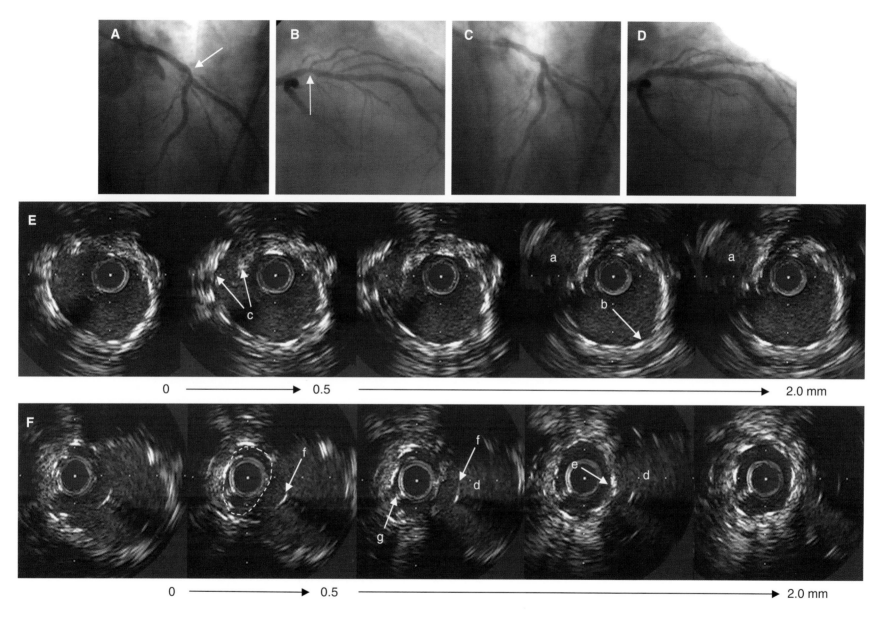

Figure 7.37 This bifurcation stenosis (white arrows in Panels A and B) was treated with bifurcation stenting using the modified T-stenting technique. A 3.5 mm stent was implanted at 18 atm into the left anterior descending, and a 3.0 mm stent was implanted at 14 atm in the diagonal. The final angiogram is shown in Panels C and D. The final IVUS of the left anterior descending is shown in Panel E; note the diagonal stent (a) as viewed from the left anterior descending stent (b) and the struts from the diagonal stent (c) protruding into the LAD stent. The final IVUS of the diagonal is shown in Panel F; note the left anterior descending stent (d) as viewed from the diagonal stent (e), the guidewire in the left anterior descending (f), and the guidewire in the diagonal (g). The left anterior descending stent CSA measured 8.8 mm^2, and the diagonal minimum lumen CSA (dashed white line in Panel F) measured 3.0 mm^2 with a minimum stent diameter of 1.5 mm

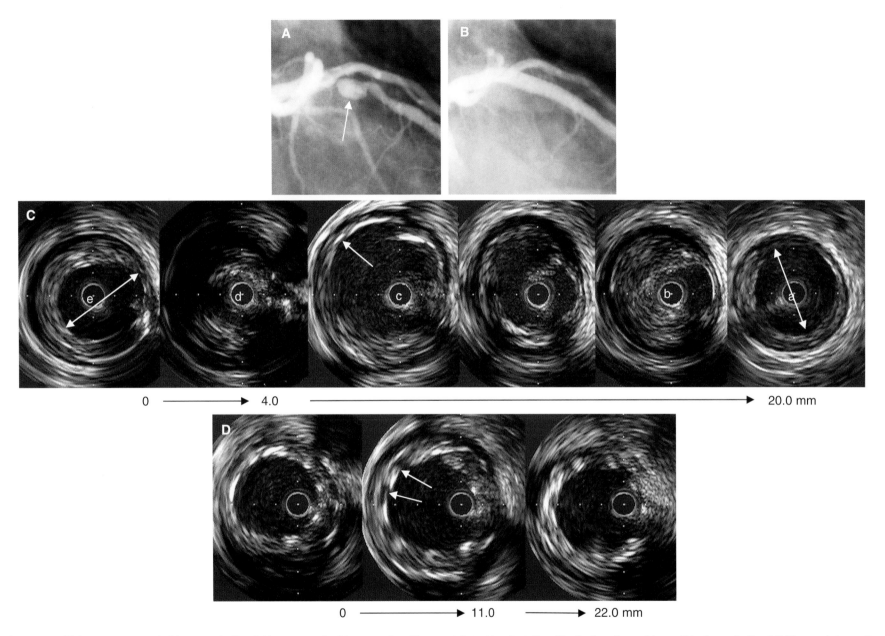

Figure 7.38 This true aneurysm (white arrow in Panel A) was treated with conventional bare-metal stent implantation. The final angiographic result is shown in Panel B. The pre-intervention IVUS (Panel C) included the distal reference (a), a distal lesion (b) with a minimum lumen CSA of 2.9 mm^2, the aneurysm (c) with all three layers intact (white arrow) and an EEM CSA of 27.6 mm^2, a proximal lesion (d) with a minimum lumen CSA of 0.9 mm^2, and the proximal reference (e) with an EEM CSA of 18.1 mm^2. The IVUS diagnosis of a true aneurysm was based on the lesion EEM CSA > 150% of the proximal reference with all three layers of arterial wall intact. Because the maximum reference-lumen diameter measured 4.0 mm (double-headed white arrows), a 4.0 mm stent was implanted at 16 atm and then post-dilated using a 4.5 mm balloon at 4 atm within the aneurysm. The final IVUS result is shown in Panel D. Note that there was only minor incomplete apposition (white arrows in Panel D)

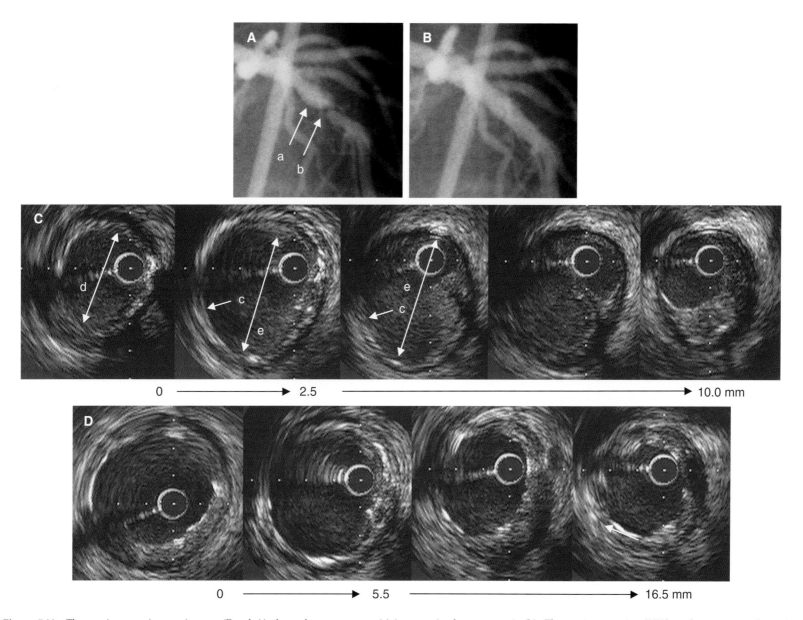

Figure 7.39   The pre-intervention angiogram (Panel A) showed an aneurysm (a) just proximal to a stenosis (b). The pre-intervention IVUS is shown in Panel C. The angiographic "aneurysm" was, in fact, a segment of normal vessel adjacent to the distal stenosis. The "aneurysm" EEM CSA measured 23.7 mm^2 with intact intima, media, and adventitia (c); this was <150% of the proximal reference EEM CSA of 18.7 mm^2, the threshold for a diagnosis of an aneurysm. The maximum reference-lumen diameter (double-headed white arrow, d, at the proximal reference) measured 3.5 mm, and the internal diameter of the "aneurysm" (double-headed white arrow, e) measured 4.5 mm. A 3.5 mm stent was implanted and post-dilated in the middle using a 4.5 mm balloon at 4 atm. The final angiographic result is shown in Panel B, and the final IVUS result is shown in Panel D

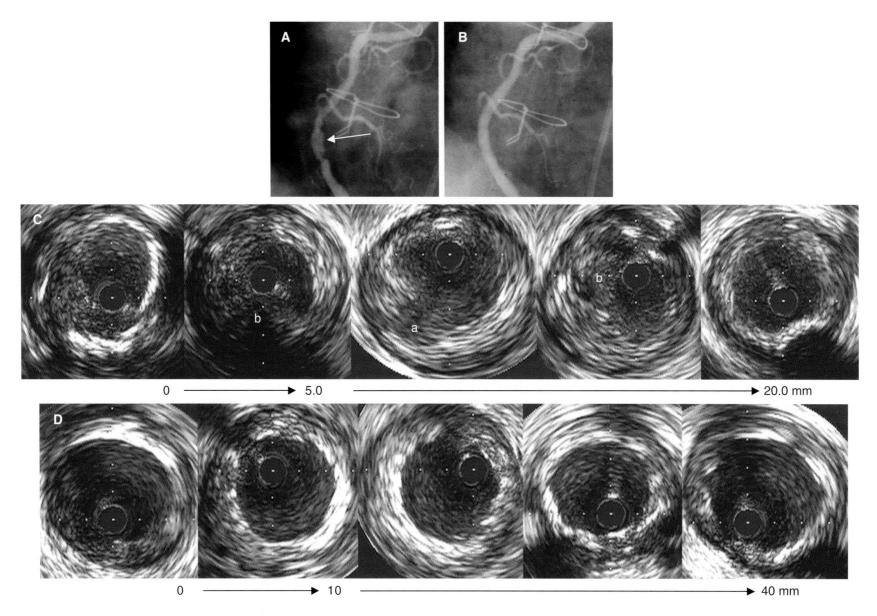

Figure 7.40 This patient presented with an acute coronary syndrome and the angiographic aneurysm (white arrow) shown in Panel A. The pre-intervention IVUS is shown in Panel C. Note the contour of the lumen (a) that, combined with the proximal and distal narrowing of the lumen by what appeared to be thrombus (b), was responsible for the angiographic "aneurysm". The entire segment was stented with a 4.0 mm stent. The angiographic and IVUS results after stent implantation are shown in Panels B and D. The minimum stent CSA measured 10.2 mm^2

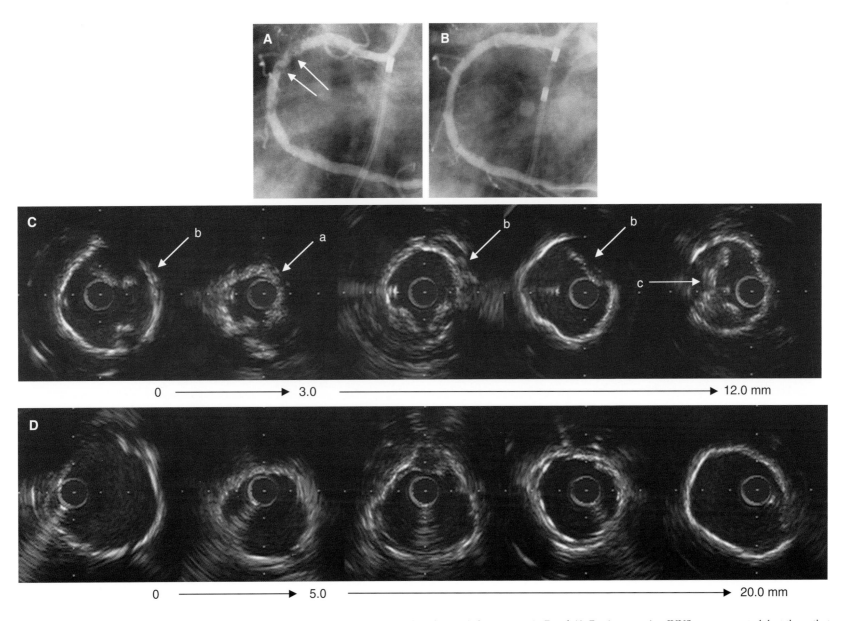

Figure 7.41   This right coronary artery contained two angiographic filling defects/complex plaques (white arrows in Panel A). Pre-intervention IVUS was attempted, but the catheter would not cross the lesions. The decision was made to perform rotational atherectomy. After a 1.75 mm burr, the IVUS catheter crossed easily. The post-rotational atherectomy IVUS is shown in Panel C. Note the extensive lesion (a) and reference (b) calcium and the fibrocalcific mass (c) that was the angiographic filling defect. The results following stent implantation are shown in Panels B and D. Note that it is difficult to distinguish stent metal from the underlying circumferential lesion calcium, particularly in the setting of full apposition

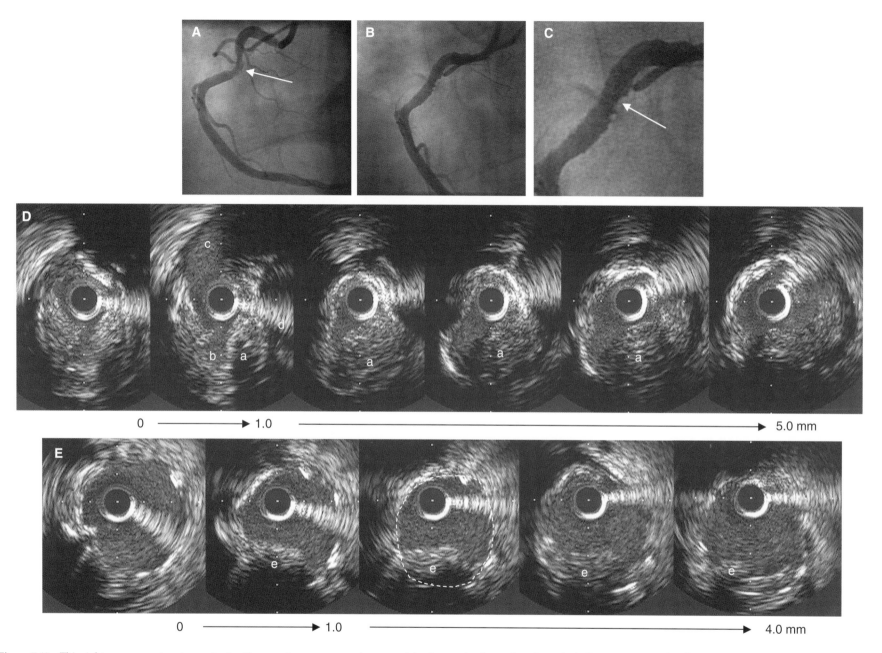

Figure 7.42 This right coronary artery in a patient with an acute coronary syndrome contained a proximal complex plaque including an angiographic filling defect (white arrow in Panel A). The pre-intervention IVUS (Panel D) showed evidence of a thrombus (a) and a ruptured plaque (b) opposite the SA nodal artery (c, which is also seen in the angiogram). The post-stent implantation angiogram is shown in Panels B and C; note the scalloped appearance in the magnified view (white arrow in Panel C). The post-stent implantation IVUS is shown in Panel E; note the plaque prolapse (e) into the stent (dashed white line)

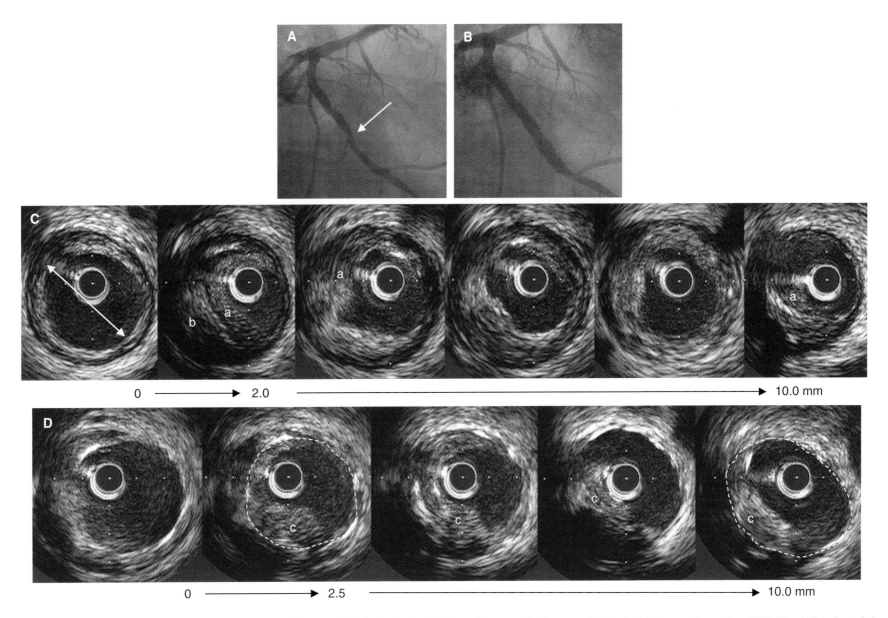

Figure 7.43 A patient presented with an acute coronary syndrome and this lesion in the left circumflex artery (white arrow in Panel A). The pre-intervention IVUS (Panel C) indicated the presence of a thrombus (a) superimposed on fibrofatty plaque (b), but no evidence of plaque rupture. The remodeling index measured 1.31. The maximum reference-lumen diameter measured 4.0 mm. The entire segment was stented (Panel B) using a 4.0 mm stent. The post-intervention IVUS shows extensive plaque prolapse (c) within the CSA of the stent (dashed white line). Note how the prolapsed plaque can obscure the stent struts

Figure 7.45 (opposite) This saphenous vein-graft lesion (white arrow in Panel A) was treated with stent implantation; the angiographic result is shown in Panel B. The pre-intervention IVUS is shown in Panel C. Note the large plaque burden (a) that is in sharp contradistinction from the lesions in Figures 7.44 and 7.46. The maximum lumen diameter (double-headed white arrow) measured 4.3 mm. A 4.0 mm stent was implanted at 10 atm and post-dilated with a 4.5 mm balloon at 8 atm. The post-intervention IVUS is shown in Panel D; note the plaque disruption (b) where the stent ended in the large, friable plaque burden

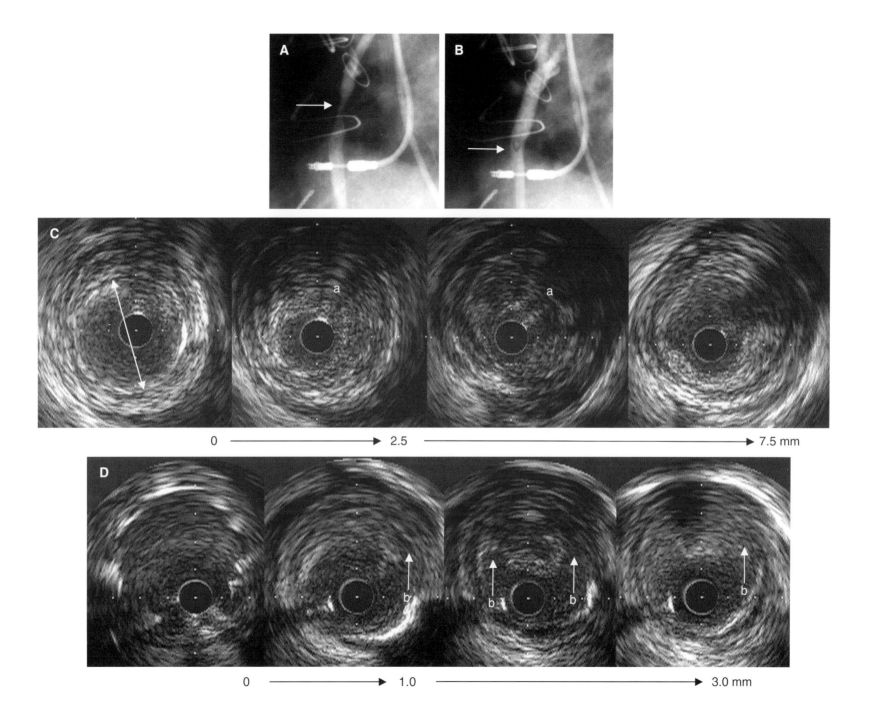

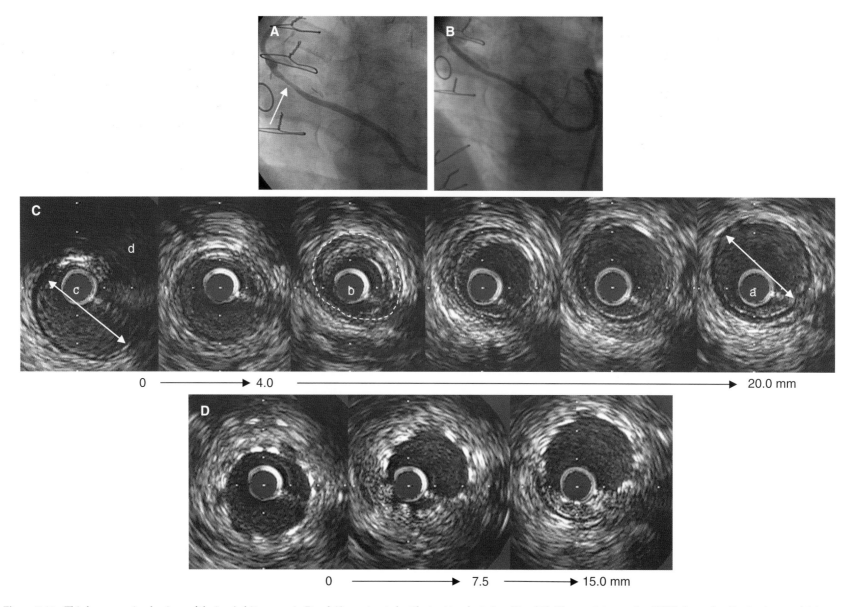

Figure 7.46 This long, proximal vein-graft lesion (white arrow in Panel A) was treated with stent implantation (Panel B). The pre-intervention IVUS showed a distal reference (a) that was nearly normal, with an EEM CSA of 10.9 mm^2 and a maximal lumen diameter of 3.2 mm; a lesion (b) with an EEM CSA of 7.8 mm^2 and a lumen CSA of 2.8 mm^2; and a nearly normal proximal reference (c), with an EEM CSA of 11.3 mm^2 and a maximum lumen diameter of 3.5 mm. Note the transition to the aorta (d). A 3.5 mm stent was implanted at 14 atm. The final IVUS result is shown in Panel D; the minimum stent CSA measured 6.5 mm^s

Penetrating the proximal fibrous cap can be very difficult. If the guidewire takes a subintimal course, the wire tends to slip into the space repeatedly to extend the medial dissection along the circumference of the artery. The most difficult step in chronic total occlusion interventions is to penetrate the distal fibrous cap and reenter the true lumen at the distal end of the lesion. In contrast to the proximal end of a chronic occlusion, a thick fibrous membrane rarely exists at the distal end. The major limitation to penetrating the distal fibrous cap is the false lumen made by the guidewire surrounding the distal true lumen. IVUS is useful for identifying the site where the wire has gone from the true to the false lumen; assessing the length, depth, and circumferential extent of the false lumen caused by the guidewire; identifying where and if the guidewire has re-entered the true lumen; and, in general, determining whether the guidewire is in the true or false lumen. The true lumen is identified by the presence of plaque or intima surrounding the IVUS catheter or from connection to side branches (side branches connect to the true lumen, not the false lumen – unless the tissue plane between them has been disrupted). Examples are shown in Figures 7.47–7.49.

COMPLICATIONS

There are very few device-specific complications, with the exception of stent thrombosis and stent dislodgement. Most complications – dissections, intramural hematomas, and perforations – can occur with any device, although the frequency and clinical settings may vary. There are also pseudocomplications – angiographic and/or IVUS findings that are benign. The recognition and diagnosis of these complications and analysis of other unusual post-intervention images is facilitated by comparison with the pre-intervention IVUS study.

Stent thrombosis

A number of studies have suggested a link between suboptimal stent implantation and stent thrombosis. However, these studies were not randomized trials; and there were significant overlaps in the IVUS findings comparing stents that thrombosed versus ones that did not. In addition, the numbers in each report were small. Many things have changed since the initial reports of stent thrombosis, including stent design, implantation technique, and adjunctive medical therapy, and the sensitivity and specificity of many of the IVUS findings is limited because the incidence of stent thrombosis is so low. Nevertheless, the IVUS observations in stent thrombosis are relatively consistent.

Moussa et al.[108] reported 19 patients (19 lesions) out of a total of 982 patients (1315 lesions) who developed stent thombosis > 24 h after implantation between 1993 and 1995. IVUS studies were available in 13 subacute thrombosis patients and in 707 non-thrombosis patients. The stent thrombosis group had a smaller minimum lumen diameter and a smaller minimum CSA (5.87 ± 1.73 mm^2 vs. 7.75 ± 2.52 mm^2, $p = 0.008$). However, a smaller stent CSA was not an independent predictor of subacute thrombosis once other procedural and angiographic variables were considered. The most significant predictor of stent thrombosis was poor flow associated with a low left ventricular ejection fraction.

Werner et al.[109] reported 6 patients with acute stent thrombosis, 4 patients with subacute stent thrombosis, and 205 without stent thrombosis. Stent thrombosis was associated with a smaller final minimum lumen diameter (2.50 ± 0.30 mm vs. 2.86 ± 0.48 mm, $p < 0.05$) and a larger residual plaque burden at the site of the minimum lumen diameter ($70.1 \pm 6.1\%$ vs. $58.4 \pm 9.8\%$, $p < 0.001$).

The multicenter POST (Predictors of Stent Thrombosis) Registry enrolled patients from 1991–1996, an era that spanned the transition from anticoagulation to antiplatelet pharmacology.[110] A total of 53 patients had subacute stent thrombosis within 4 weeks of implantation. Of the 53 patients, 50 received aspirin: 15 received aspirin alone, while 6 received aspirin+warfarin and 29 received aspirin+ticlopidine. The minimum stent CSA measured 7.7 ± 2.8 mm^2, and 26 (49%) had stent underexpansion defined as a minimum stent CSA less than 80% of the mean reference lumen. Stent malapposition (at least one stent strut not in contact with the arterial wall intima, with blood speckle behind the stent strut) was seen in 49%. There was the suggestion of thrombus in 23%, plaque protrusion in 19%, and edge tears or dissections in 26%. Two abnormalities were seen in 38% and three abnormalities in 30%. This study did not have a true control arm; however, the authors compared these patients with the following multicenter studies: STRUT, CRUISE, and AVID. Compared with the STRUT registry (Stent Treatment Region assessed by Ultrasound Tomography, $n = 111$), there was no difference in stent underexpansion, but there was more malapposition (49% vs. 22%, $p < 0.001$), more edge tears or dissection (26% vs. 14%, $p < 0.05$), and more evidence of thrombus (23% vs. 0%, $p < 0.0001$). When patients with acute thrombosis (< 24 h) were compared with those with subacute thrombosis, patients with acute thrombosis tended to have less underexpansion (36% vs. 50%), more malapposition (64% vs. 45%), more edge tears or dissections (47% vs. 27%), and more intra-stent thrombosis (24% vs. 9%); however none of these differences reached statistical significance.

Cheneau et al.[111] compared 23 stent thrombosis lesions with a matched group of 69 lesions without stent thrombosis. The most notable pre-intervention finding was that stent thrombosis lesions were rarely calcified. The most notable post-

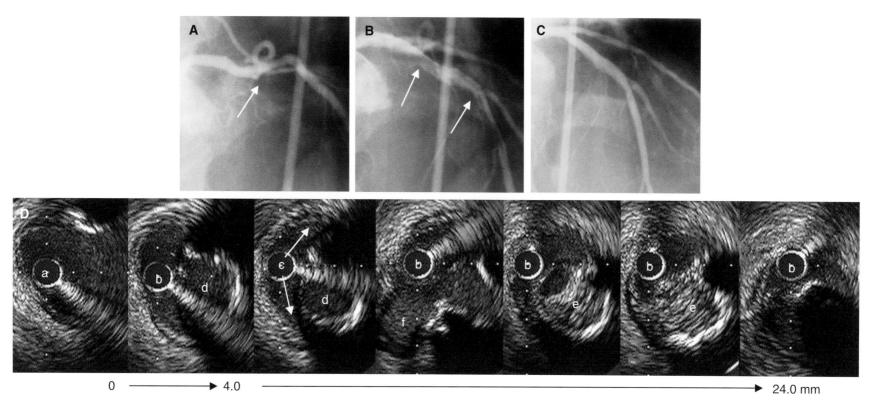

Figure 7.47 This left anterior descending chronic total occlusion (white arrow in Panel A) was crossed with a guidewire and pre-dilated (Panel B); the final angiogram after additional balloon angioplasty is shown in Panel C. The IVUS in Panel D was recorded after pre-dilation. Proximally, the IVUS transducer was in the true lumen (a); however, thereafter, the IVUS transducer was in the false lumen of a medial dissection plane (b). The guidewire and transducer re-entered the true lumen more distally (not shown). Note the circumferential extent of the medial dissection (c). There was a residual true lumen (d) within the proximal several millimeters of the total occlusion, but a residual lumen was not seen distally (e). Note the location of the diagonal branch (f) that connected with the true lumen while the IVUS catheter was in the false lumen. In this example, the true lumen was identified by the intima (at a and d), by the presence of occlusive plaque (e), and by connection to the diagonal branch (f). At the level of the diagonal branch, the tissue plane separating the true from the false lumen surrounds the IVUS catheter

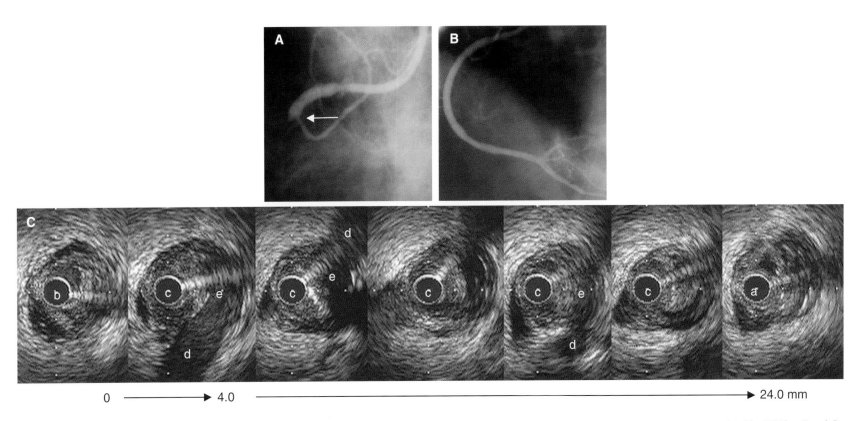

Figure 7.48   This right coronary artery chronic total occlusion (white arrow in Panel A) was crossed, dilated, and stented. The final angiogram is shown in Panel B. The IVUS in Panel C was recorded after the occlusion was crossed and pre-dilated. The transducer was in the true lumen distally (a) and proximally (b); note that the transducer was surrounded by plaque when it was in the true lumen but not when it was in the false lumen (c). Note several side branches (d) connected with the true lumen (e), which was parallel to the false lumen

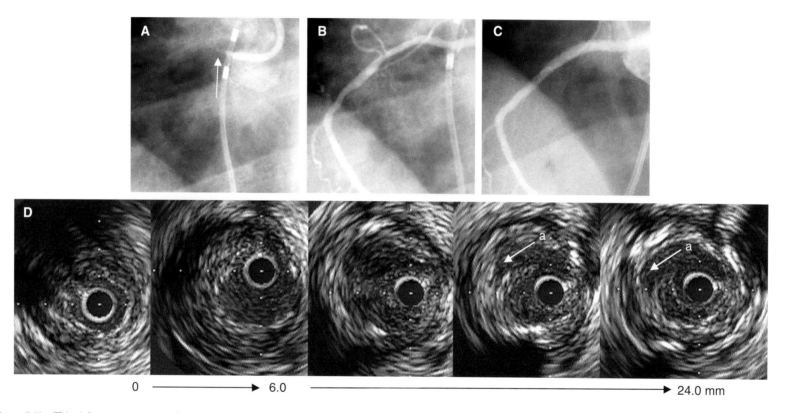

0 ———→ 6.0 ——————————————————————→ 24.0 mm

Figure 7.49 This right coronary artery chronic total occlusion (white arrow in Panel A) was crossed and dilated (Panel B) and then stented (Panel C). The IVUS in Panel D was recorded after the occlusion was crossed and dilated. The transducer was in the true lumen throughout the length of the occlusion; the IVUS lumen was always surrounded by plaque. Note the dissection in the plaque (a)

intervention finding was that residual lumen dimensions were smaller than the matched group. When quantitative measurements and qualitative findings (malapposition, dissection, thrombus, tissue protrusion, etc.) were combined, at least one abnormality was seen in 78% of stent thrombosis lesions (vs. 33% of matched lesions, $p = 0.0002$)). Multiple abnormalities were seen in 48% (vs. 3%, $p < 0.0001$).

Alfonso *et al.*[112] recently presented a series of stent thrombosis lesions. Most patients showed evidence of severe underexpansion and none fulfilled standard criteria for optimal stent implantation with frequent malapposition, residual dissections, and inflow or outflow disease.

Examples of stent thrombosis are shown in Figures 7.50—7.53 illustrates the IVUS findings in acute thrombosis during a stent-implantation procedure.

Stent "loss"

Stents can become dislodged from the delivery balloon. This may not be detected by angiography. The stent may be lost into the aorta and peripheral circulation and never be located, or it may become stuck in the coronary artery proximal or distal to the stenosis. A dislodged stent may cause recurrent ischemia even in the absence of a stenosis – presumably by being a nidus for platelet aggregation and embolization. If a dislodged stent is imaged, it has the appearance of a never-expanded stent with a diameter of less than 1.0 mm. Sometimes a stent is partially expanded before it is lost, in which case it has the appearance of a partially expanded stent. Once a stent has been lost within a coronary artery, recrossing the lesion alongside the stent and inflating a balloon can crush the stent against the vessel wall. Examples are shown in Figures 7.54–7.56.

Dissections

Dissections are tears in the plaque that are parallel to the vessel wall with visualization of blood flow in the false lumen (confirmed, if necessary, with saline or contrast injection). Dissections can be described as proximal or distal to the lesion; epicardial or myocardial; and according to length, circumferential arc, depth, lumen compromise (and contact with the IVUS catheter), and bulkiness and mobility of the flap. Examples are shown in Figures 7.57–7.65.

The following have been associated with an increased risk of dissection propagation or abrupt closure: free-wall (i.e. pericardial as opposed to myocardial side, where the surrounding muscle may constrain propagation); large mobile flaps; and medial tears occupying > 50% of vessel circumference. Nishida *et al.*[15] suggested that a lumen CSA less than 40% of the EEM CSA at the site of the dissection best predicted in-hospital major adverse events with a sensitivity and specificity of 68%.

Dissections tend to occur at the junction of plaque or arterial elements of different compliance: calcific versus non-calcific plaque, fibrotic versus non-fibrotic plaque, and plaque versus normal vessel wall. This also explains the tendency of dissections to occur at the edges of stents. IVUS has a higher sensitivity than angiography in detecting post-intervention dissections. Negative contrast imaging can increase the frequency of IVUS detection of dissections.[113]

Honye *et al.*[9] reported four morphologic patterns of dissection in 66 lesions after balloon angioplasty. Type A consisted of a linear, partial tear of the plaque from the lumen towards the media (seven lesions). Type B was defined by a split in the plaque that extended to the media (12 lesions). Type C demonstrated a dissection behind the plaque that subtended an arc of < 180° (18 lesions). Type D subtended an arc of > 180° (four lesions). However, this classification did not gain widespread acceptance.

Hong *et al.*[88] reported minor stent edge dissections detected by IVUS in 67 out of 348 stented lesions, only 12 of which were angiographically evident. Sheris *et al.*[89] reported minor edge dissections in 16 out of 150 stented lesions, none of which were seen angiographically. Minor edge dissections were defined as (1) non-flow-limiting or no lumen compromise, (2) arc of dissection < 90°, and (3) freely mobile plaque protruding into the lumen, but not directed toward the center of the lumen.[88,114]

There are a number of limitations of IVUS in assessing dissections and other complications. In particular, a dissection plane "behind" calcium will be shadowed. However, the appearance of the vessel at the edge of the arc of calcium can provide a clue as to its presence, although it may be impossible to assess its length, depth, and circumference (Figure 7.64). A thin dissection flap that is "propped up" by the IVUS catheter may be difficult to detect, particularly if the near-field gain settings are low or if the flap occurs within the zone of uncertainty adjacent to the transducer (for examples, see Figures 7.25 and 7.57)

Intramural hematomas

Intramural hematomas are a variant of a dissection. They tend to occur in arcs of normal vessel wall proximal or distal to a lesion or in arcs of normal vessel wall opposite the plaque in an eccentric lesion. The EEM expands outward and the internal elastic membrane or intima is pushed inward and straightened to cause lumen compromise. Blood accumulates in the space caused by the split in the media. The accumulated blood becomes static and echogenic, if not completely thrombotic. The hematoma can propagate antegrade or retrograde, but tends to

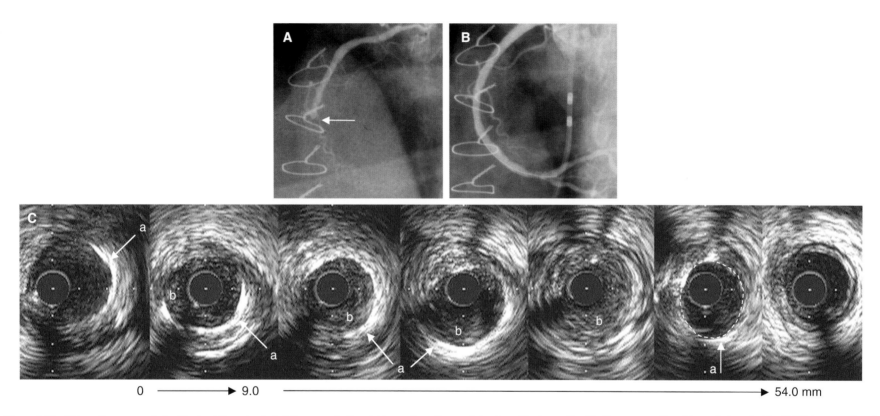

Figure 7.50 This patient presented with stent thrombosis (white arrow in Panel A) one day after receiving two Gianturco–Roubin II stents totalling 54 mm in length. The IVUS image in Panel C showed the typical slice-to-slice variation in the metallic arcs of this stent design (a). The minimum stent CSA (dashed white line) measured 4.8 mm^2. Note the mottled, heterogeneous, hypoechoic in-stent tissue (b) representing acute thrombosis. The patient was treated with tubular slotted stents, and the angiographic result is shown in Panel B

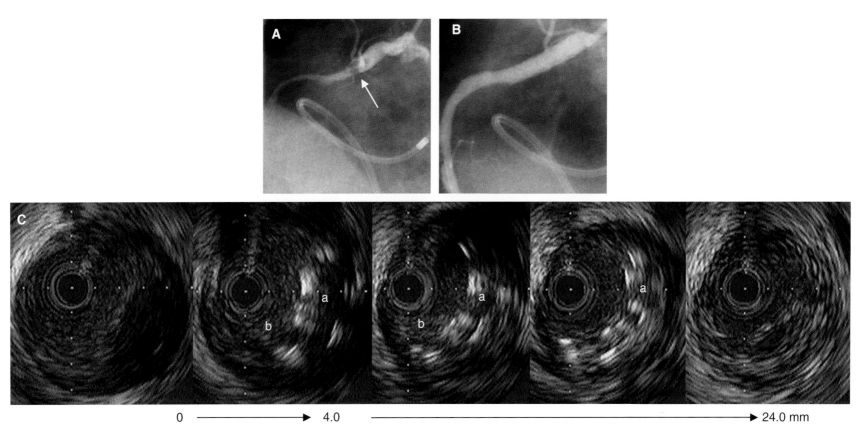

Figure 7.51 This patient presented with stent thrombosis (white arrow in Panel A) 2 weeks post-intervention. The IVUS imaging run (Panel C) showed that the stent (a) was crushed against one side of the vessel wall. During stent implantation, wire position was lost. In rewiring the vessel in order to post-dilate the stent, the guidewire passed alongside not through the middle of the stent. Balloon dilation then crushed the partially expanded stent against one side of the arterial wall. This partially expanded and partially crushed stent became a nidus for thrombus (b). Another stent was implanted, and the final result is shown in Panel B

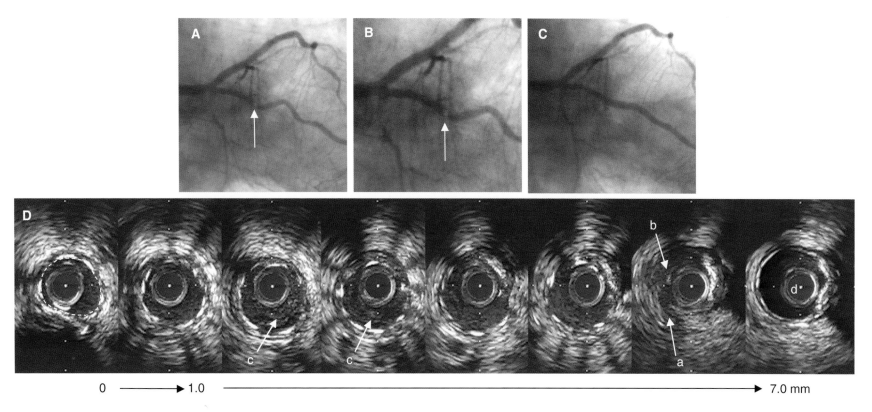

Figure 7.52 This patient presented with thrombosis of a 2.5 mm drug-eluting stent 4 days after implantation. Note the filling defect (white arrows) in the ramus branch in Panel A and in the magnified view (Panel B). IVUS imaging (Panel D) showed a perforation in the arterial wall (a) and a dissection plane (b) abutting the IVUS catheter (b) just distal to the distal edge of the stent as well as the mottled, heterogeneous, hypoechoic in-stent tissue (c) representing stent thrombosis. (The dissection flap b is difficult to see because it abuts the IVUS catheter.) The minimum stent CSA (dashed white line) measured 3.5 mm^2 with a minimum diameter of 2.0 mm. (The distal reference lumen CSA (d) measured 5.0 mm^2.) Thus, there was stent underexpansion plus outflow obstruction. Another stent was implanted, overlapping the first and extending distally; the result is shown in Panel C

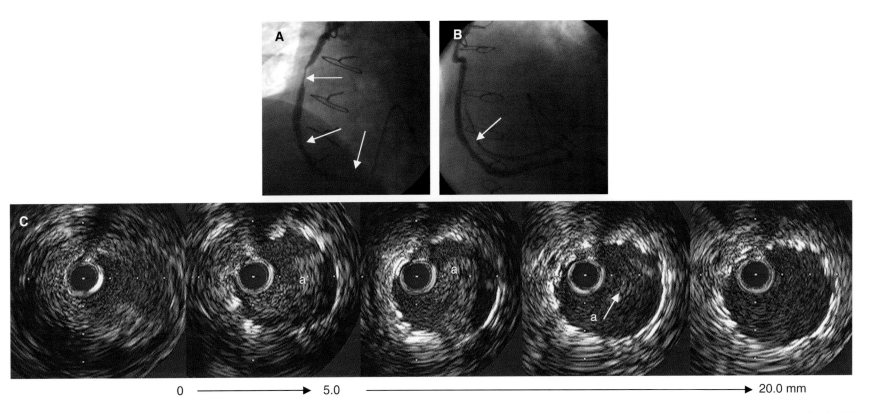

Figure 7.53 During stenting of these multiple vein-graft lesions (white arrows in Panel A), the graft developed a hazy appearance (white arrow in Panel B). The ACT was found to be 214 s. IVUS showed an irregular, mobile intraluminal mass (a) that presumably represented acute thrombosis

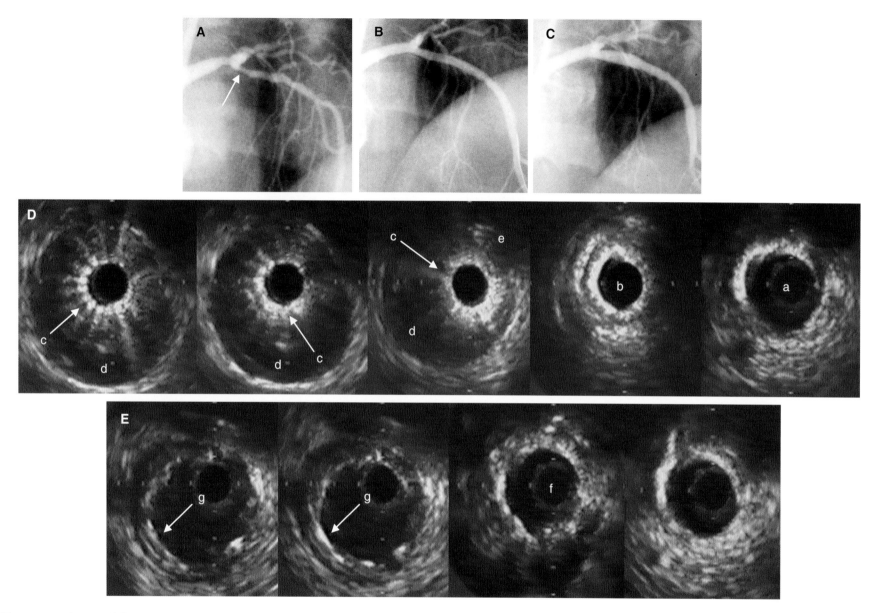

Figure 7.54 This ostial left anterior descending stenosis (white arrow in Panel A) was treated with rotational atherectomy and stent implantation with the result shown in Panel B. At this point, IVUS (Panel D) showed the distal vessel (a), an unstented calcified ostium of the left anterior descending (b), and an unexpanded stent (c) in the left main (d). (Note the left circumflex, e.) Presumably, contact of the stent with the calcified ostial left anterior descending lesion stripped the stent from the balloon. The unexpanded stent (c) stayed in the left main (d) while the balloon was advanced into the anterior descending artery. The angiographic improvement in the proximal left anterior descending lesion was the result of balloon dilation, not stent implantation. The ostial lesion was then vigorously pre-dilated, a stent was delivered successfully, and the stent in the left main was expanded against the vessel wall. The final result is shown in Panels C and E. Note the stented ostial left anterior descending (f) and the expanded stent in the left main artery (g) without malapposition

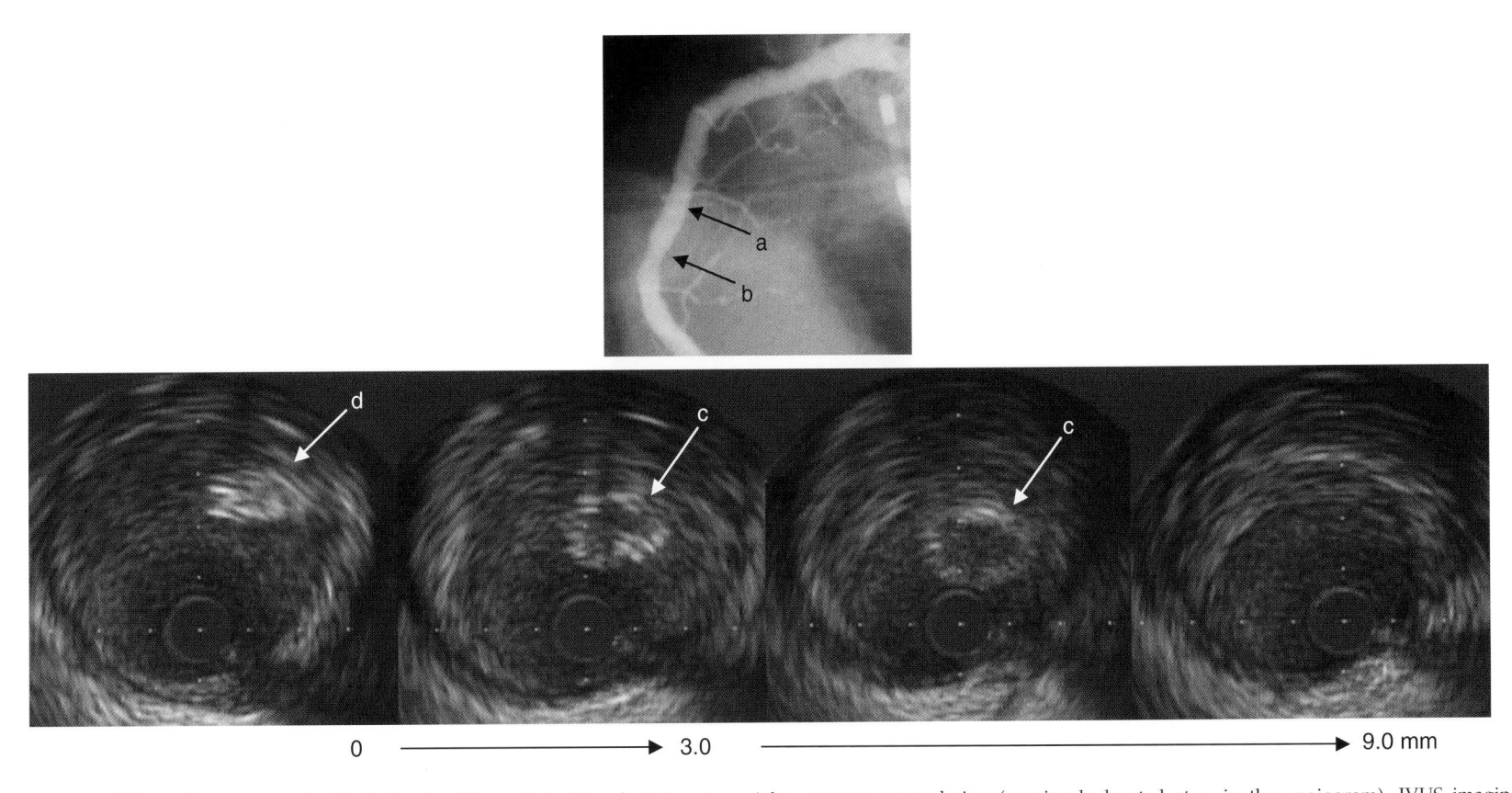

Figure 7.55 This patient presented with ischemia 48 h post-stent implantation in a right coronary artery lesion (previously located at a, in the angiogram). IVUS imaging (corresponding to b in the angiogram) showed an underexpanded, stripped stent (c) that presumably came off the balloon during the stent implantation procedure. Note that the proximal portion of this stripped stent (d) is crushed. There was no flow-limiting stenosis. Presumably, the unexpanded stent metal was a nidus for platelet aggregation/adhesion and embolization that was responsible for the ischemia

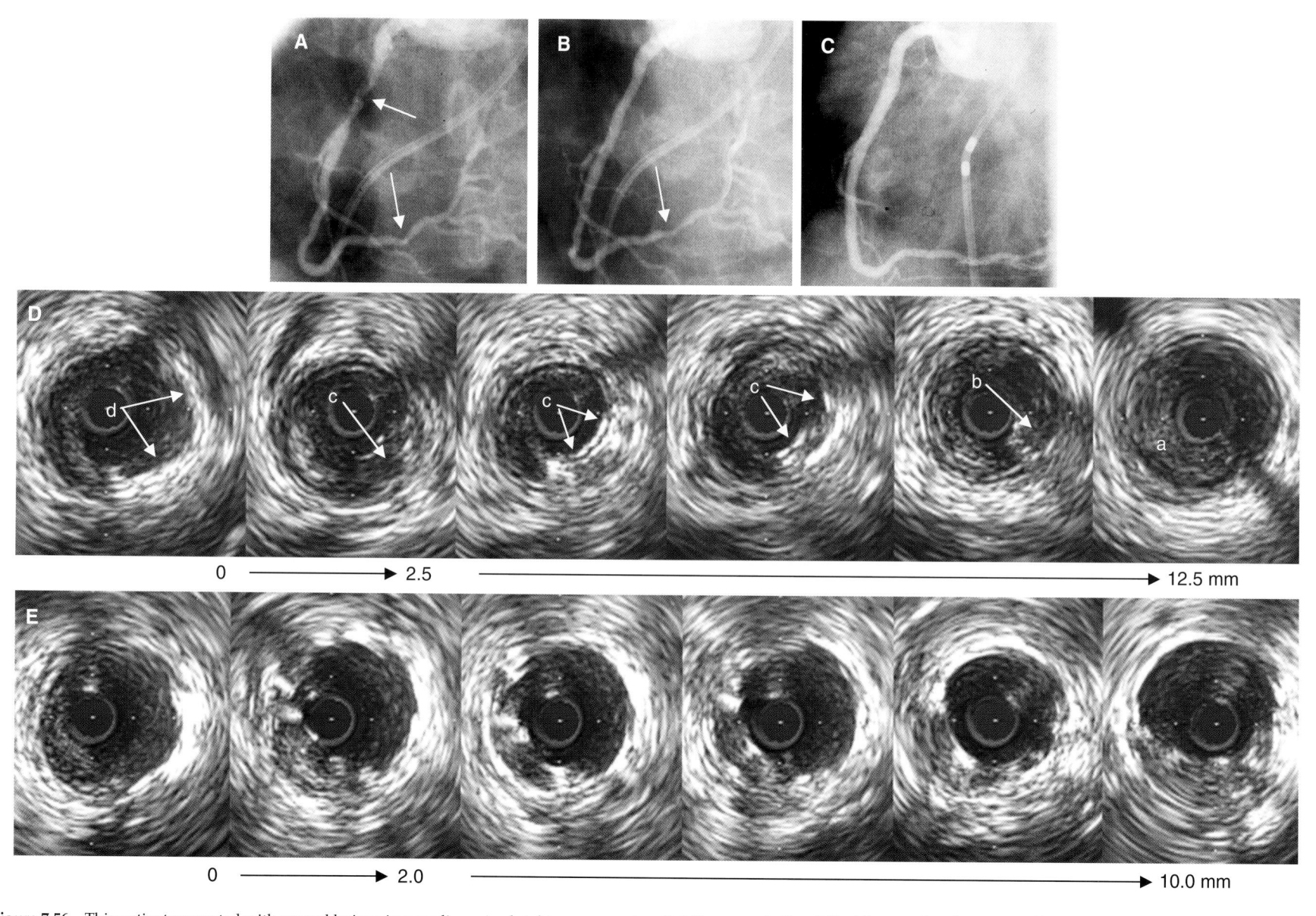

Figure 7.56   This patient presented with several lesions in a medium-sized right coronary artery (white arrows in Panel A). After stenting the proximal lesion, it was difficult to deliver multiple different stents to the distal lesion (white arrow in Panel B). IVUS imaging of the distal lesion (Panel D) showed a distal intramural hematoma (a), a stripped unexpanded distal edge of a stent (b), a partially expanded, partially crushed middle and proximal part of a stent (c), and an expanded, fully crushed proximal part of the stent (d). Another stent was implanted, and the final angiogram (Panel C) and final IVUS (Panel E) of this lesion are shown

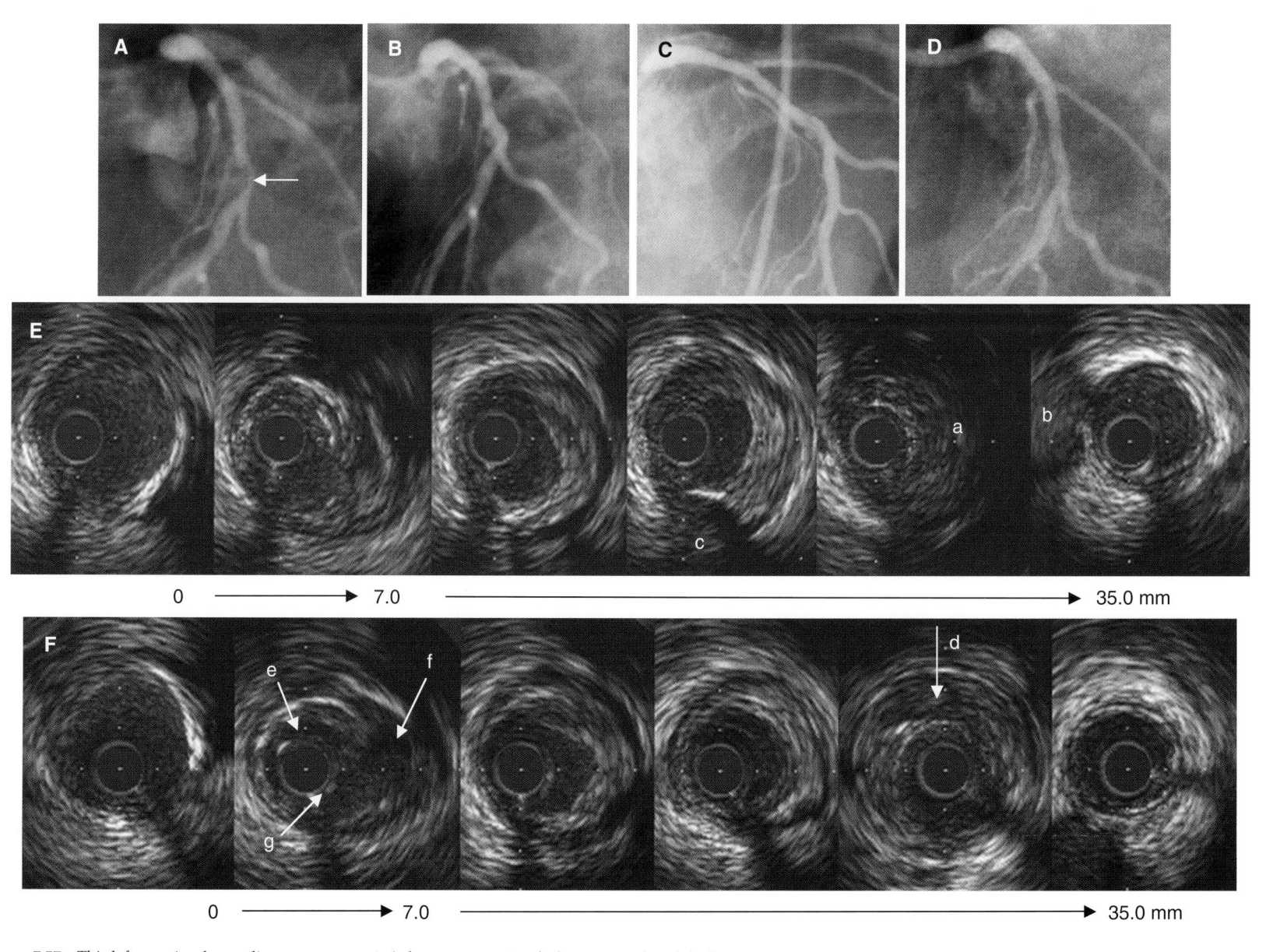

Figure 7.57   This left anterior descending artery stenosis (white arrow in Panel A) was treated with balloon angioplasty (Panels B and C). The pre-intervention IVUS is shown in Panel E; note the eccentric plaque (a) opposite the diagonal branch (b) and the septal perforator (c) at the proximal end of the stenosis. The post-balloon angioplasty IVUS is shown in Panel F. There was one superficial, intraplaque dissection at the lesion (d), where the minimum lumen CSA measured 3.6 mm^2, and another superficial, intraplaque dissection proximally, where the true lumen CSA (e) measured 2.7 mm^2; the false lumen CSA (f) measured 2.8 mm^2, and the dissection flap (g) abutted the IVUS catheter. Stents were implanted, with the final result shown in Panel D

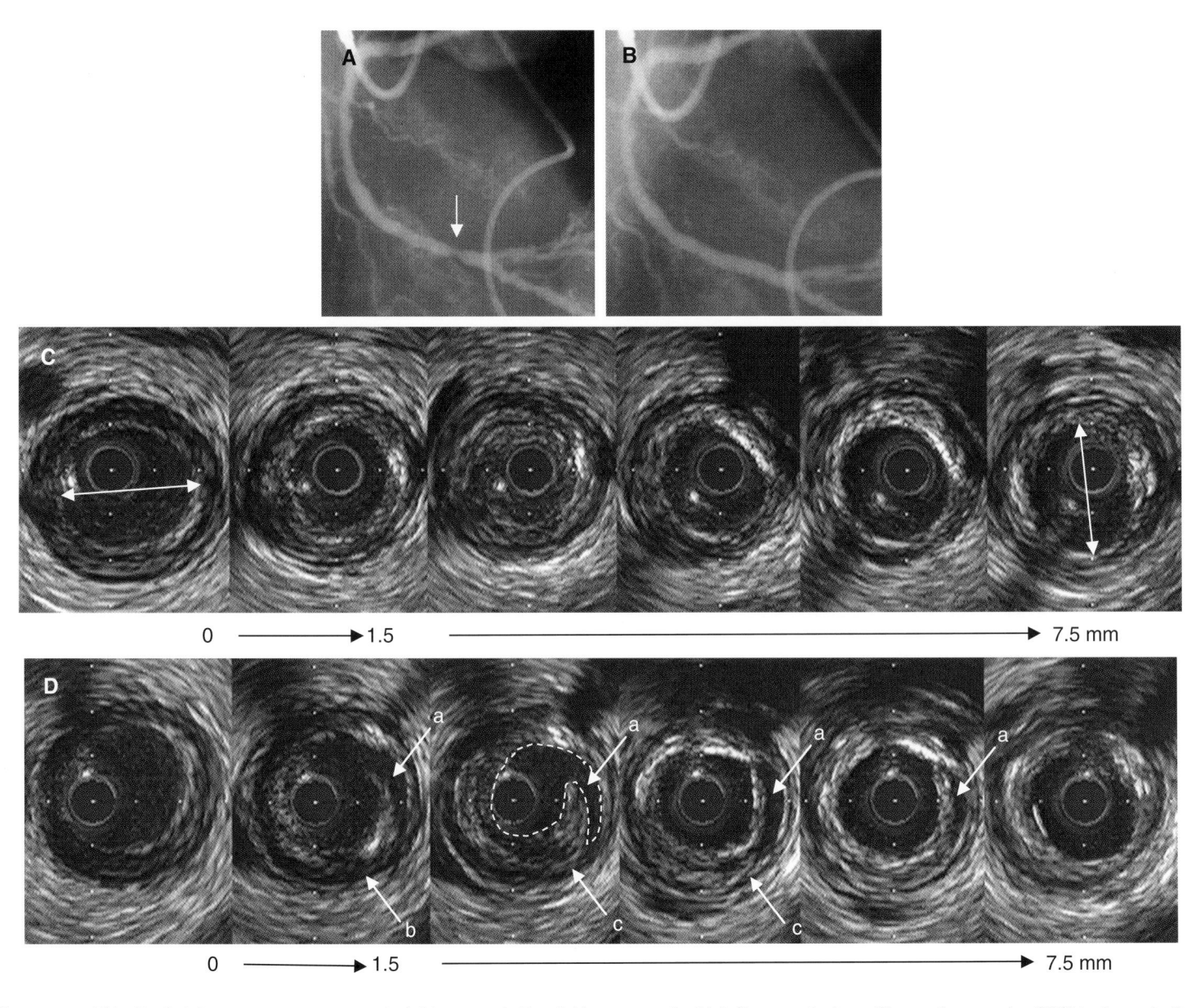

Figure 7.58   This distal right coronary artery stenosis (white arrow in Panel A) was treated with balloon angioplasty. The pre-intervention IVUS is shown in Panel C; note the negative remodeling (remodeling index = 0.83). The post-balloon angioplasty IVUS is shown in Panel D; even including the dissection plane (a), the minimum lumen CSA (dashed white line) measured only 3.6 mm^2, i.e. 28% of the EEM CSA and 55% of the mean reference-lumen CSA. The dissection extended down to the media proximally (b), but not distally (the dissection plane does not communicate with the media, c). Based on the pre-intervention maximum reference-lumen diameter (which measured 3.0 mm both proximal and distal to the lesion, double-headed white arrows in Panel C), a 3.0 mm stent was implanted at 18 atm. The final angiogram is shown in Panel B. The final stent CSA (not shown) measured 6.0 mm^2, i.e. 92% of the mean reference-lumen CSA

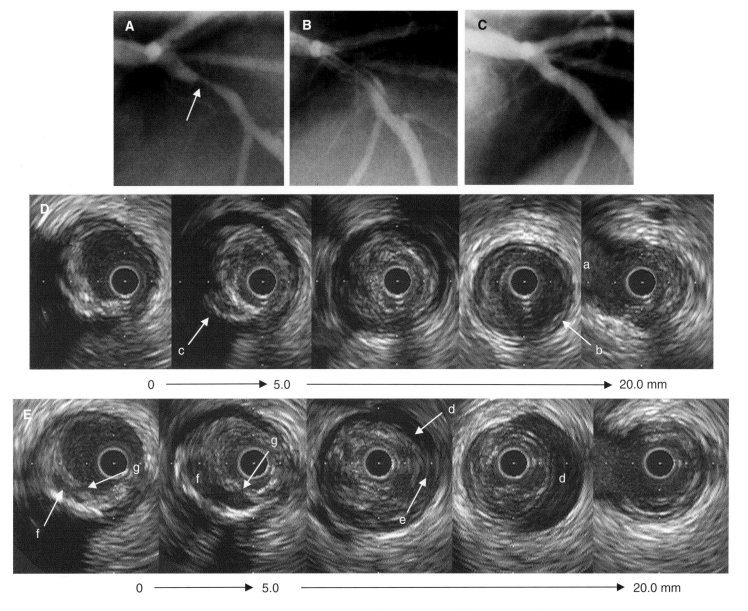

Figure 7.59 This left anterior descending artery stenosis (white arrow in Panel A) was treated with balloon angioplasty (Panel B). The pre-intervention IVUS is shown in Panel D; note the large septal perforator (a), an arc of near-normal vessel wall (b) distal to the stenosis, and deep calcium (c) proximal to the stenosis. The post-balloon angioplasty IVUS is shown in Panel E; note the extensive medial dissection (d) at the site of the pre-intervention normal vessel wall with its entrance (e) and the intraplaque dissection (f) with its entrance (g) at the site of the pre-intervention deep calcium. A 5.0 mm stent was implanted at 16 atm with the final angiogram as shown in Panel C and an IVUS final lumen CSA of 8.2 mm^2 (not shown)

Figure 7.60 (opposite)   Pre-dilation of these two lesions in the right coronary artery (white arrows in Panel A) caused an extensive dissection between the white arrows in Panel B. Three stents were implanted, with the result shown in Panel C. At this point, IVUS imaging (Panel E) showed a long, severe dissection between the proximal stent (a) and the middle stent (b). There was a bulky dissection flap (c) caused by plaque that had detached from the arterial wall at the level of the media (d) and curled around the IVUS catheter (e). A fourth stent was implanted, and the IVUS was repeated (Panel F). Although much shorter, there was still a dissection plane (f) that separated the narrowed true lumen (g) from the false lumen (h). The true lumen (dashed white line) measured only 2.7 mm^2. A fifth stent was implanted that totally covered the dissection; the final angiogram is shown in Panel D

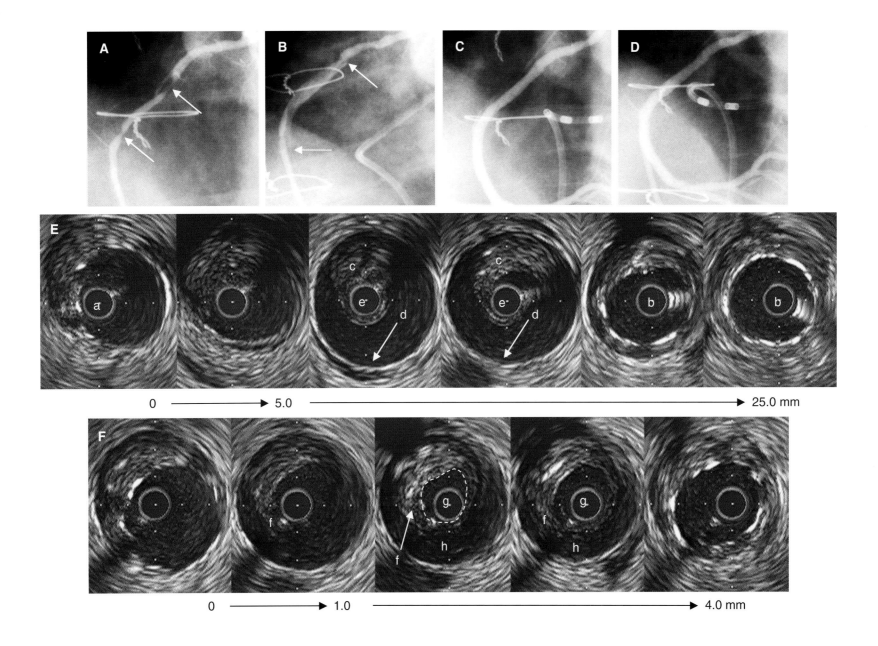

Figure 7.61 (opposite)   This ostial major marginal branch stenosis (white arrow in Panel A) was pre-dilated, with the angiographic result shown in Panels B and C. At this point, the IVUS (Panel E) showed a true lumen (a), a false lumen that contained echolucent contrast or saline (b) and blood stasis (c) proximally, and the tissue plane (d) that separated the true lumen from the false lumen and that wrapped around the IVUS catheter. The IVUS catheter was in the true lumen in each image slice, even when the lumen was occlusive (e). Also note the break in the vessel wall (f) with extravasation of echolucent contrast or saline (g). 3.5 mm stents were implanted at 18 atm, with the final angiographic result as shown in Panel D and the final IVUS as shown in Panel F. The minimum stent CSA (dashed white line) at the ostium of the major marginal branch measured only 5.3 mm^2 at the end of the procedure. Note the large plaque burden (h) at the site of the minimum stent CSA and the residual extravasated contrast or saline (i) outside of the vessel

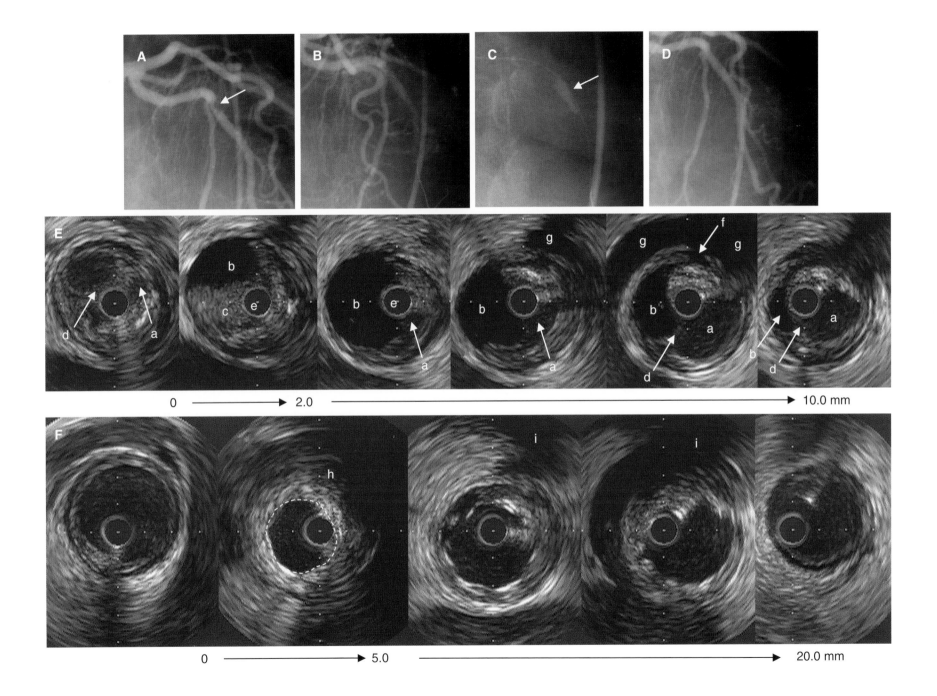

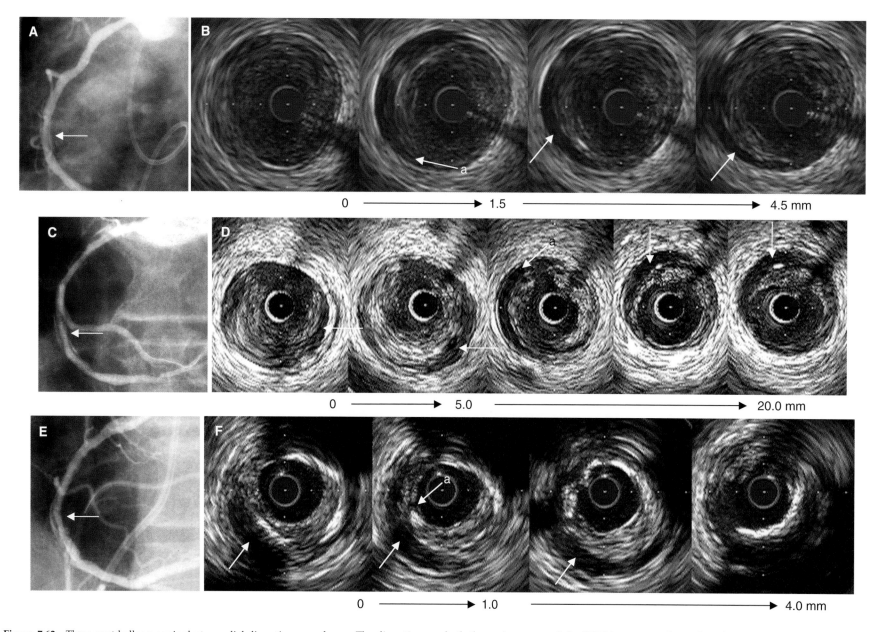

Figure 7.62 Three post-balloon angioplasty medial dissections are shown. The dissections on both the angiograms and the IVUS images are shown by white arrows. It may be difficult to distinguish a medial dissection from a thick-appearing media. Two helpful hints are (1) to search for an entrance point to the dissection (shown by a in all three examples) and (2) to look for blood speckle in the dissection

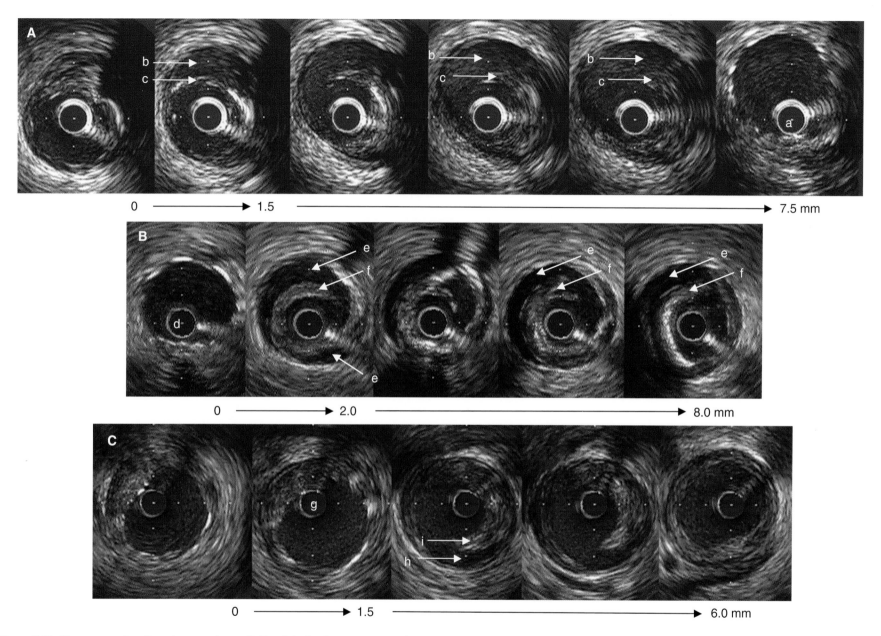

Figure 7.63 Three stent edge dissections are shown. In Panel A, the dissection was at the proximal edge of the stent (a). Note the dissection plane (b) and the tissue flap (c). The lumen CSA measured 4.5 mm², which is less than half of the CSA of the distal edge of the stent (10.9 mm²). Another stent was implanted. In Panel B, the dissection was at the distal edge of the stent (d). Note the dissection plane (e) and the mobile tissue flap (f) that curled around the IVUS catheter. Another stent was implanted. In Panel C, the dissection was also at the distal edge of the stent (g). Note the dissection plane (h) and the tissue flap (i). The tissue flap was short, non-mobile, occupied less than 90° of the arterial circumference, and did not compromise the lumen (the lumen CSA measured 7.5 mm²). Another stent was not implanted. In Panels A and B, part of the dissection plane was shadowed by calcium; nevertheless, this did not preclude detection and assessment of the stent edge dissection

Figure 7.64 (opposite)   This figure shows two examples of dissection between fibrocalcific plaque and either non-fibrocalcific plaque or undiseased vessel wall. The right coronary artery in Panel A was treated with rotational atherectomy and balloon angioplasty. The IVUS (Panel B) showed calcium proximally (a) and distally (b) that made assessment of the dissection difficult. However, between these two calcific deposits, there was a short segment of artery where careful interrogation showed two dissection planes (c and d). In the second example, the left anterior descending lesion (white arrow in Panel C) was dilated, with the angiographic result shown in Panel D. The IVUS (Panel E) showed a dissection at the junction of fibrocalcific plaque and normal vessel wall. Note that the outward expansion of the normal vessel wall (e) compared with the edges of the fibrocalcific plaque (f) caused a separation between the plaque and the vessel wall (g) at the level of the media that tracked distally (h and i). It is probable that the dissection was also present in the segment of vessel that was shadowed (j) by the calcium. Both lesions were stented

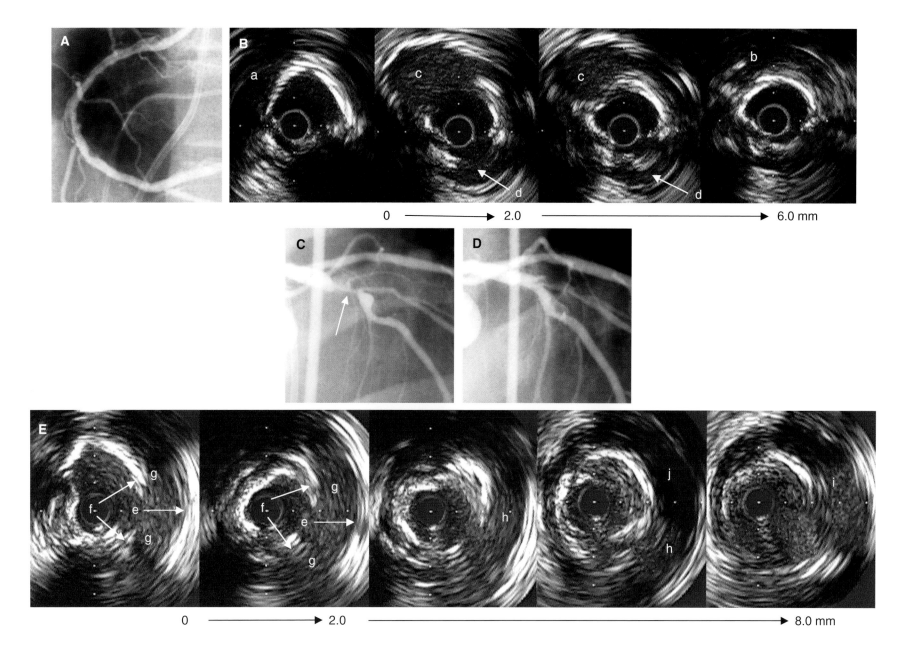

Figure 7.66 (opposite)   A patient presented with this ostial left anterior descending lesion (white arrow in Panel A). Pre-intervention IVUS imaging of the left anterior descending artery (Panel D) showed an eccentric fibrocalcific lesion (a) with superficial calcium (b) opposite the left circumflex (c). Note the calcific plaque (d) that appeared to narrow the ostium of the left circumflex (e) just distal to the left main artery (f). Owing to concern about the ostium of the left circumflex, the guidewire was repositioned into the circumflex to perform another IVUS imaging run. IVUS of the circumflex (Panel E) showed a fibrocalcific mass (g) at the ostium. Although the minimum lumen CSA was difficult to measure, it was felt to be adequate. Note the relationship of the left anterior descending (h) and the left main (i). The patient was first treated with rotational atherectomy. The angiographic result is shown in Panel B. Note the hazy appearance at the origin of the left circumflex (j), the dissection into the proximal circumflex (k), and the narrowing of the distal left main (l). IVUS was performed (see Panel A in Figure 7.67). Stents were implanted into both the left circumflex (first) and the left anterior descending (second), and IVUS was repeated (see Figure 7.67). The final angiographic result is shown here in Panel C

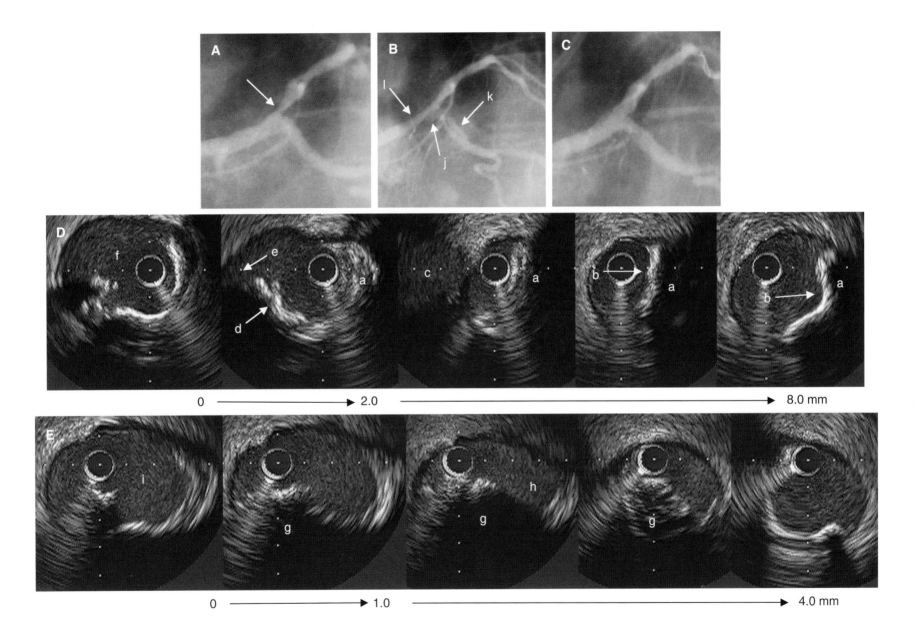

Figure 7.67 (opposite)   The post-intervention IVUS sequence of the patient in Figure 7.66 is shown. Panel A (which corresponds to Panel B in Figure 7.66) was recorded from the left anterior descending artery back into the left main. In the left anterior descending, IVUS showed the reverberations typical of rotational - atherectomy-treated calcium (a) and a dissection into the plaque (b) opposite to the left circumflex (c). Throughout the left main, IVUS showed an intramural hematoma (d) that was associated with straightening of the intimal border (e) and a reduction in lumen dimensions compared with pre-intervention (see Figure 7.66). At this point, the left circumflex was not imaged. Instead, a stent was first implanted into the left circumflex. IVUS (Panel B) showed a dissection in the proximal circumflex (f) covered by the stent as well as the dissection within the normal intima of the left main (h) that created the intramural hematoma. Note the location of the left anterior descending (g). A stent was then placed into the left anterior descending. IVUS (Panel C) showed stenting of the left anterior descending (i) across the left circumflex (j) back into the left main artery (k). The final angiographic result is shown in Figure 7.66

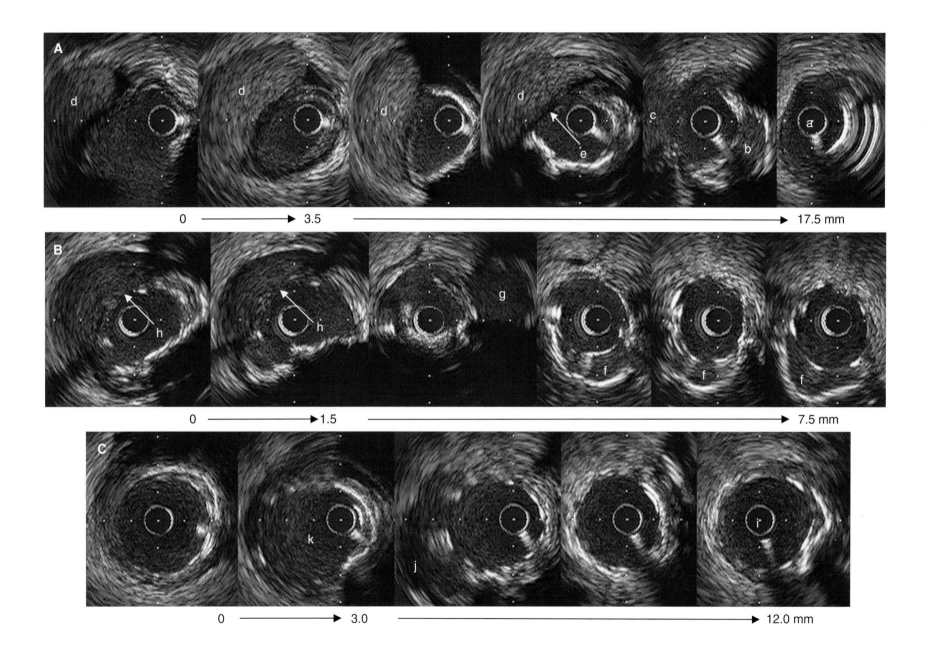

Figure 7.68 (opposite)   This patient presented with a proximal left anterior descending stenosis (white arrow in Panel A) distal to the major diagonal branch. Pre-intervention IVUS (Panel D) showed a lesion with fibrocalcific plaque (a) and shadowing (b) distal to the major diagonal branch (c). The minimum lumen CSA measured 3.1 mm². The distal-reference maximum lumen diameter (double-headed white arrow) measured 3.5 mm. Note that the distal reference contained large arcs of normal vessel wall (d). A 3.5 mm stent was implanted. The angiographic result is shown in Panel B; note the appearance of a severe stenosis distal to the original stenosis. IVUS imaging (Panel E) showed an intramural hematoma (e) distal to the stent (f). The hematoma developed in the arc of normal vessel wall opposite the calcific plaque (g). Note that the calcific plaque (h) also caused asymmetry of the distal end of the stent (i), that the hematoma stopped at the edge of the calcium, and that the hematoma caused straightening of the intima (white arrow in Panel E). The minimum lumen CSA measured 2.3 mm². Another stent was implanted with the final angiographic result shown in Panel C

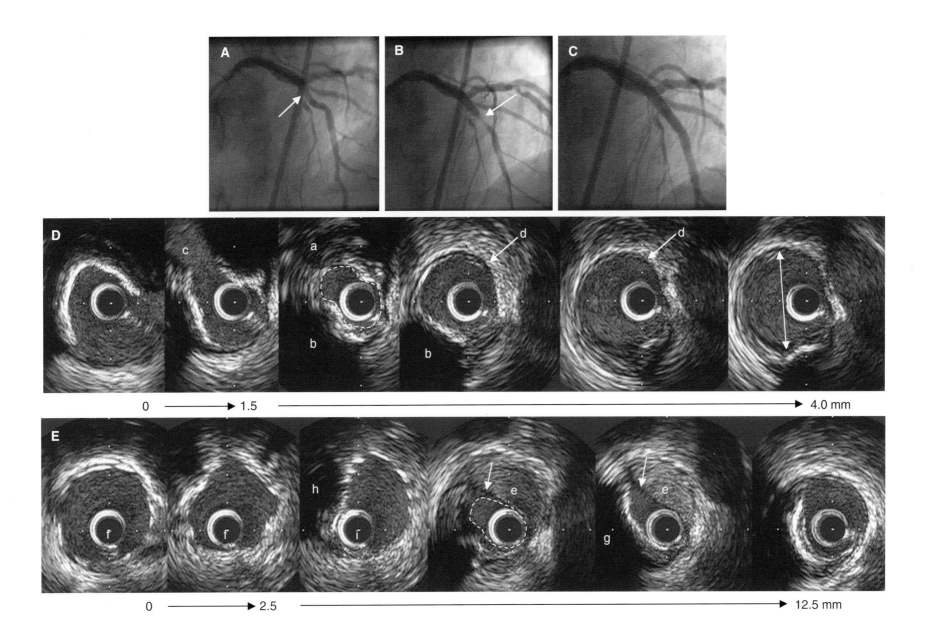

Figure 7.69 (opposite)   Three examples of an intramural hematoma are shown: Panel A after stent implantation, Panel B after cutting balloon, and Panel C after rotational atherectomy. Note in each case the hematoma (a), loss of the normal echolucent medial stripe that defines the junction between media and adventitia, causing an indistinct border between the hematoma and the adjacent peri-advential structures (b), and straightening of the intima (c). These findings are consistent whenever an intramural hematoma occurs

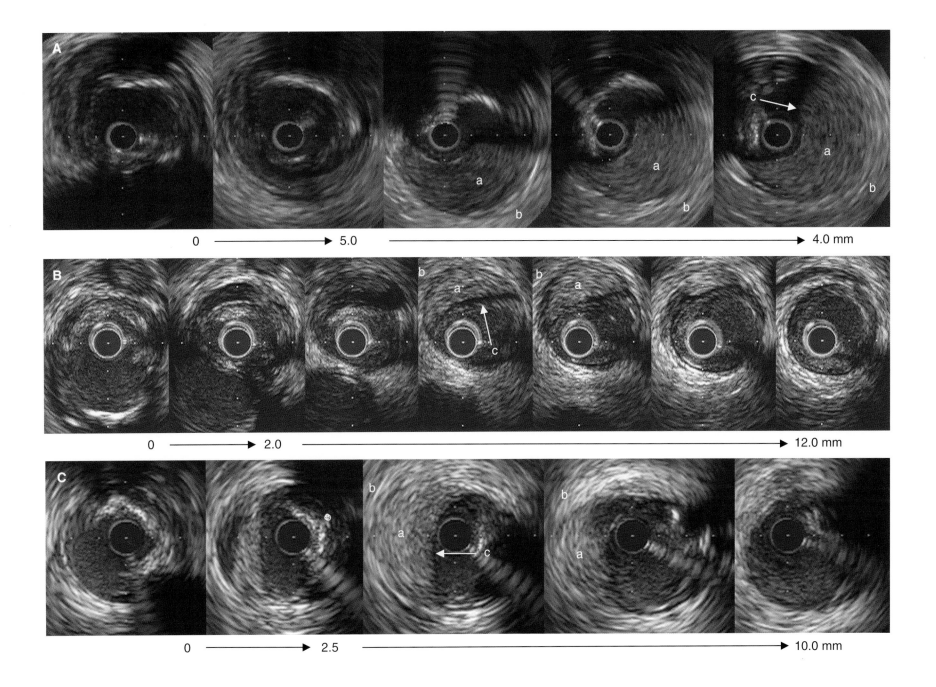

Figure 7.70 (opposite)   These four intramural hematomas were associated with angiographic contrast staining. Each IVUS image shows a split in the media, with an echogenic hematoma and a sharply defined echolucent zone indicating trapped contrast, saline, or (potentially) serum. The higher the transducer frequency, the greater is the intensity of the blood stasis and the less is its granular appearance; this causes the hematoma to become visually more continuous with the peri-advential structures. In Panel A, the hematoma occurred at the distal edge of a stent (a). Note the entrance to the hematoma (b), accumulated blood stasis (c), and the trapped contrast and/or saline (d). The hematoma occupied the newly created space in the media to separate the intima (e) from the adventitia (f). In Panel A, the hematoma tracked distally, but stopped at the diagonal branch (g). In Panel B, a very short segment of artery is displayed in order to illustrate the "to-and–fro" motion of the interface between the static blood (h) and the trapped contrast and/or saline (i). Notice that the loss of the echolucent media causes the interface between the hematoma (h) and the peri-adventitia (j) to become blurred. This hematoma developed during balloon angioplasty. The intramural hematoma in Panel C also developed during balloon angioplasty. Note the entrance to the hematoma (k), a second small dissection (l), the accumulated blood (m), the visually continuous peri-adventitial structures (n), a small amount of trapped contrast (o), and the straightening of the intimal border (p). The somewhat atypical hematoma in Panel D occurred at the proximal end of a stent (q). Note the small, unusually shaped accumulation of blood (r), the echolucent zone (s), and the bowed intimal border (t). The narrowed lumen is outlined by a dashed white line

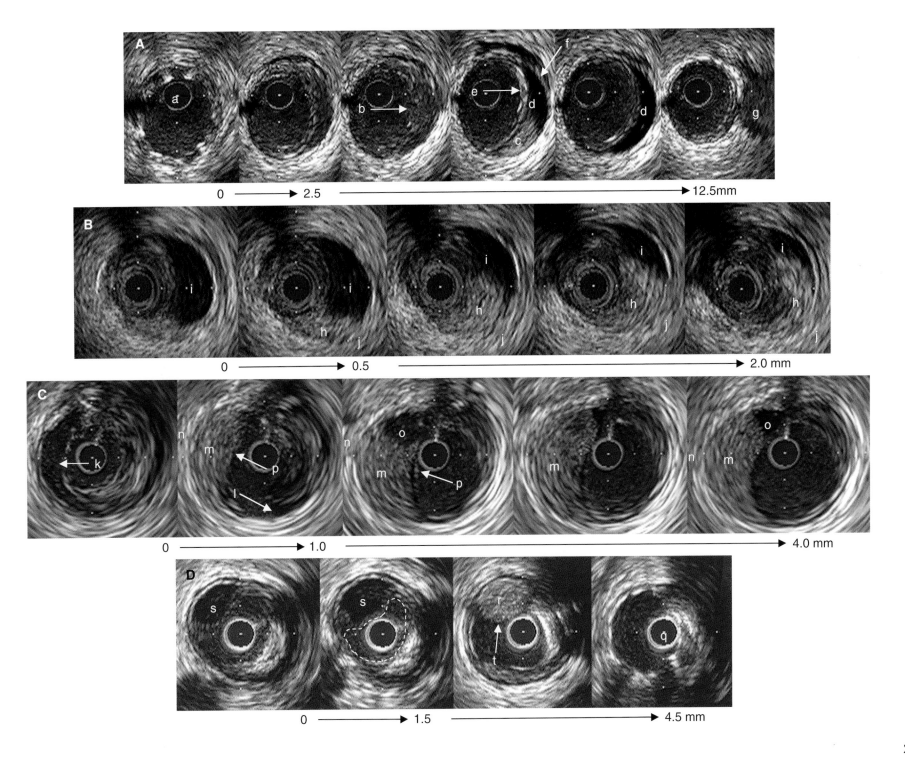

Figure 7.71 (opposite)   These angiographic series from four patients (#1–#4) illustrate different angiographic appearances of an intramural hematoma. Row A shows the pre-intervention angiogram, with the lesion indicated by a white arrow. The lesion in the left circumflex from Patient #1 and the lesion in the left anterior descending from Patient #2 were both treated with balloon angioplasty; the lesion in the left anterior descending from Patient #3 and the ostial right coronary artery lesion in Patient #4 were both treated with stent implantation. The site of each hematoma is shown by the white arrows in Row B. The final results after implantation of initial or additional stents is shown in Row C

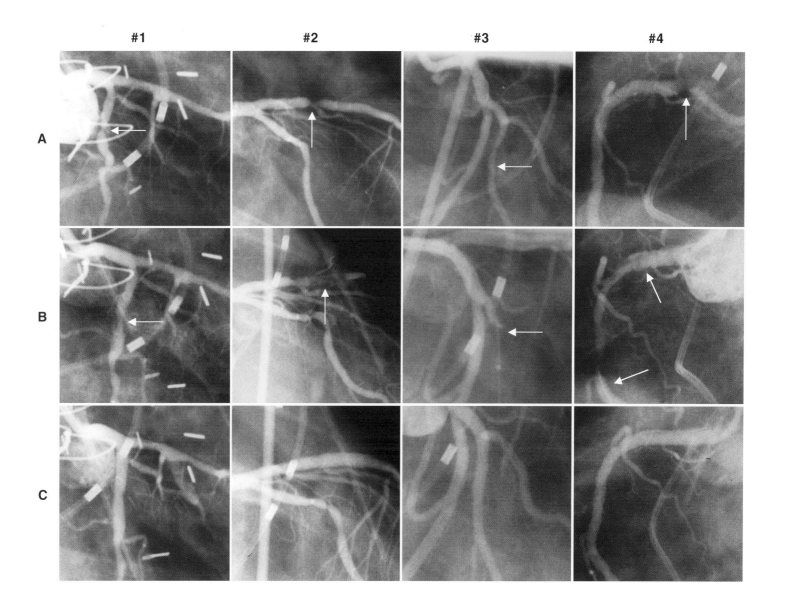

Figure 7.72 (opposite) This ostial left anterior descending artery lesion (white arrow in Panel A) was treated with excimer laser angioplasty, resulting in a perforation. Note the contrast extravasation in Panel B (white arrows). The pre-intervention IVUS is shown in Panel D. Note the distal reference (a), where the lumen CSA and EEM CSA measured 5.2 mm^2 and 13.8 mm^2, respectively, the left circumflex artery (b); and an ostial lesion that contained hypoecholic plaque (c), an echolucent zone (d), and an arc of normal vessel wall (e). Post-laser angioplasty IVUS (Panel E) showed a gap in the EEM (f) at the distal end of the lesion and in the adjacent reference segment; extravasation of blood (g) that tracked distally (h); and at i (compared with the equivalent pre-intervention image slide, a), a reduction in the lumen CSA to 2.6 mm^2 and in the EEM CSA to 11.2 mm^2, caused by compression of the artery by the extravasated blood. The perforation occurred in the arc of normal vessel wall noted in the pre-intervention IVUS study. Two overlapping conventional bare-metal stents were implanted, and the final angiogram is shown in Panel C. Note the residual extravasated contrast (white arrow)

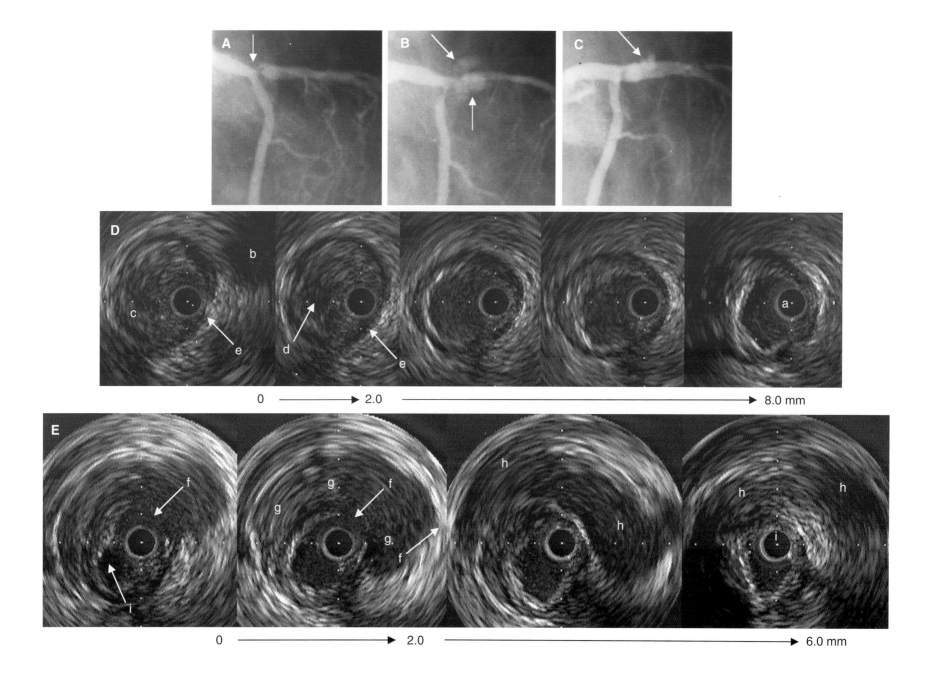

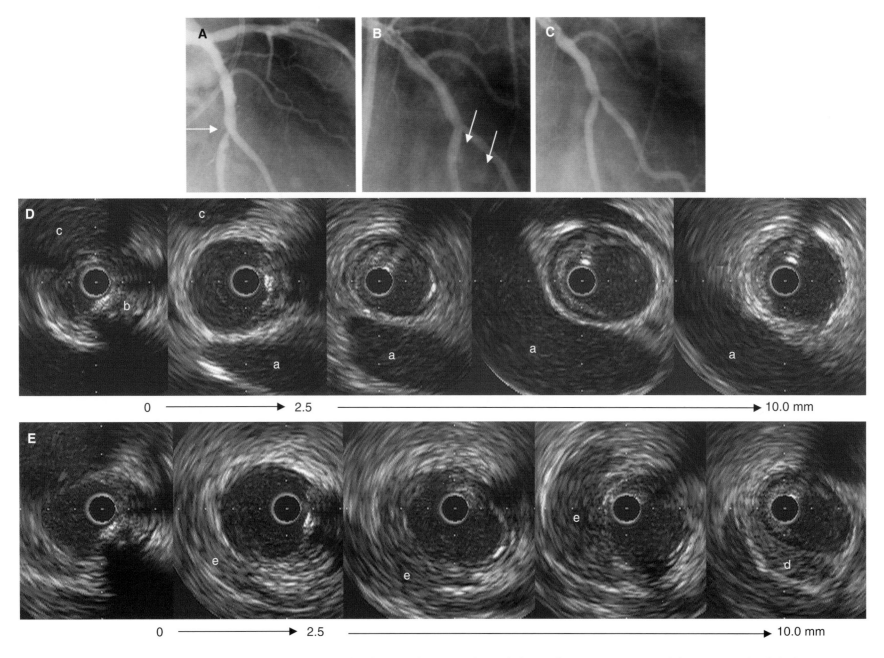

Figure 7.73 This left circumflex lesion (white arrow in Panel A) was treated with excimer laser angioplasty, which caused contrast extravasation (white arrows in Panel B). The pre-intervention IVUS is shown in Panel D; note the cardiac vein (a), the eccentric plaque (b), and the circumflex proximal to the bifurcation (c). The IVUS in Panel E corresponds to the angiogram in Panel B. Note the extramural hematoma (d) and blood extravasation (e), although the exact site of perforation is not seen. Conventional bare-metal stents were implanted (Panel C)

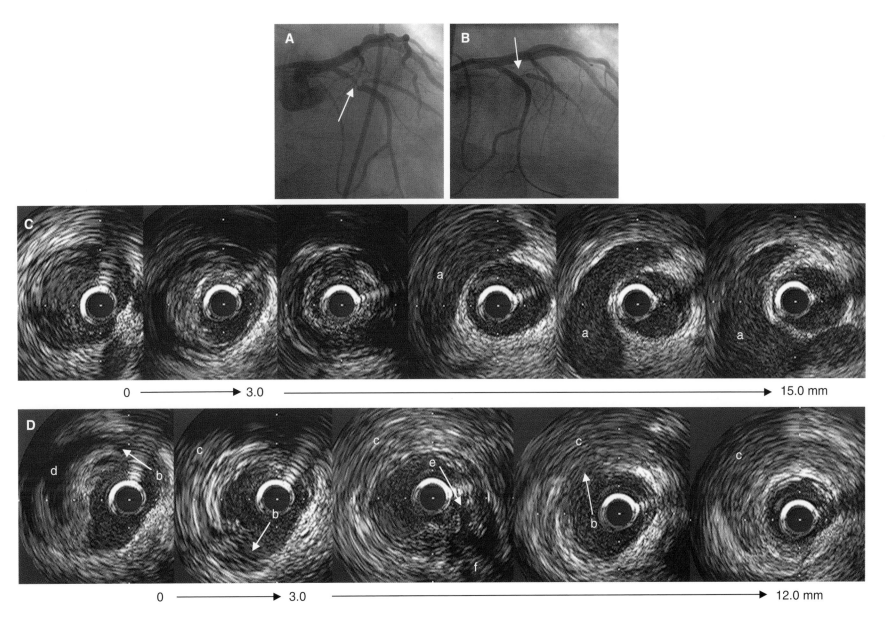

Figure 7.74 This left circumflex lesion (white arrow in Panel A) was treated with cutting balloon angioplasty, causing contrast extravasation (the angiogram is not shown). The pre-intervention IVUS is shown in Panel C; note the great cardiac vein (a). the post cutting ballon IVUS is shown in Panel D. The cutting balloon caused breaks in the arterial wall (b), resulting in extravasation of blood (c) and contrast or saline (d), probably into the cardiac vein as well as into the peri-adventitial spaces. Note the radial dissection into plaque (e) at the site of the marginal branch (f). Multiple conventional bare-metal stents were implanted (Panel B); there was compromise of the marginal branch at the end of the procedure (white arrow in Panel B)

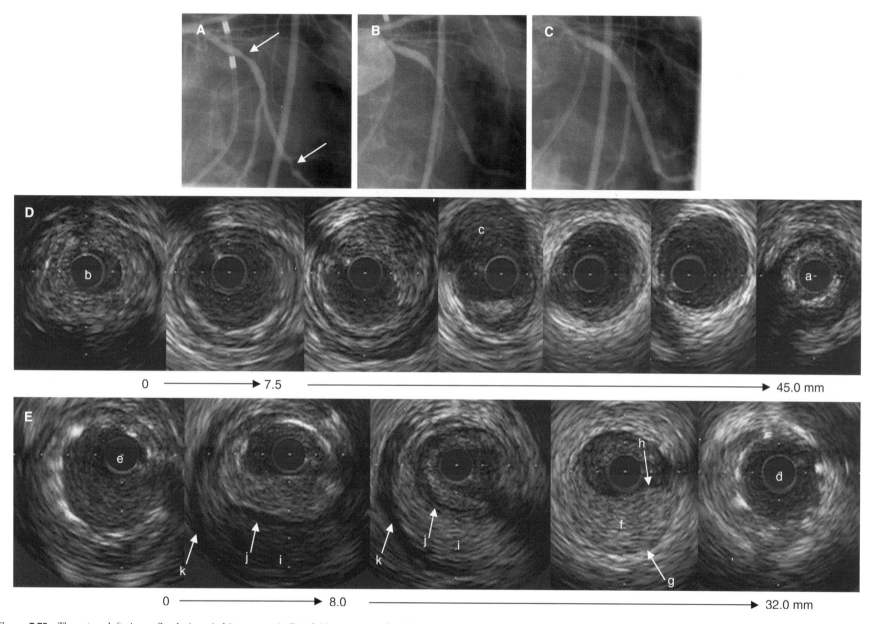

Figure 7.75 These two left circumflex lesions (white arrows in Panel A) were treated with stent implantation, resulting in the angiogram shown in Panel B. The pre-intervention IVUS in Panel D showed a distal, negatively remodeled lesion (a) and a proximal, positively remodeled lesion (b); note the location of the continuation of the left circumflex in the atrioventricular groove (c). Panel E shows the IVUS corresponding to the angiogram in Panel B; note the distal stent (d) and the proximal stent (e). Between the two stents, there was an intramural hematoma (f) that displaced the EEM (g) outward and the intima (h) inward to almost completely occlude the lumen; an extramural hematoma (i) that displaced the EEM (j) inward; and a new echolucent interface (k) that was not present pre-intervention and that, based on examples such as Figure 7.77, may represent contrast or saline extravasation. Additional stents were implanted, with the final result shown in Panel C

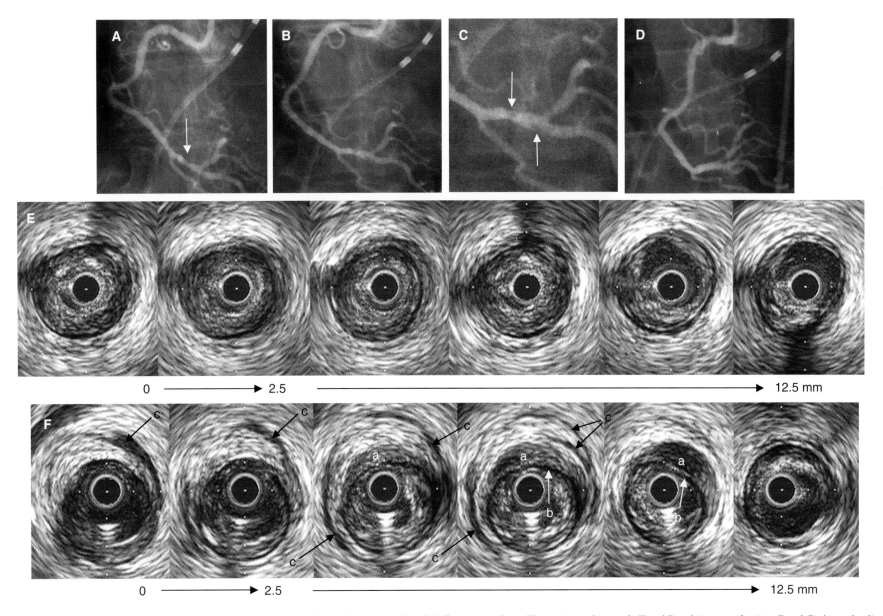

Figure 7.76   This distal right coronary artery lesion (white arrow in Panel A) was treated with balloon angioplasty. The angiographic result (Panel B and its magnification, Panel C) showed a dissection and a subtle filling defect (white arrows). The pre-intervention IVUS is shown in Panel E; and the post-balloon angioplasty IVUS (corresponding to the angiograms in Panels B and C) is shown in Panel F. Note the extramural hematoma (a) that displaced the media and EEM (b) inward and a new, peri-adventitial echolucent interface (c) that was not evident in the pre-intervention IVUS. Based on examples such as Figure 7.77, this new echolucent interface appears to represent contrast extravasation. A 3.0 mm stent was implanted, with the result shown in Panel D

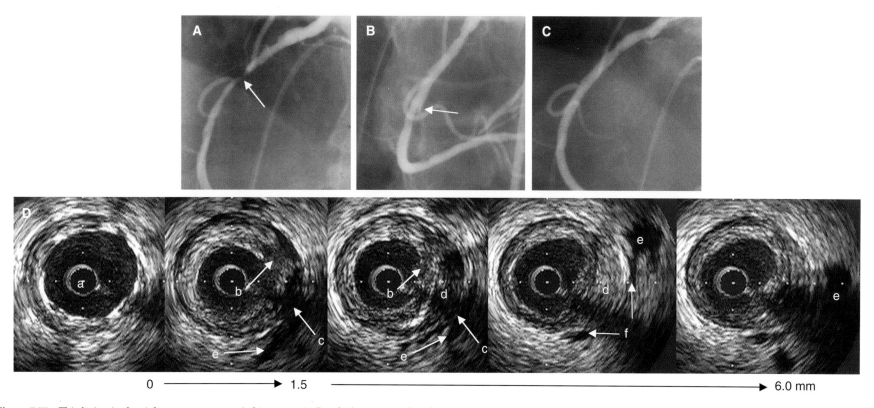

Figure 7.77   This lesion in the right coronary artery (white arrow in Panel A) was treated with stent implantation, after which there was angiographic evidence of perforation (white arrow in Panel B). The IVUS showed the distal edge of the stent (a), disruption of the plaque (b) through to the EEM (c), development of an intramural hematoma (d), and extravasation of contrast (e). The extravasated contrast created a peri-adventitial echolucent layer (f) similar to that shown in Figures 7.75 and 7.76. Another conventional bare-metal stent was implanted, and the angiographic result is shown in Panel C

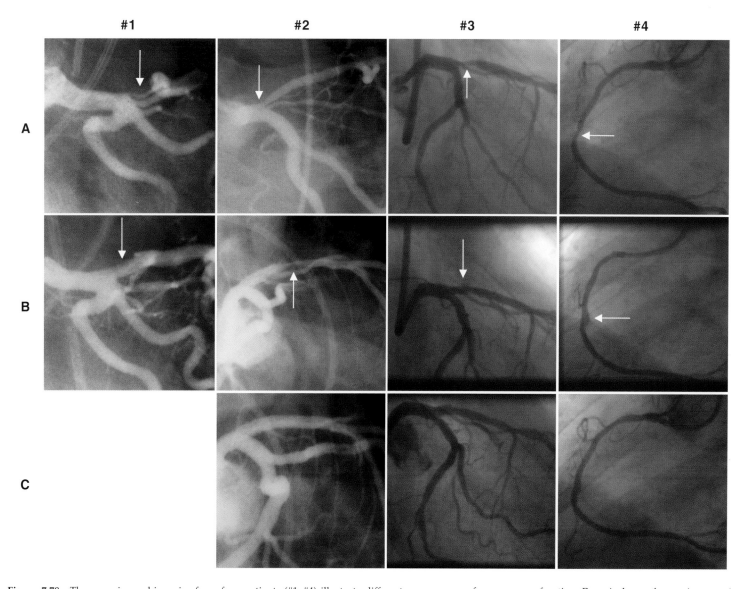

Figure 7.78   These angiographic series from four patients (#1–#4) illustrate different appearances of coronary perforation. Row A shows the pre-intervention angiogram, with the lesion indicated by a white arrow. The lesions in the left anterior descending from Patients #1–#3 were all treated with directional coronary atherectomy; the lesion in the right coronary artery from Patient #4 was treated with the cutting balloon. The site of each perforation is shown by the white arrows in Row B. The results after stent implantation in Patients #2–#4 are shown in Row C

Figure 7.79 (opposite) This right coronary artery (Panel A) contained two lesions (a) and (b). Stents were implanted into both (Panel B). There was "haziness" at the end of the distal stent (3.5 mm diameter implanted at 16 atm) – at the distal bifurcation of the right coronary artery (white arrow in Panel B). A magnification of this segment is shown in Panel C. The pre-intervention IVUS of the distal lesion is shown in Panel D. (The pre- and post-intervention IVUS of the more proximal lesion are shown in Figure 7.80.) In Panel D, note the hypoechoic, eccentric lesion (a) with a ruptured plaque (b); this lesion had positive remodeling characteristics and a maximum reference-lumen diameter (double-headed white arrow) of 3.3 mm. The post-intervention IVUS of the distal lesion is shown in Panel E. Note the bifurcation of the distal right coronary artery (c), the posterior left ventricular branch (d), and the distal end of the stent (e). Despite the angiographic appearance, there was no lumen compromise at the distal edge of the stent. The minimum lumen CSA measured 8.6 mm^2. Compare the pre-intervention IVUS of this distal lesion with the more proximal lesion shown in Figure 7.80. Even in the same artery in the same patient, two different lesions will often have different pre-intervention features such as remodeling, eccentricity, and plaque composition

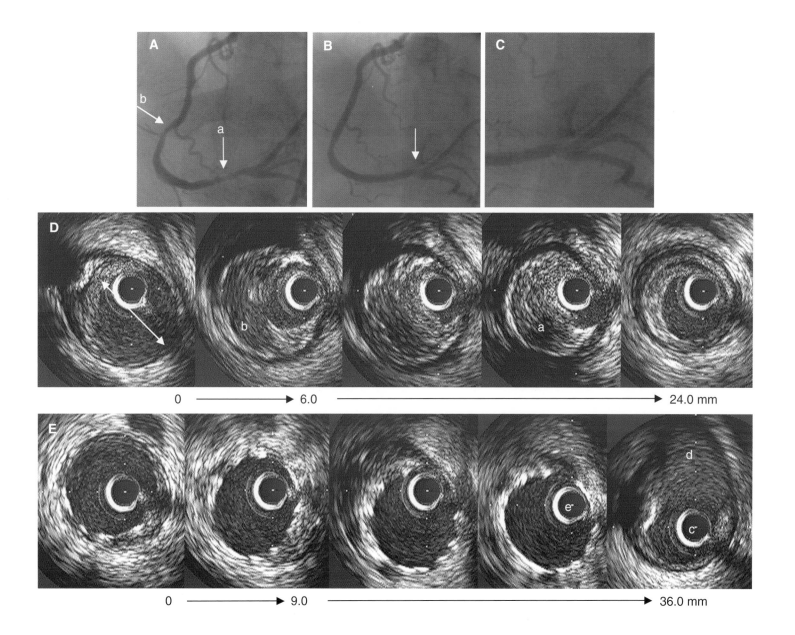

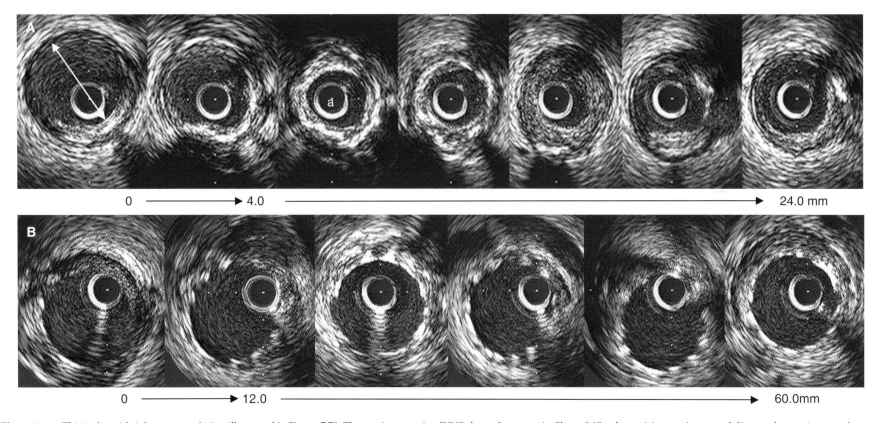

Figure 7.80 This is the mid right coronary lesion illustrated in Figure 7.79. The pre-intervention IVUS showed concentric, fibrocalcific plaque (a), negative remodeling, and a maximum reference-lumen diameter of 3.4 mm. A 3.5 mm stent was implanted at 16 atm, and the post-intervention IVUS is shown in Panel B. The minimum lumen CSA measured 9.0 mm^2. Even in the same artery in the same patient, two different lesions will often have different pre-intervention features such as remodeling, eccentricity, and plaque composition. In fact, the concordance is typically only 50%. Compare this lesion with the one illustrated in Figure 7.79

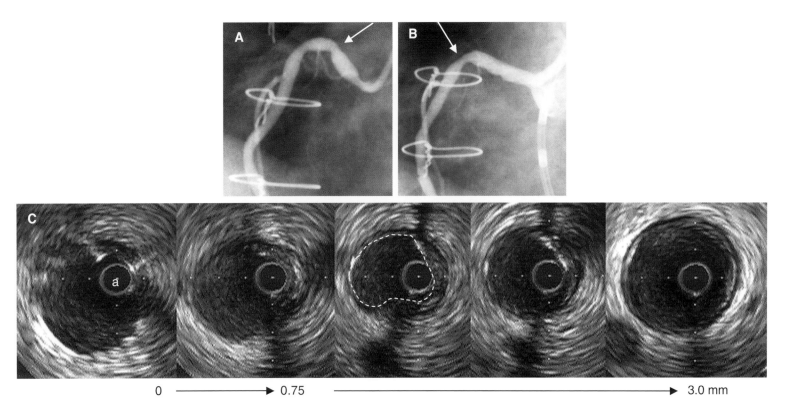

Figure 7.81 This very proximal right coronary artery lesion (white arrow in Panel A) was treated with stent implantation. The post-intervention angiogram showed angiographic evidence of a decrease in lumen dimensions at the distal end of the stent at the bend in the artery (white arrow in Panel B). The post-intervention IVUS (Panel C) showed no evidence of lumen compromise, dissection, or significant plaque burden distal to the distal edge of the stent (a). The lumen CSA (dashed white line) measured 6.3 mm^2 and the plaque burden measured 35%

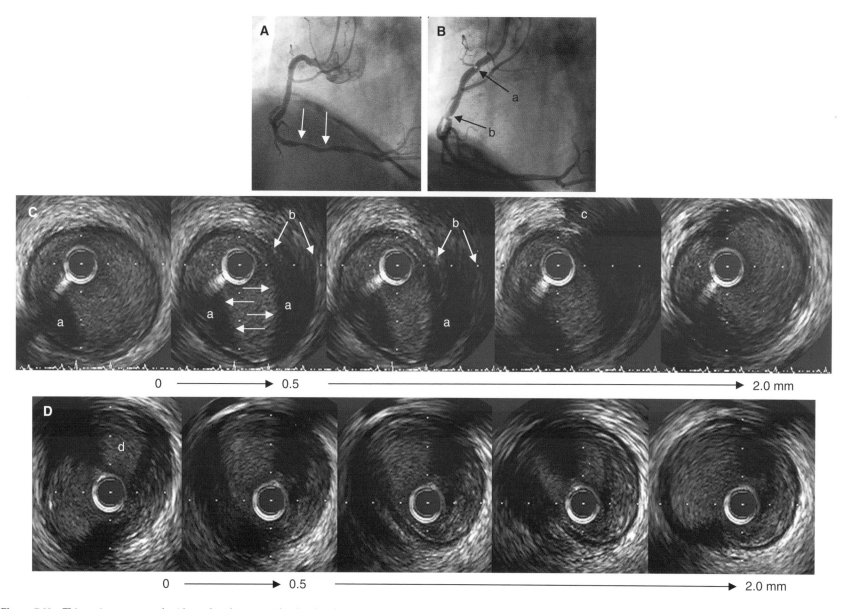

Figure 7.82 This patient presented with tandem lesions in the distal right coronary artery (white arrows in Panel A). After wiring the artery, two new lesions appeared in the proximal and mid right coronary artery (a and b in Panel B). The IVUS in Panel C corresponded to lesion a in Panel B, and the IVUS in Panel D corresponded to lesion b in Panel B. As seen in Panel C, over a very short distance, there was narrowing of the lumen, straightening of a normal-appearing intima (white arrows), behind which there was an echolucent zone (a) that extended almost entirely to the EEM without shadowing or attenuation of the EEM, and (b) a discontinuity of the EEM caused by the fold in the artery. The beam width of the IVUS transducer allowed the adventitia on both sides of the fold to be visualized simultaneously to create this appearance of discontinuity. Note the small atrial branch (c). The IVUS findings in Panel D were identical although unlabeled; note the location of the right ventricular branch (d). This has been called a wrinkled or accordion appearance; it is caused by straightening of the artery, usually by a stiff guidewire (This example was courtesy of Satoru Sumitsuji)

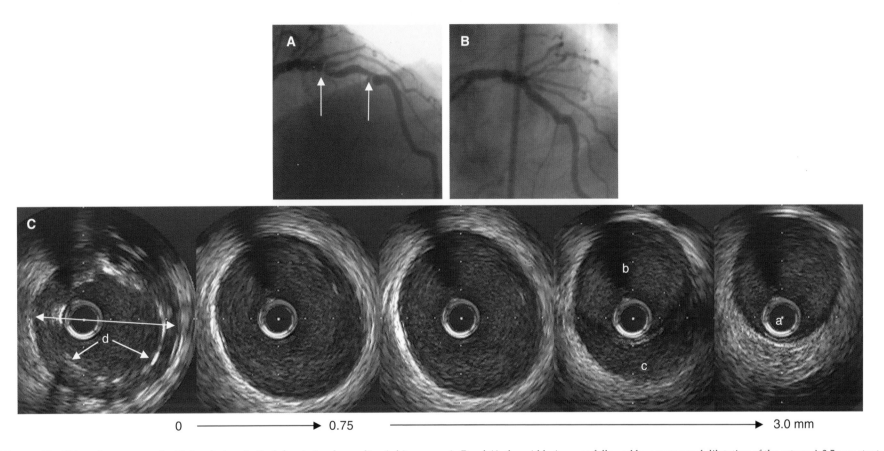

Figure 7.83 This patient presented with two lesions in the left anterior descending (white arrows in Panel A); the mid lesion was followed by aneurysmal dilatation of the artery. A 3.5 mm stent was implanted and post-dilated to 4.0 mm at 18 atm (Panel B). The post-intervention IVUS (Panel C) showed a normal distal reference (a), a slice through the artery at which the oblique angle of the transducer imaged both the true lumen (b) and part of the "aneurysm", creating the false impression of an intramural hematoma (c), and malapposition of the very distal end of the stent (d). As shown by the double-headed white arrow, it would have taken a 5.0 mm balloon to appose the stent to the intima

REFERENCES

1. Colombo A, Hall P, Nakamura S, et al. Intracoronary stenting without anticoagulation accomplished with intravascular ultrasound guidance. Circulation 1995; 91: 1676–88
2. Ahmed JM, Mintz GS, Weissman NJ, et al. Mechanism of lumen enlargement during intracoronary stent implantation: an intravascular ultrasound study. Circulation 2000; 102: 7–10
3. von Birgelen C, Mintz GS, Eggebrecht H, et al. Preintervention arterial remodeling affects vessel stretch and plaque extrusion during coronary stent deployment as demonstrated by three-dimensional intravascular ultrasound. Am J Cardiol 2003; 92: 130–5
4. Tobis JM, Mallery JA, Gessert J, et al. Intravascular ultrasound cross-sectional arterial imaging before and after balloon angioplasty in vitro. Circulation 1989; 80: 873–82
5. Davidson CJ, Sheikh KH, Kisslo KB, et al. Intracoronary ultrasound evaluation of interventional technologies. Am J Cardiol 1991; 68: 1305–9
6. Potkin BN, Keren G, Mintz GS, et al. Arterial responses to balloon coronary angioplasty: an intravascular ultrasound study. J Am Coll Cardiol 1992; 20: 942–51
7. Tenaglia AN, Buller CE, Kisslo KB, et al. Mechanisms of balloon angioplasty and directional coronary atherectomy as assessed by intracoronary ultrasound. J Am Coll Cardiol 1992; 20: 685–91
8. Braden GA, Herrington DM, Downes TR, et al. Qualitative and quantitative contrasts in the mechanisms of lumen enlargement by coronary balloon angioplasty and directional coronary atherectomy. J Am Coll Cardiol 1994; 23: 40–8
9. Honye J, Mahon DJ, Jain A, et al. Morphological effects of coronary balloon angioplasty in vivo assessed by intravascular ultrasound imaging. Circulation 1992; 85: 1012–25
10. Mintz GS, Pichard AD, Kent KM, et al. Axial plaque redistribution as a mechanism of percutaneous transluminal coronary angioplasty. Am J Cardiol 1996; 77: 427–30
11. Kearney P, Erbel R, Rupprecht HJ, et al. Differences in the morphology of unstable and stable coronary lesions and their impact on the mechanisms of angioplasty. An in vivo study with intravascular ultrasound. Eur Heart J 1996; 17: 721–30
12. Fitzgerald PJ, Ports TA, Yock PG. Contribution of localized calcium deposits to dissection after angioplasty. An observational study using intravascular ultrasound. Circulation 1992; 86: 64–70
13. Lee RT, Richardson G, Loree HM, et al. Prediction of mechanical properties of human atherosclerotic tissue by high-frequency ultrasound imaging. An in vitro study. Arterioscler Thromb 1992; 12: 1–5
14. Lee RT, Loree HM, Cheng GC, et al. Computational structural analysis based on intravascular ultrasound imaging before in vitro angioplasty: prediction of plaque fractures. J Am Coll Cardiol 1993; 21: 777–82
15. Nishida T, Colombo A, Briguori C, et al. Outcome of nonobstructive residual dissections detected by intravascular ultrasound following percutaneous coronary intervention. Am J Cardiol 2002; 89: 1257–62
16. Schroeder S, Baumbach A, Mahrholdt H, et al. The impact of untreated coronary dissections on acute and long-term outcome after intravascular ultrasound-guided PTCA. Eur Heart J 2000; 21: 92–4
17. Meerkin D, Tardif JC, Bertrand OF, et al. The effects of intracoronary brachytherapy on the natural history of postangioplasty dissections. J Am Coll Cardiol 2000; 36: 59–64
18. Stone GW, Hodgson JMcB, St Goar FG, et al. Improved procedural results of coronary angioplasty with intravascular ultrasound-guided balloon sizing; the CLOUT Pilot Trial. Circulation 1997; 95: 2044–52
19. Stone GW, Frey A, Linnemeier T, et al. 2.5 year follow-up of the CLOUT study – long-term implications for an aggressive IVUS-guided balloon angioplasty study. J Am Coll Cardiol 1999; 33: 81A
20. Abizaid A, Pichard AD, Mintz GS, et al. Acute and long-term results of an IVUS-guided PTCA/provisional stent implantation strategy. Am J Cardiol 1999; 84: 1381–4
21. Schroeder S, Baumbach A, Haase KK, et al. Reduction of restenosis by vessel size adapted percutaneous transluminal coronary angioplasty using intravascular ultrasound. Am J Cardiol 1999; 83: 875–9
22. Baumbach A, Schroeder S, Athanasiadis A, et al. Ultrasound guidance: technique and results of aggressive-guided PTCA. The UPSIZE Pilot Trial. Int J Cardiovasc Intervent 2001; 4: 115–19
23. Schiele F, Meneveau N, Gilard M, et al. Intravascular ultrasound-guided balloon angioplasty compared with stent: immediate and 6-month results of the multicenter, randomized Balloon Equivalent to Stent Study (BEST). Circulation 2003; 107: 545–51
24. Frey AW, Hodgson JMcB, Muller C, et al. Ultrasound-guided strategy for provisional stenting with focal balloon combination catheter: results from the randomized Strategy for Intracoronary Ultrasound-guided PTCA and Stenting (SIPS) Trial. Circulation 2000; 102: 2497–502
25. Barath P, Fishbein MC, Vari S, et al. Cutting balloon: a novel approach to percutaneous angioplasty. Am J Cardiol 1991; 68: 1249–52
26. Okura H, Hayase M, Shimodozono S, et al. Mechanisms of acute lumen gain following cutting balloon angioplasty in calcified and noncalcified lesions: an intravascular ultrasound study. Catheter Cardiovasc Interv 2002; 57: 429–36
27. Hara H, Nakamura M, Asahara T, et al. Intravascular ultrasonic comparisons of mechanisms of vasodilatation of cutting balloon angioplasty versus conventional balloon angioplasty. Am J Cardiol 2002; 89: 1253–6
28. Liao CK, Bonneau HN, Yock PG, et al. Arterial response during cutting balloon angioplasty: a volumetric intravascular ultrasound study. J Formos Med Assoc 2002; 101: 756–61
29. Rizik DG, Popma JP, Leon MB, et al. Benefits of cutting balloon before stenting. J Invasive Cardiol 2003; 15: 624–8
30. Mintz GS, Pichard AD , Kovach JA, et al. Impact of pre-intervention intravascular ultrasound imaging on transcatheter treatment stategies in coronary artery disease. Am J Cardiol 1994; 73: 423–30
31. Matar FA, Mintz GS, Farb A, et al. The contribution of tissue removal to lumen improvement after directional coronary atherectomy. Am J Cardiol 1994; 74: 647–50
32. Umans VA, Baptista J, DiMario C, et al. Angiographic, ultrasonic, and angioscopic assessment of the coronary artery wall and lumen area configuration after directional atherectomy: the mechanism revisited. Am Heart J 1995; 130: 217–27
33. Popma JJ, Mintz GS, Satler LF, et al. Clinical and angiographic outcome after directional coronary atherectomy: a qualitative and quantitative analysis using coronary arteriography and intravascular ultrasound. Am J Cardiol 1993; 72: 55E–64E
34. Matar FA, Mintz GS, Pinnow E, et al. Multivariate predictors of intravascular ultrasound endpoints after directional coronary atherectomy. J Am Coll Cardiol 1995; 25: 318–24
35. Mintz GS, Pichard AD, Popma JJ, et al. Preliminary experience with adjunct directional coronary atherectomy following high-speed rotational atherectomy in the treatment of calcific coronary artery disease. Am J Cardiol 1993; 71: 799–804
36. Foreman DW, Mitchell JC, Baker PB. Physical chemical evidence of structural weakness in coronary arterial calcification. Cardiovasc Res 1989; 23: 64–9
37. Marisco F, Kubica J, De Servi S, et al. Influence of plaque morphology on the mechanism of liminal enlargement after directional coronary atherectomy and balloon angioplasty. Br Heart J 1995; 74: 134–9
38. Bauman R, Yock PG, Fitzgerald PJ, et al. "Reference cut" method of intracoronary ultrasound-guided directional coronary atherectomy: initial and six months results. Circulation 1995; 92: I-546
39. Mintz GS, Popma JJ, Pichard AD, et al. Intravascular ultrasound predictors of restenosis following percutaneous transcatheter coronary revascularization. J Am Coll Cardiol 1996; 27: 1678–87
40. The GUIDE trial investigators. IVUS-determined predictors of restenosis in PTCA and DCA: Final report from the GUIDE Trial. J Am Coll Cardiol 1996; 27: 156A
41. Lansky AJ, Mintz GS, Popma JJ, et al. Remodeling after directional coronary atherectomy (with and without adjunctive percutaneous coronary angioplasty): a serial angiographic and intravascular ultrasound analysis from the Optimal Atherectomy Restenosis Study. J Am Coll Cardiol 1998; 32: 329–37
42. Suzuki T, Hosakawa H, Katoh O, et al. Effects of adjunctive balloon angioplasty after intravascular ultrasound-guided directional coronary atherectomy: the results of Adjunctive Balloon Angioplasty After Coronary Atherectomy Study (ABACAS). J Am Coll Cardiol 1999; 343: 1028–35

43. Hong MK, Mintz GS, Lee CW, et al. Incidence, mechanism, predictors, and long-term prognosis of late stent malapposition after bare-metal stent implantation. Circulation 2004; 109: 881–6

44. Kiesz RS, Rozek MM, Mego DM, et al. Acute directional coronary atherectomy prior to stenting in complex coronary lesions: ADAPTS Study. Catheter Cardiovasc Interv 1998; 45: 105–12

45. Moussa I, Moses J, DiMario C, et al. Stenting after optimal lesion debulking (SOLD) resigtry. Angiographic and clinical outcome. Circulation 1998; 98: 1604–9

46. Hu F-B, Tamai H, Kosuga K, et al. Intravascular ultrasound-guided directional coronary atherectomy for unprotected left main coronary stenosis with distal bifurcation involvement. Am J Cardiol 2003; 92: 936–40

47. Park SJ, Hong MK, Lee CW, et al. Elective stenting of unprotected left main coronary artery stenosis: effect of debulking before stenting and intravascular ultrasound guidance. J Am Coll Cardiol 2001; 38: 1054–60

48. Kovach JA, Mintz GS, Pichard AD, et al. Sequential intravascular ultrasound characterization of the mechanisms of rotational atherectomy and adjunct balloon angioplasty. J Am Coll Cardiol 1993; 22: 1024–32

49. Dussaillant GR, Mintz GS, Pichard AD, et al. Effect of rotational atherectomy in noncalcified atherosclerotic plaque: a volumetric intravascular ultrasound study. J Am Coll Cardiol 1996; 28: 856–60

50. Whitbourn RJ, Sethi R, Pomerantsev EV, et al. High-speed rotational atherectomy and coronary stenting: QCA and QCU analysis. Catheter Cardiovasc Interv 2003; 60: 167–71

51. Moussa I, Di Mario C, Moses J, et al. Coronary stenting after rotational atherectomy in calcified and complex lesions. Angiographic and clinical follow-up results. Circulation 1997; 96: 128–36

52. Hoffmann R, Mintz GS, Popma JJ, et al. Treatment of calcified coronary lesions with Palmaz–Schatz stents. An intravascular ultrasound study. Eur Heart J 1999; 19: 1224–31

53. Henneke KH, Regar E, Konig A, et al. Impact of target lesion calcification on coronary stent expansion after rotational atherectomy. Am Heart J 1999; 137: 93–9

54. Dussaillant GD, Mintz GS, Pichard AD, et al. Mechanisms and acute and long term results of adjunctive directional atherectomy after rotational atherectomy. J Am Coll Cardiol 1996; 27: 1390–7

55. Hoffmann R, Mintz GS, Kent KM, et al. Comparative early and 9-month results of rotational atherectomy, stents, and the combination for calcified lesions in large coronary arteries. Am J Cardiol 1998; 81: 552–7

56. Kobayashi Y, De Gregorio J, Kobayashi N, et al. Lower restenosis rate with stenting following aggressive versus less aggressive rotational atherectomy. Catheter Cardiovasc Interv 1999; 46: 406–14

57. Mintz GS, Kovach JA, Javier SP, et al. Mechanisms of lumen enlargement after excimer laser coronary angioplasty: An intravascular ultrasound study. Circulation 1995; 92: 3408–14

58. Honye J, Mahon DJ, Nakamura S, et al. Intravascular ultrasound imaging after excimer laser angioplasty. Cathet Cardiovasc Diagn 1994; 32: 213–22

59. Isner JM, Rosenfield K, Losordo DW. Excimer laser atherectomy (The greening of Sisyphus). Circulation 1990; 81: 2018–20

60. van Leeuwen TG, van Erven L, Meertens JH, et al. Origin of arterial wall dissections induced by pulsed excimer and mid-infrared laser ablation in the pig. J Am Coll Cardiol 1992; 19: 1610–18

61. van Leeuwen TG, Meertens JH, Velema E, et al. Intraluminal vapor bubble induced by excimer laser pulse causes microsecond arterial dilation and invagination leading to extensive wall damage in the rabbit. Circulation 1993; 87: 1258–63

62. Maehara A, Takagi A, Okura H, et al. Longitudinal plaque redistribution during stent expansion. Am J Cardiol 2000; 86: 1069–72

63. Prati F, Pawlowski T, Gil R, et al. Stenting of culprit lesions in unstable angina leads to a marked reduction in palque burden: a major role of plaque embolizaion? A serial intravacular ultrasound study. Circulation 2003; 107: 2320–5

64. Kotani J, Mintz GS, Pregowski J, et al. Volumetric intravascular ultrasound evidence that distal embolization during acute infarction intervention contributes to inadequate myocardial perfusion grade. Am J Cardiol 2003; 92: 728–32

65. Tanaka A, Kawarabayashi T, Nishibori Y, et al. No-reflow phenomenon and lesion morphology in patients with acute myocardial infarction. Circulation 2002; 105: 2148–52

66. Fukuda D, Tanaka A, Shimada K, et al. Predicting angiographic distal embolization following percutaneous coronary intervention in patients with acute myocardial infarction. Am J Cardiol 2003; 91: 403–7

67. Watanabe T, Nanto S, Uematsu M, et al. Prediction of no-reflow phenomenon after successful percutaneous coronary intervention in patients with acute myocardial infarction: intravascular ultrasound findings. Circ J 2003; 67: 667–71

68. Kotani J, Mintz GS, Castagna MT, et al. Usefulness of preprocedural coronary lesion morphology as assessed by intravasuclar ultrasound in predicting thrombolysis in myocardial infarction frame count after percutaneous coronary intervention in patients with Q-wave acute myocardial infarction. Am J Cardiol 2003; 91: 870–2

69. Kotani J, Mintz GS, Castagna MT, et al. Relation of plaque morphology to thrombolysis in myocardial infarction flow in acute myocardial infarction determined by intravascular ultrasound. Am J Cardiol 2003; 91: 1096–9

70. Ziada KM, Tuzcu EM, De Franco AC, et al. Intravascular ultrasound assessment of the prevalence and causes of angiographic "haziness" following high-pressure coronary stenting. Am J Cardiol 1997; 80: 116–21

71. Stone GW, St Goar FG, Hodgson JM, et al. Analysis of the relation between stent implantation pressure and expansion. Optimal Stent Implantation (OSTI) Investigators. Am J Cardiol 1999; 83: 1397–400

72. Iakovou I, Mintz GS, Dangas G, et al. Increased CK-MB release is a "trade-off" for optimal stent implantation: an intravascular ultrasound study. J Am Coll Cardiol 2003; 42: 1900–5

73. Morino Y, Honda Y, Okura H, et al. An optimal diagnostic threshold for minimal stent area to predict target lesion revascularization following stent implantation in native coronary lesions. Am J Cardiol 2001; 88: 301–3

74. Ziada KM, Kapadia SR, Belli G, et al. Prognostic value of absolute versus relative measures of the procedural result after successful coronary stenting: importance of vessel size in predicting long-term freedom from target vessel revascularization. Am Heart J 2001; 141: 823–31

75. Sonoda S, Morino Y, Ako Y, et al. Impact of final stent dimensions on long-term results following sirolimus-eluting stent implantation: serial IVUS analysis from the SIRIUS Trial. J Am Coll Cardiol 2004; 43: 1959–63

76. Gilutz H, Russo RJ, Tsameret I, et al. Comparison of coronary stent expansion by intravascular ultrasounic imaging in younger versus older patients with diabetes mellitus. Am J Cardiol 2000; 85: 559–62

77. Syeda B, Wexberg P, Gyongyosi M, et al. Mechanism of lumen gain during coronary stent deployment in diabetic patients compared with non-diabetic patients. Coron Artery Dis 2002; 13: 263–8

78. Castagna MT, Mintz GS, Pinnow E, et al. Do intravascular ultrasound predictors for target lesion revascularization apply to saphenous vein grafts? J Am Coll Cardiol 2002; 39: 55A

79. Iakovou I, Dangas G, Abizaid A, et al. In saphenous vein grafts bigger is not significantly better: an intravascular ultrasound study. J Am Coll Cardiol 2002; 39: 74A

80. Colombo A, De Gregorio J, Moussa I, et al. Intravascular ultrasound-guided percutaneous transluminal coronary angioplasty with provisional spot stenting for treatment of long coronary lesion. J Am Coll Cardiol 2001; 38: 1427–33

81. de Feyter PJ, Kay P, Disco C, et al. Reference chart derived from post-stent-implantation intravascular ultrasound predictors of 6-month expected restenosis on quantitative coronary angiography. Circulation 1999; 100: 1777–83

82. Oemrawsingh PV, Mintz GS, Schalij MJ, et al. Intravascular ultrasound guidance improves angiographic and clinical outcome of stent implantation for long coronary artery stenoses: final results of a randomized comparison with angiographic guidance (TULIP Study). Circulation 2003; 107: 62–7

83. Hong MK, Park SW, Lee CW, et al. Long-term outcomes of minor plaque prolapsed within stents documented with intravascular ultrasound. Catheter Cardiovasc Interv 2000; 51: 22–6

84. Maehara A, Mintz GS, Bui AB, et al. Morphologic and angiographic features of coronary plaque rupture detected by intravascular ultrasound. J Am Coll Cardiol 2002; 40: 904–10

85. Baim DS, Wahr D, George B, et al. Randomized trial of a distal embolic protection device during percutaneous intervention of saphenous vein aorto-coronary bypass grafts. Circulation 2002; 105: 1285–90

86. Stone GW, Rogers C, Hermiller J, et al. Randomized comparison of distal protection with a filter-based catheter and a balloon occlusion and aspiration system during percutaneous intervention of diseased saphenous vein aorto-coronary bypass grafts. Circulation 2003; 108: 548–53

87. Nakamura S, Colombo A, Gaglione A, et al. Intracoronary ultrasound observations during stent implantation. Circulation 1994; 89: 2026–34

88. Hong MK, Park SW, Lee NH, et al. Long-term outcomes of minor dissection at the edge of stents detected with intravascular ultrasound. Am J Cardiol 2000; 86: 791–5

89. Sheris SJ, Canos MR, Weissman N. Natural history of intravascular ultrasound-detected edge dissections from coronary stent deployment. Am Heart J 2000; 139: 59–63

90. Fitzgerald PJ, Oshima A, Hayase M, et al. Final results of the Can Routine Ultrasound Influence Stent Expansion (CRUISE) study. Circulation 2000; 102: 523–30

91. Russo RJ, Attubato MJ, Davidson CJ, et al. Angiography versus intravascular ultrasound-directed stent placement: final results from AVID. Circulation 1999; 100: I–234

92. Nagai T, Luo H, Atar S, et al. Intravascular ultrasound imaging of ruptured atherosclerotic plaques in coronary arteries. Am J Cardiol 1999; 83: 135–7

93. Choi JW, Goodreau LM, Davidson CJ. Resource ultilization and clinical outcomes of coronary stenting: a comparison of intravascular ultrasound and angiographical guided stent implantation. Am Heart J 2001; 142: 112–18

94. Sousa A, Abizaid A, Mintz GS, et al. The influence of intravascular ultrasound guidance on the in-hospital outcomes after stent implantation: results from the Brazilian Society of Interventional Cardiology Registry – CENIC. J Am Coll Cardiol 2002; 39: 54A

95. Gaster AL, Slothuus U, Larsen J, et al. Cost-effectiveness analysis of intravascular ultrasound guided percutaneous coronary intervention versus conventional percutaneous coronary intervention. Scand Cardiovasc J 2001; 35: 80–5

96. Gaster AL, Slothuus U, Skjoldborg U, Larsen J, et al. Continued improvement of clinical outcome and cost effectiveness following intravascular ultrasound guided PCI: insights from a prospective, randomised study. Heart 2003; 89: 1043–9

97. Schiele F, Meneveau N, Seronde MF, et al. Medical costs of intravascular ultrasound optimization of stent deployment. Results of the multicenter randomized 'REStenosis after Intravascular ultrasound STenting' (RESIST) Study. Int J Cardiovasc Intervent 2000; 3: 207–13

98. Gercken U, Lansky AJ, Buellesfeld L, et al. Results of the Jostent coronary stent graft implantation in various clinical settings: procedural and follow-up results. Catheter Cardiovasc Interv 2002; 56: 353–60

99. Stankovic G, Colombo A, Presbitero P, et al. Randomized evaluation of polytetrafluoroethylene-covered stent in saphenous vein grafts: the Randomized Evaluation of polytetrafluoroethylene COVERed stent in Saphenous vein grafts (RECOVERS) Trial. Circulation 2003; 108: 37–42

100. Takebayashi H, Kobayashi Y, Mintz GS, et al. Intravascular ultrasound assessment of lesions with sirolimus-eluting stent failure. J Am Coll Cardiol 2004; 43: 65A

101. Lemos PA, Hoye A, Goedhart D, et al. Clinical, angiographic, and procedural predictors of angiographic restenosis after sirolimus-eluting stent implantation in complex patients: an evaluation from the Rapamycin-Eluting Stent Evaluated At Rotterdam Cardiology Hospital (RESEARCH) study. Circulation 2004; 109: 1366–70

102. Mintz GS, Tinana A, Hong MK, et al. Impact of preinterventional arterial remodeling on neointimal hyperplasia after implantation of (non-polymer-encapsulated) paclitaxel-coated stents: a serial volumetric intravascular ultrasound analysis from the ASian Paclitaxel-Eluting Stent Clinical Trial (ASPECT). Circulation 2003; 108: 1295–8

103. Colombo A, Moses JW, Morice MC, et al. Randomized study to evaluate sirolimus-eluting stents implanted at coronary bifurcation lesions. Circulation 2004; 109: 1244–9

104. Hoffmann R, Mintz GS, Dussaillant GR, et al. Patterns and mechanisms of in-stent restenosis: a serial intravascular ultrasound study. Circulation 1996; 94: 1247–54

105. Mudra H, Regar E, Klauss V, et al. Serial follow-up after optimized ultrasound-guided deployment of Palmaz-Schatz stents. In-stent neointimal proliferation without significant reference segment response. Circulation 1997; 95: 363–70

106. Hong MK, Park SW, Lee CW, et al. Intravascular ultrasound comparison of chronic recoil among different stent designs. Am J Cardiol 1999; 84: 1247–50

107. Gatzoulis L, Watson RJ, Jordan LB, et al. Three-dimensional forward-viewing intravascular ultrasound imaging of human arteries in vitro. Ultrasound Med Biol 2001; 27: 969–82

108. Moussa I, DiMario C, Reimers B, et al. Subacute thrombosis in the era of intravascular ultrasound-guided coronary stenting without anticoagulation: frequency, predictors, and clinical outcome. J Am Coll Cardiol 1997; 29: 6–12

109. Werner GS, Gastmann O, Ferrari M, et al. Risk factors for acute and subacute stent thrombosis after high-pressure stent implantations: a study by intracoronary ultrasound. Am Heart J 1998; 135: 300–9

110. Uren NG, Schwarzacher SP, Metz JA, et al. Predictors and outcomes of stent thrombosis: an intravascular ultrasound registry. Eur Heart J 1997; 23: 124–32

111. Cheneau E, Leborgne L, Mintz GS, et al. Predictors of subacute stent thrombosis: results of a systematic intravascular ultrasound study. Circulation 2003; 108: 43–7

112. Alfonso F, Suarez A, Angiolillo DJ, et al. Findings of intravascular ultrasound during acute stent thrombosis. J Am Coll Cardiol 2004; 43: 55A

113. Honye J, Saito S, Takayama T, et al. Clinical utility of negative contrast intravascular ultrasound to evaluate plaque morphology before and after coronary interventions. Am J Cardiol 1999; 83: 687–90

114. Schwarzacher SP, Metz JA, Yock PG, et al. Vessel tearing at the edge of intracoronary stents detected with intravascular ultrasound imaging. Cathet Cardiovasc Diagn 1997; 40: 152–5

115. Maehara A, Mintz GS, Bui AB, et al. Incidence, morphology, angiographic findings, and outcomes of intramural hematomas after percutaneous coronary interventions: an intravascular ultrasound study. Circulation 2002; 105: 2037–42

8
Mechanisms, prevention, and treatment of restenosis

Serial IVUS studies were fundamental to understanding the restenosis process. Previously, histologic studies or analysis of retrieved atherectomy specimens focused on plaque elements and postulated that restenosis in non-stented lesions was the result of intimal hyperplasia.[1,2] (Of note, subsequent histologic studies confirmed that a late decrease in arterial dimensions was an important component of the restenosis process in non-stented lesions and that this process also impacted adjacent reference segments.[3–14])

Angiographic studies are only able to analyze changes in lumen dimensions. For example, early studies comparing angiograms at stent implantation (in which full balloon inflation was erroneously equated with complete stent expansion) with follow-up IVUS studies (which showed stent underexpansion) suggested that chronic stent recoil was an important component of restenosis in stented lesions. Serial IVUS studies showed that in-stent restenosis was almost exclusively from intimal hyperplasia and only rarely from stent recoil.

METHODOLOGIC CONSIDERATIONS IN ASSESSING RESTENOSIS

Several methodologic decisions are important. The first decision is whether to perform planar or volumetric analysis.

Planar analysis

In performing planar analysis, the next decisions include (1) whether to analyze only one or multiple anatomic slices; (2) which anatomic slice to measure: smallest lumen pre-intervention, smallest post-intervention lumen, or smallest follow-up lumen; and (3) whether or not to average multiple slices. In general, restenosis studies should always analyze the anatomic location of the smallest follow-up lumen

cross-sectional area (CSA) since this is the site of restenosis. The anatomic slice with the same axial location (not the anatomic slice with the minimum lumen CSA regardless of its location) should be analyzed on serial studies; this is discussed in more detail in Chapter 2. In non-stented lesions, the site of the minimum lumen CSA can migrate significantly from pre-intervention to post-intervention to follow-up. In one study, the location of the smallest follow-up lumen CSA was more than 2 mm from the smallest pre-intervention lumen CSA in 67% of lesions and more than 2 mm from the smallest post-intervention lumen CSA in 78% of lesions.[15]

Volumetric analysis

In performing volumetric analysis, decisions include whether to analyze a fixed segment length (e.g. a 20 mm-long segment in all patients) or whether to analyze the entire length of the lesion in each patient. In stent restenosis studies, the entire stented length should be measured. Because longer lesions (and stents) have larger volumes, volumetric analysis should be accompanied by mean CSA analysis (volume divided by length). Some volumetric studies also include analysis of subsegments (e.g. five 3 mm-long subsegments within a 15 mm-long lesion or stent). This analysis assumes that adjacent subsegments behave independently with regard to changes in external elastic membrane (EEM), plaque & media (P&M), lumen, stent, and intimal hyperplasia – an assumption that may not be valid. In addition, the anatomic slice that corresponds to the follow-up minimum lumen area should also be reported.

Although there is no clear evidence that edge effects are confined to a 5 mm-long segment, for practical reasons, at least 5 mm-long proximal and distal reference segments (edges) should be measured and analyzed. Proximal and distal edges should be analyzed and reported separately – not combined and analyzed together since – there is no evidence that proximal versus distal edges always behave similarly or differently. Some studies report volumetric (or mean planar) analysis; others report CSA analysis mm-by-mm over a specified reference segment length. Because edge effects can be very focal and change over short distances, it is preferable to analyze studies mm-by-mm over the length of the edge/reference segment. This requires very careful "registration" of serial (post-intervention and follow-up) images. Good examples of the discrepancy between volumetric (or mean planar) analysis versus mm-by-mm edge analysis include the various Isostent studies and reports from drug-eluting stent studies where major changes occur only within the first 1–2 mm from stent edges. When assessing edge or reference-segment effects, it is important to determine the relationship between the injured segment, the treatment strategy, and the IVUS images; angiographic–IVUS comparisons may work in stented lesions, but are more problematic in non-stented lesions.

It is also important to look at individual cases, not just average changes in EEM, lumen, P&M, stent, or intimal hyperplasia CSA or volume.

Non-stented lesions and stent edges

Using IVUS, changes in lumen dimensions in non-stented lesions and arterial segments (including stent edges) can be separated into four components: increase or decrease in EEM and increase or decrease in P&M (Figure 8.1). In practice, the inclusion of the media into the P&M is not important. The media represents only a very small fraction of the P&M complex and does not change measurably during serial studies. IVUS cannot determine the plaque components responsible for changes in the P&M complex – i.e. IVUS cannot differentiate plaque progression from intimal hyperplasia or thrombus formation.

The change in EEM CSA during follow-up has unfortunately been termed "remodeling", the term that is also used to describe changes in the EEM during atherogenesis (see Chapter 5). The interchangeable use of the term remodeling to describe these two scenarios has led to the misconception that the two pathophysiologic processes are the same; this is not likely. Furthermore, the changes in EEM CSA that are observed during follow-up may merely reflect perivascular trauma, hematoma formation, and scar contraction as suggested by some histopathologic studies – although this conclusion is beyond the current imaging capability of IVUS.[6,9,10] Therefore, in this chapter, the term remodeling will not be used to describe changes in EEM CSA (vessel shrinkage or expansion) that occur as a consequence of intervention.

Stented lesions

Using IVUS, late lumen loss in stented lesions (whether *de novo* stenting or treatment of in-stent restenosis) can be separated into four components: increase or decrease in stent dimensions and increase or decrease in intimal hyperplasia (Figure 8.2). However, chronic stent recoil is rare; an increase in stent dimensions occurs only with self-expanding stents; a decrease in intimal hyperplasia leading to an increase in lumen dimensions only occurs after treatment of in-stent restenosis; and an increase in lumen dimensions in *de novo* stenting occurs only with late stent malapposition. Therefore, intra-stent lumen loss is directly related to intimal hyperplasia; and only small patient numbers are required to assess intra-stent effects.

Conversely, stent-edge and reference-segment effects can be separated into an increase or decrease in EEM versus a decrease or increase in P&M (presumably intimal hyperplasia that has spilled over from the stent into the contiguous reference segments) as noted above (Figure 8.1). Because there is a wider range of potential edge effects, larger patient numbers are required to assess edge and reference-segment changes as apposed to intra-stent changes. Meticulous collection and comparison of both IVUS and angiographic studies is necessary to determine the relationship between the injured segment, the treatment strategy, and the IVUS images.

Lesions that are totally occluded at follow-up present a challenge. While it is possible to cross a total occlusion with the IVUS catheter, this is rarely done. In totally occluded balloon-expandable, tubular-slotted, multicellular stents that were imaged at implantation, the amount of intimal hyperplasia can be determined from post-implantation stent measurements and "zero" follow-up lumen dimensions since stent dimensions do not change after implantation. This approach is not possible in non-stented lesions or self-expanding or coiled stents.

When quantifying the amount of intimal hyperplasia, it is important to pay attention to machine settings. As discussed in Chapter 1 (see particularly Figure 1.21), excessive reduction in near-field intensity (in an attempt to reduce blood speckle, ring-down, or other near-field artifacts) can blank out echolucent neointima tissue to produce a lumen artificially. It is also not possible to differentiate conclusively intimal hyperplasia from thrombus or chronic tissue prolapse, although thrombus and chronic tissue prolapse are less common than intimal hyperplasia.

Compliance

One disappointing reality of IVUS, particulary with multicenter studies, is site compliance. It was initially thought that volumetric IVUS methodology would result in a marked reduction in sample size needed for restenosis studies. However, this assumption did not anticipate the reality of a low data acquisition rate. In general, studies requiring both post-intervention and follow-up IVUS imaging using motorized transducer pullback for volumetric analysis have complete data in approximately 60% of patients. This is the result of a 75–80% compliance rate at index and a 75–80% compliance rate at follow-up. Some notable exceptions include MVP (MultiVitamins and Probucol), TAXUS-II, the various Isostent studies, HIPS (Heparin Infusion Prior to Stenting), the original (but not the subsequent) WRIST (Washington Radiation In-stent Restenosis) study, CART-1 (Canadian Antioxidant Restenosis Trial-1), various small first-in-man drug-eluting stent studies, ASPECT (Asian Paclitaxel-Eluting Stent Clinical Trial), ENDEAVOR-1, and DANTE (Diabetes Abciximab steNT Evaluation). In these studies, there was a greater than 90% compliance at baseline and at follow-up, and volumetric analysis was possible in over 80% of the lesions. In general, studies with good compliance have the following in common: limited numbers of sites (sometimes only one); site-specific substudies with sites selected for their interest and experience in routine use of IVUS; real interest in the IVUS data or use of IVUS as the primary endpoint; and (often) dedicated personnel to oversee IVUS data collection. The most common reasons for not having analyzable volumetric IVUS studies include:

- Lack of angiographic follow-up;
- Not performing either the index or follow-up IVUS study despite not imaging the entire lesion and reference segment – particularly distally;
- Problems with motorized pullback – the accuracy of the pullback can be checked against the known length of the stent and repeated if necessary, and there should be only a minimal difference in measured stent lengths between serial studies (core labs will routinely exclude patients with significant differences between post-intervention and follow-up stent lengths);
- Artifacts;
- Poor image quality.

In general, it is always easier to find an excuse not to do IVUS – particularly at follow-up. However, IVUS can be performed on an outpatient basis using 6-Fr guiding catheters and adequate, but not excessive anticoagulation with or without an access-closure device. Beyond this, all other problems are minimized with experience and proper attention to detail.

RESTENOSIS IN NON-STENTED LESIONS

Mechanisms of restenosis in non-stented lesions

In our initial study of 221 non-stented lesions, we analyzed the image slice with the smallest lumen CSA at follow-up (since this was the restenosis lesion) and compared it with the same anatomic location post-intervention.[16] The change in lumen CSA correlated more strongly with the change in EEM CSA ($r = 0.75$) than with the change in P&M CSA ($r = 0.28$). Restenotic lesions (> 50% angiographic diameter stenosis at follow-up) had a greater decrease in EEM CSA and lumen CSA than non-restenotic lesions, but only a trend towards a greater increase in P&M CSA. The decrease in EEM CSA (arterial shrinkage) contributed three-quarters of late lumen loss, while the increase in P&M CSA contributed only 25%. However, 22% of the 221 lesions had an *increase* in EEM CSA during follow-up. Lesions with a sustained late increase in EEM CSA showed a decreased incidence of angiographic restenosis and more frequent late lumen gain *despite* a greater increase in P&M CSA. This may explain why some non-stented lesions "look better" at follow-up than post-intervention (Figure 8.1).

There was one exception to these findings: diabetic patients. In diabetic patients, the increase in P&M CSA was greater than in non-diabetics (Figure 8.1). In some non-diabetics, there was an increase in EEM CSA that prevented lumen loss despite an increase in P&M CSA; this was not seen in diabetics.[17]

Numerous other studies have substantiated the importance of a decrease in EEM to the restenosis process, although the relative magnitude of the decrease in EEM versus intimal hyperplasia varied from study to study.[18–30] The Optimal Atherectomy Restenosis Study (OARS) also showed that the decrease in EEM CSA extended into the reference segments. The decrease in reference-segment EEM CSA could be correlated with but was only half of the decrease in lesion-site EEM CSA.[31] This finding may explain why some restenotic lesions are longer compared with pre-intervention (Figure 8.3).

In the remarkable SURE (Serial Ultrasound REstenosis) trial, patients were treated with balloon angioplasty or directional coronary atherectomy and studied pre-intervention, immediately post-intervention, 24 h post-intervention, after 1 month of follow-up, and after 6 months of follow-up.[32] The SURE study averaged two image slices: the anatomic location with the smallest lumen CSA pre-intervention and the slice with the smallest lumen CSA at follow-up. Throughout the duration of the SURE trial, changes in lumen CSA could be correlated more strongly with changes in EEM CSA ($r = 0.7–0.8$) than with changes in P&M CSA ($r = 0.3–0.4$). However, the unique finding in the SURE trial was an early (1 month) increase in EEM CSA that was followed by a late (1–6 month) decrease in EEM CSA (Figures 8.4 and 8.5). Critics of previous studies suggested that the decrease in EEM CSA was just passive elastic recoil or creep that was not seen until follow-up.[33] However, because the decrease in EEM CSA was a late event and was *preceded* by a 1-month *increase* in EEM CSA, late EEM CSA decrease was not merely passive elastic recoil or creep. Furthermore, in individual patients, the follow-up EEM CSA was often smaller than pre-intervention (Figures 8.3 and 8.5), which also argues against passive elastic recoil or creep as an explanation for these changes. In SURE, as in OARS, there were reference-segment changes in EEM CSA that paralleled lesion-site changes, but that were quantitatively less. This late decrease in EEM was confirmed in another small serial IVUS study with long-term follow-up[23] and was supported by one animal study.[14]

Most of the IVUS studies cited above used planar analysis. However, these planar analyses were later supported by volumetric IVUS studies.[26,34] Directional coronary atherectomy-treated lesions in OARS and SURE were submitted to independent volumetric IVUS analysis. When 20 mm-long segments were measured post-intervention and at follow-up, lumen volume decrease was the result of a decrease in EEM volume with no change in P&M volume; the change in lumen volume could be correlated with the change in EEM volume, not with the change in P&M volume.[34]

The impact of the increase or decrease in EEM on restenosis is also substantiated by numerous studies of strategies to reduce restenosis. In general, strategies that successfully reduced restenosis in non-stented lesions (or reduced edge effects in stented lesions) reported increases in EEM as a primary reason for success. These studies are discussed below.

Fate of dissections

Of 94 patients enrolled in the IVUS substudy of the MVP trial, 28 patients had post-angioplasty dissections. At 6-month follow-up, only one patient had an unhealed, residual dissection.[35] An example of dissection healing is shown in Figure 8.5.

IVUS predictors of restenosis in non-stented lesions

Several studies have shown that the residual plaque burden and residual lumen dimensions determined by IVUS predicted restenosis.[20,24,26,36–40] Both the GUIDE and MVP trials indicated that a residual plaque burden of 67% best predicted restenosis after balloon angioplasty.[37,38] Comparison of restenosis rates versus the residual plaque burdens in CAVEAT (Coronary Angioplasty Versus Excision Atherectomy Trial), GUIDE, OARS, and ABACAS (Adjunct Balloon Angioplasty Coronary Atherectomy Study) substantiated the importance of the residual plaque burden after directional coronary atherectomy. Taken together, these studies suggested that the lower the post-atherectomy residual plaque burden, the lower the restenosis rate – ideally, a residual plaque burden of less than 40%. However, the predictive power of the residual plaque burden was not confirmed in balloon angioplasty patients in PICTURE (Post-IntraCoronary Treatment Ultrasound Result Evaluation).[41] Using multivariate analysis, PICTURE failed to identify any predictors of restenosis, including diabetes, the final angiographic minimum lumen diameter or diameter stenosis, and the residual plaque burden.

There are several explanations for the importance of the residual plaque burden. One plausible explanation is that the residual plaque burden acts as an amplifier of the changes in EEM CSA; a small decrease in EEM CSA would have a greater impact on lumen dimensions in a lesion with a large residual plaque burden compared with a lesion with a small residual plaque burden.[36] In one directional coronary atherectomy study, lesions with a large residual plaque burden had a late *decrease* in EEM CSA, while lesions with a low residual plaque burden had a late *increase* in EEM CSA; a plaque burden of 40% was the cut-off between a late increase or decrease in EEM CSA, and a late increase in EEM CSA militates against restenosis.[15,16,20] The amount of subsequent intimal hyperplasia has been correlated with the residual plaque burden[24], and larger residual plaque burden has been associated with more early lumen loss (or recoil) within 1 h of successful balloon angioplasty.[42]

Pre-intervention remodeling has been identified as a predictor of target-lesion revascularization after non-stent interventions.[43–45] Lesions with positive remodeling had more revascularization events despite a larger post-intervention lumen CSA. Positive remodeling lesions may be more biologically active, and this may cause both an unstable clinical presentation (see Chapter 5) and more late events. In one study, positive remodeling lesions had a greater early increase in EEM CSA and a greater late decrease in EEM CSA.[45] In another study, intimal hyperplasia had a greater impact on late lumen loss in positive remodeling lesions.[25]

Other predictors of restenosis have included absence of post-angioplasty dissections[26], particularly deep dissections.[22,46] In one study of lesions with deep vessel wall injury (dissections into the media), late lumen loss could be correlated with the decrease in EEM CSA; conversely, in lesions without deep vessel wall injury, late lumen loss could be correlated with intimal hyperplasia.[22] Gray-scale plaque composition has not been shown to be a predictor of restenosis[26,47].

Preventing restenosis in non-stented lesions

Pre-treatment with probucol reduced restenosis after balloon angioplasty by promoting a late increase in EEM CSA, while the increase in P&M CSA was similar to placebo.[48] The CART-1 trial studied AGI-1067 and probucol versus placebo. While some balloon angioplasty patients were included in CART-1, they were not reported separately from the overall cohort of stented patients.

Brachytherapy

The data on irradiation of non-stented lesions are limited to BERT (Beta Energy Restenosis Trial). One study showed no change in lesion EEM, lumen, or P&M CSA from post-irradiation to follow-up.[49] However, in this report, only one image slice per lesion was studied, the location of this image slice was not specified, and edges were not analyzed. A second study was an extensive and detailed ECG-gated volumetric analysis of 30 mm-long lesion segments and contiguous 5 mm-long edges.[50] There was a significant increase in lesion EEM volume that was roughly equal to the increase in lesion P&M volume; as a result, lesion lumen volume remained unchanged. However, these "beneficial" effects did not extend to the edges, where there was an increase in P&M but no increase in EEM, resulting in net lumen loss.

In another report from BERT, the irradiated segments (but not the edges) were analyzed in 2 mm-long subsegments.[51] There were three independent predictors of the absolute P&M volume at follow-up: plaque volume post-irradiation, minimum effective dose delivered to 90% of the adventitia, and the type of plaque (hard versus soft).

The impact of brachytherapy on the healing of post-angioplasty dissections was also reported from BERT. In one study, IVUS dissections were seen in 16 of 22 patients; at follow-up, 6 patients had no evidence of healing, and 2 patients had partial healing. The calculated dose was similar in healed and unhealed dissections.[52] In another report of 16 patients with post-angioplasty dissections in BERT, 7 patients had not healed.[35]

The Proliferation Reduction with Vascular Energy Trial (PREVENT) included patients treated with just balloon angioplasty. They were not reported separately.

Treatment of restenosis in non-stented lesions

There have been no specific IVUS studies addressing restenotic non-stented lesions – from either a morphologic or a quantitative standpoint. Unusual restenotic non-stented lesion morphology should be assessed pre-intervention as discussed in Chapter 6. In the study by Maehara, 35 out of 77 angiographic aneurysms were in previously treated lesions. Of the 35, 31% were true aneurysms, 9% were pseudoaneurysms, 17% were complex plaques, and 43% were normal-appearing segments adjacent to one or more significant stenoses (Figure 8.6).

MECHANISMS OF IN-STENT RESTENOSIS IN BARE-METAL STENTS

Bare-metal stents reduce restenosis by achieving a larger post-intervention lumen CSA and by opposing the post-intervention decrease in EEM CSA seen in non-stented lesions. This accommodates the exaggerated neointimal hyperplasia that occurs after stent implantation.[53] In START (STent versus Directional Coronary Atherectomy Randomized Trial), although the post-procedural lumen dimensions were similar, serial IVUS revealed that intimal proliferation was significantly larger in the stent arm than in the directional coronary atherectomy arm.[54]

IVUS restenosis findings in tubular-slotted or multicellular stents can be summarized as in the following paragraphs.

Tubular-slotted or multicellular stents only rarely exhibit chronic recoil (Figure 8.7); therefore, late lumen loss is almost entirely neointimal hyperplasia (Figures 8.8 and 8.9).[55–58] In most cases of suspected chronic stent recoil, careful review of the post-stent implantation IVUS will show inadequate initial stent expansion or poor imaging technique, such that the entire stent was never visualized. (Conversely, stents can acutely recoil – or show plastic deformation – during the very initial part of balloon deflation. However, the stent configuration that becomes "locked" during balloon deflation is stable and does not change during follow-up.)

There is a non-statistically significant trend for greater neointimal hyperplasia to occur in the middle of a bare-metal stent, but no other regional predilection, although there is significant patient-to-patient variation (Figure 8.7).[55,56,59]

Intimal hyperplasia volume divided by stent volume (often called %intimal hyperplasia or %stent volume obstruction) is normally distributed and averages approximately 30% when the results of many trials are considered.[56,59–62]

Stenting has an impact on adjacent reference segments, with progressively more EEM decrease and progressively less P&M (or intimal hyperplasia) increase at greater distances from the edge of the stent, although there is significant patient-to-patient variation (Figure 8.7).[55,59,61]

In patients who are clinically stable and who do not present with symptomatic restenosis, the neointima remains stable or regresses from 6 months to 1 year, substantiating similar angiographic and angioscopic reports.[63,64]

For any given stent type, intimal hyperplasia thickness is independent of stent size. (However, larger stents have a larger circumference; and the same neointima thickness distributed over a larger circumference will necessarily result in a larger intimal hyperplasia CSA, but not more restenosis.) Thus, intimal hyperplasia thickness may be a useful stent-size-independent measure of restenosis.[65–67]

Lesions treated with two stents showed the same intra-stent and edge findings compared with lesions treated with one stent. When there was a gap between the two stents, there was no significant difference in final or follow-up lumen dimensions, late lumen loss, ΔEEM, or intimal hyperplasia compared with stents that overlapped. When native vessel and saphenous vein-graft lesions were normalized for post-intervention stent CSA, intimal hyperplasia was similar in both types of lesions.[55]

Figure 8.1 (opposite)   Three examples of post-intervention and follow-up IVUS imaging after directional coronary atherectomy of right coronary artery lesions are shown. In all three examples, the anatomic site of the smallest follow-up lumen CSA was measured post-intervention and at follow-up.

In the top example, the post-intervention and follow-up angiograms and the post-intervention and follow-up IVUS images are shown from left to right. The restenotic lesion (a) is shown on the follow-up angiogram. The residual plaque burden measured 47%. At follow-up, the EEM CSA (outer dashed white line on the post-intervention and follow-up IVUS images) decreased from 24.6 to 16.8 mm^2, the lumen CSA (inner dashed white line on each study) decreased from 13.0 to 2.6 mm^2, and the P&M CSA increased from 11.6 to 14.2 mm^2. Therefore, 75% of late lumen loss was from a decrease in EEM CSA, while 25% of late lumen loss was from an increase in P&M CSA. Note how the small calcific deposit (b) with shadowing helped to locate the same anatomic image slice on each study. Thus, arterial shrinkage caused restenosis.

In the middle example, the post-intervention and follow-up angiograms and the post-intervention and follow-up IVUS images are shown from left to right. The restenotic lesion (c) is shown on the follow-up angiogram. The residual plaque burden measured 59%, and there is a superficial dissection (d). At follow-up, the EEM CSA (outer dashed white line on each study) decreased from 28.3 to 26.1 mm^2, the lumen CSA (inner dashed white line on each study) decreased from 10.7 to 1.3 mm^2, and the P&M CSA increased from 16.6 to 24.8 mm^2. Therefore, 23% of late lumen loss was from a decrease in EEM CSA, while 77% of late lumen loss was from an increase in P&M CSA. Note how the small calcific deposit (e) helped to locate the same anatomic image slice on each study. This patient was an insulin-treated diabetic. Thus, intimal hyperplasia caused restenosis.

In the bottom example, the pre-intervention, post-intervention, and follow-up angiograms and the post-intervention and follow-up IVUS images are shown from left to right. The pre-intervention lesion (f) is shown on the baseline angiogram. The residual plaque burden measured 50%. At follow-up, the EEM CSA (outer dashed white line on both the post-intervention and follow-up IVUS images) decreased from 40.1 to 45.3 mm^2, and the lumen CSA (inner dashed white line on each study) increased from 20.0 to 23.0 mm^2 despite a P&M CSA increase from 20.1 to 22.3 mm^2. Note how the small calcific deposit (g) helped to ensure that the same anatomic slice was identified on each study. Thus, arterial enlargement caused lumen enlargement

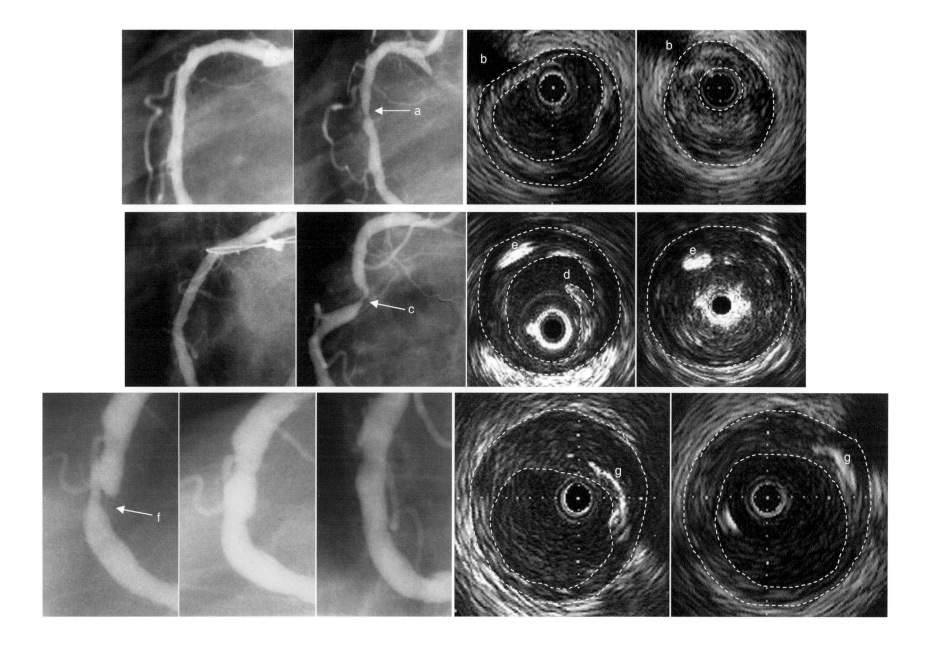

Figure 8.2 (opposite) Two examples of in-stent restenosis after implantation of Palmaz–Schatz stents into ostial lesions are shown (white arrows on the angiograms). In the top example, the pre-intervention, post-intervention, and follow-up angiograms and the post-intervention and follow-up IVUS images are shown from left to right; the post-intervention and follow-up studies were acquired 11 months apart. The baseline and restenotic lesions are shown by the white arrows on the pre-intervention and follow-up angiograms. Stent CSA measured $9.1 \, mm^2$ at implantation (a) and at follow-up (b); therefore, all of the late lumen loss (from 9.1 to $1.3 \, mm^2$, the size of the IVUS catheter) was due to intimal hyperplasia (c). Thus, intimal hyperplasia caused in-stent restenosis. The bottom example shows a rare case of chronic stent recoil. The pre-intervention, post-intervention, and follow-up angiograms and the post-intervention and follow-up IVUS images are shown from left to right; the post-intervention and follow-up studies were acquired 3 months apart. The baseline and restenotic lesions are shown by the white arrows on the pre-intervention and follow-up angiograms. Stent CSA measured $9.3 \, mm^2$ at implantation. While the exact minimum stent CSA was difficult to measure at follow-up, there has been a considerable decrease in minimum stent CSA from baseline (d) to follow-up (e), together with significant stent deformation. This example will be discussed in more detail in Figure 8.12

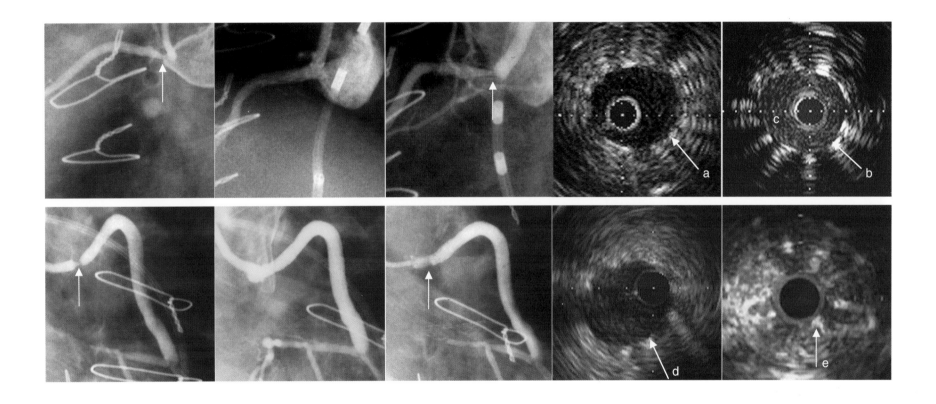

Figure 8.3 (opposite) Pre-intervention (top panel), post-intervention (middle panel), and 5-month follow-up (bottom panel) are IVUS images from the directional atherectomy treatment of a focal, near ostial left anterior descending stenosis. Each imaging run shows an identical series of five image slices including distal reference (a), center of lesion (b), and ostial left anterior descending (c, note the left circumflex d). The EEM volume increased from 114.2 mm^3 pre-atherectomy to 122.4 mm^3 post-intervention and decreased to 91.2 mm^3 at follow-up; the lumen volume increased from 31.1 mm^3 pre-atherectomy to 59.6 mm^3 post-intervention and decreased to 24.0 mm^3 at follow-up; and the P&M volume decreased from 83.1 mm^3 pre-atherectomy to 64.4 mm^3 post-intervention and increased to 68.7 mm^3 at follow-up. Thus, overall, 87% of the late lumen volume loss was from a decrease in EEM volume; and only 13% was from an increase in P&M volume. However, at the center of the lesion (b), all of the lumen CSA decrease was from a decrease in EEM CSA; while the decrease in distal reference EEM CSA (a) was 48% of the decrease in lesion site EEM CSA (a). Thus, arterial shrinkage caused restenosis and this extended to the distal reference. Note that the follow-up EEM volume and EEM CSA at the center of the lesion were smaller than pre-intervention. The EEM is shown by the dashed white line e, and the lumen is shown by the dashed white line f

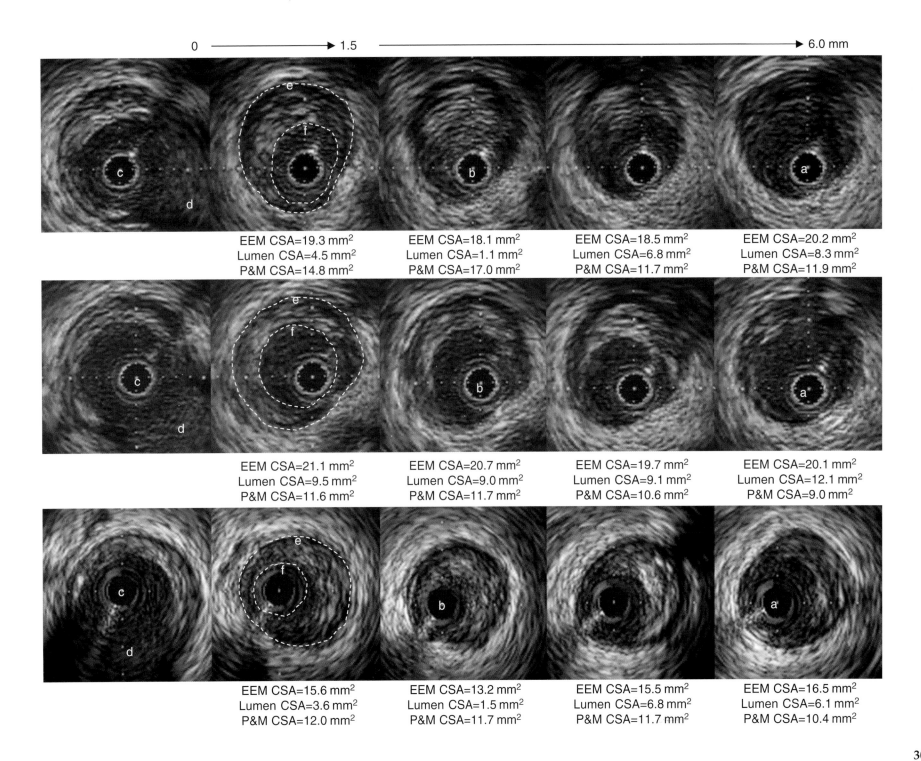

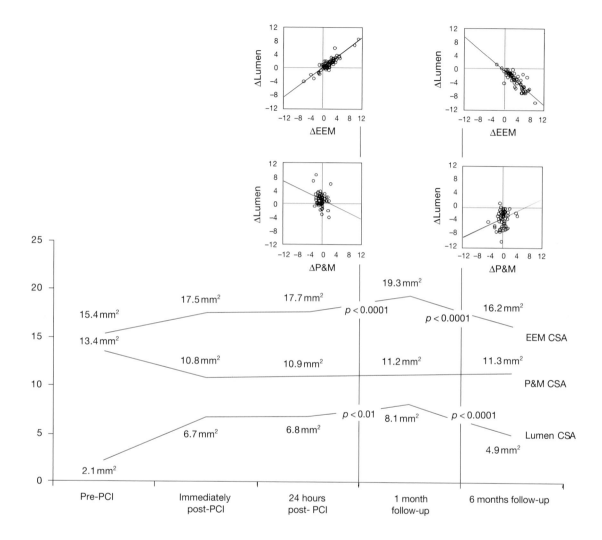

Figure 8.4 The results of the lesion-site analysis from the SURE trial are shown. Although, in the SURE trial, the anatomic slices corresponding to both the minimum lumen area pre-percutaneous coronary intervention (PCI) and the minimum lumen area at follow-up were selected, measured, and averaged, in this illustration only the analysis of the image slices corresponding to the minimum lumen CSA at follow-up are shown. There was an early (24 h to 1 month) increase in lumen CSA and EEM CSA and a late (1–6 months) decrease in lumen CSA and EEM CSA. As shown by the insets, from 24 h to 1 month, the increase in lumen CSA correlated better with the increase in EEM CSA ($r = 0.63$, $p < 0.0001$) than with the change in P&M CSA ($r = 0.25$, $p = 0.05$); and from 1 month to 6 months, the decrease in lumen CSA correlated better with the decrease in EEM CSA ($r = 0.84$, $p < 0.0001$) than with the increase in P&M CSA ($r = 0.27$, $p = 0.04$). (Adapted from Kimura T *et al.*[32])

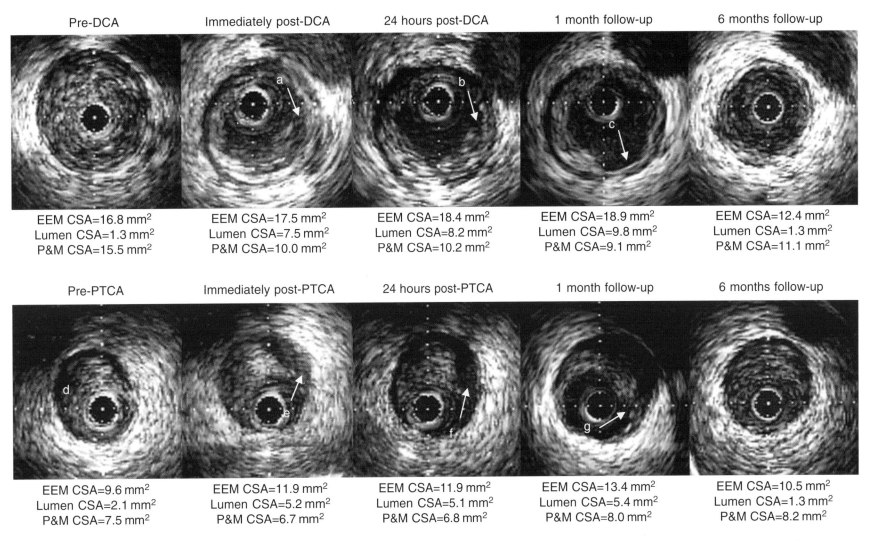

Figure 8.5 This patient, who was enrolled in the SURE trial, had a proximal left anterior descending lesion treated with directional coronary atherectomy (DCA, top panel) and a mid left anterior descending lesion treated with balloon angioplasty (PTCA, bottom panel). The EEM, lumen, and P&M CSA measurements for each image slice are shown. Note in the proximal lesion, there was a superficial dissection (a) that had improved by 24 h (b) and disappeared by 1 month (c). Also note in the mid lesion, the eccentric plaque pre-intervention (d) and the dissection between plaque and normal vessel wall down to the media (e) that persisted at 24 h (f), partially healed at 1 month (g), and totally healed at 6 months. In both lesions, the late decrease in EEM CSA caused most of the late decrease in lumen CSA. In the proximal lesion, the 6-month follow-up EEM CSA was smaller than pre-intervention. Thus, arterial shrinkage caused restenosis of the proximal lesion and both arterial shrinkage and intimal hyperplasia caused restenosis of the mid lesion

Figure 8.6 (opposite) This patient with a left anterior descending and major diagonal branch bifurcation stenosis (white arrow in Panel A) was treated with directional coronary atherectomy of both branches. The post-intervention angiogram is shown in Panel B, the 2-month angiogram is shown in Panel C, and the 6-month angiogram is shown in Panel D. Note the progressive increase in lumen diameter proximal to the bifurcation (white arrows in Panels C and D); the bifurcation itself appears free of restenosis. The IVUS study at 2 months is shown in Panel E, and the IVUS study at 6 months is shown in Panel F. At the lesion site (a), there has been no change in EEM CSA or lumen CSA (8.2 mm^2 in both studies), while proximal to the lesion, there has been an increase in maximum EEM CSA (outer dashed white lines) from 28.7 to 35.2 mm^2 and an increase in maximum lumen CSA (inner dashed white lines) from 12.4 to 19.2 mm^2

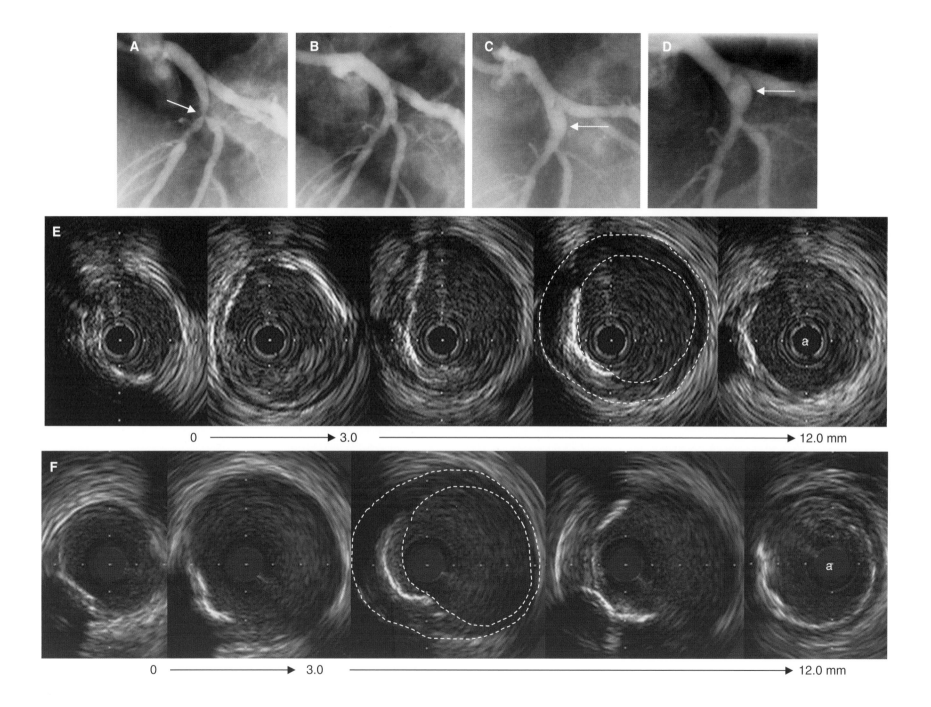

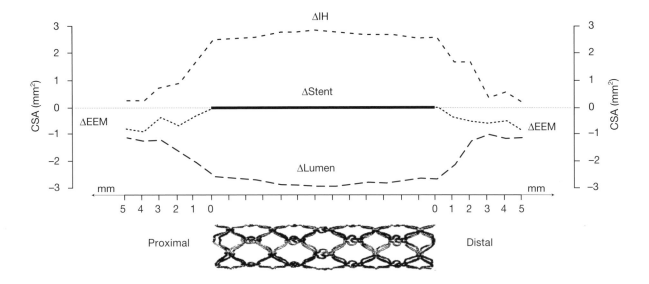

Figure 8.7 This illustration shows paired (post-intervention and follow-up) IVUS analysis from HIPS performed mm-by-mm throughout the length of the stent as well as 5 mm proximal and distal to the stent (into the contiguous reference segments or stent edges). Within the stent, the stent, lumen, and intimal hyperplasia (IH = stent minus lumen), CSA were measured and the differences calculated; in the adjacent non-stented 5 mm-long segment, EEM, lumen, and P&M CSA were measured and the differences calculated. A total of 179 patients were enrolled; each patient had one focal, *de novo*, stenosis in a native coronary artery treated with 1.2 ± 0.6 Palmaz–Schatz stents per vessel. Follow-up angiography was obtained in 159 patients at 6.4 ± 1.9 months after stent deployment. IVUS was performed in 146 of these patients; 140 paired studies were suitable for volumetric analysis. On average across all patients, there was no predilection for the amount of intimal hyperplasia to occur within any one segment of the stent; however, there was substantial patient-to-patient variability in the distribution of the intimal hyperplasia. The greatest edge lumen loss occurred within the first 2 mm proximal and distal to the stent edge and was primarily due to an increase in P&M CSA (presumably intimal hyperplasia that spilled over from the stent). Beyond 2 mm from the stent edge, lumen loss was less severe and due to a combination of an increase in P&M CSA and a decrease in EEM CSA, although the decrease in EEM CSA contributed more to lumen loss distally than it did proximally. As with intimal hyperplasia within the stent, there was a high degree of variability of the increase in P&M CSA within the adjacent reference segments; the standard deviation for changes in P&M CSA within the first 2 mm proximal and distal to the stent edge ranged from 2.05 to 3.17, larger than the mean change in P&M CSA. The increase in P&M CSA in the first 2 mm proximal and distal to the stent could be correlated with IH CSA within the stent edge both proximally ($r = 0.66$, $p = 0.03$) and distally ($r = 0.71$, $p = 0.01$). Conversely, more than 2 mm proximal and distal to the stent edge, there was no relationship between the increase in P&M CSA versus IH CSA within the stent. (Adapted from Weissman NJ *et al.*[59])

IVUS is also useful for differentiating intra-stent restenosis from stent edge restenosis and determining whether edge restenosis is caused by intimal hyperplasia or a decrease in EEM CSA (Figures 8.10 and 8.11).

The diagnosis of chronic stent recoil requires complete post-intervention and follow-up IVUS imaging to document proper expansion at the time of implantation. A rare example is shown in Figure 8.12.

In many cases of in-stent restenosis, the stent-implantation angiograms are not available or the angiograms poorly document the procedure. IVUS findings can be surprising and assist in patient management (Figure 8.13).

If a patient presents with in-stent restenosis and IVUS shows either a small stent CSA or another mechanical complication, the odds are overwhelming that this occurred at the time of implantation and did not develop during the intervening period. Castagna *et al.*[68] studied 1090 patients who presented with in-stent restenosis. In 49 lesions (4.5%), there were mechanical complications that contributed to restenosis. Examples included (1) missing the lesion, (2) stent "crush", and (3) having the stent stripped off the balloon during the implantation procedure. In the remaining 1051 patients, 65% had a minimum stent CSA < 7.5 mm^2, 38% had a minimum stent CSA < 6.0 mm^2, and 20% had a minimum stent CSA < 5.0 mm^2. Thus, because stents do not recoil, there was an important contribution of inadequate stent expansion to restenosis. In general, mechanical problems (including stent underexpansion) are more common in patients who present with early in-stent restenosis. Examples of chronic stent underexpansion are shown in Figures 8.14–8.17. Figure 8.18 is an example where the stent missed the lesion and this, potentially, contributed to early in-stent restenosis. Figures 8.19–8.21 are examples of in-stent restnosis because of stent crush or stent dislodgement from the delivery balloon.

Peri-stent increase in EEM CSA

The vascular response to stent implantation is not limited to the luminal side of the stent or to the proximal and distal reference segments. There is an increase in peri-stent (or abluminal) P&M associated with an increase in EEM CSA.[69–71] This, presumably, reflects peri-stent neointimal hyperplasia. However, studies differ on whether the increase in peri-stent EEM CSA is associated with more or less intra-stent intimal hyperplasia. In some studies, increases in peri-stent EEM CSA and P&M CSA are associated with more intra-stent intimal hyperplasia; in other studies, they are associated with less intra-stent intimal hyperplasia. In one study, a lower residual peri-stent plaque burden predicted an increase in EEM CSA.[71]

The most common cause of late stent malapposition (discussed below) is an increase in EEM that is greater than the increase in peri-stent P&M. This suggests that, in some patients, the increase in EEM CSA is not necessarily a response to peri-stent intimal hyperplasia, but can occur independently, leading to late stent malapposition.

Late stent malapposition

Late stent malapposition (also called late incomplete apposition) is defined as separation of at least one stent strut from the intima, not overlapping a side branch, with evidence of blood flow (speckling) behind the strut, and where post-implantation IVUS revealed complete apposition of the stent to the vessel (Figure 8.22). However, most of the time, only follow-up IVUS is available (Figure 8.23); therefore, it is not clear whether malapposition occurred at implantation or was a late event. Malapposition at implantation can resolve or persist. In general, there is minimal intimal hyperplasia at the site of late (or persistent) stent malapposition (Figure 8.23), and patients with late stent malapposition rarely require revascularization.[72–74] Late stent malapposition occurs in 4–5% of electively implanted bare-metal stents, increasing to 10–12% after directional coronary atherectomy or primary infarct intervention.[72,73] This was substantiated in the DESIRE (Debulking and Stenting in Restenosis Elimination) trial, in which most of the late malapposition cases occurred in the pre-stent atherectomy group.[74] There are three possible mechanisms for late stent malapposition: chronic stent recoil without any change in EEM or P&M, increase in EEM without an equal increase in P&M, and a reduction in P&M (i.e. apoptosis or thrombus dissolution) without an equal decrease in EEM. Serial IVUS studies have indicated that an increase in EEM without an equal increase in P&M is the main mechanism of late stent malapposition except in infarct lesions, where thrombus dissolution is the presumed mechanism.[74,75]

It is easy to fix late stent malapposition. An appropriately sized balloon is expanded at low pressures to fully appose the stent struts to the vessel wall (see Figure 7.20). However, bare-metal stents that present with malapposition at 6 months are not associated with increased complications at long-term follow-up (3 years), indicating that this is not a clinical problem that requires treatment.[73,74]

Diabetes mellitus

There is more intimal hyerplasia in diabetics compared with non-diabetics.[17] There is also more intimal hyperplasia in patients with hyperinsulinemia during an oral glucose tolerance test.[76] In addition, the final lumen CSA is smaller in insulin-treated diabetics compared with non-diabetics or non-insulin-treated diabetics.[77] Thus, the increased rate of in-stent restenosis in diabetics appears to be a combination of a smaller final stent CSA – presumably reflecting smaller reference-segment lumen dimensions, diffuse disease, or less lesion compliance – on top of which is superimposed more neointimal hyperplasia.

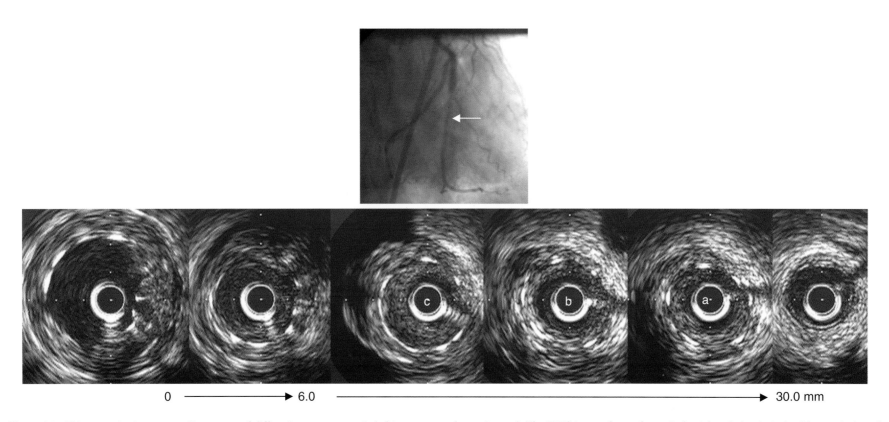

Figure 8.8 This example shows an ordinary case of diffuse in-stent restenosis (white arrow on the angiogram). The IVUS image shows the typical axial variation in intimal hyperplasia and lumen compromise. At a, the stent CSA measured 7.0 mm^2, the lumen CSA measured 2.5 mm^2, and the intimal hyperplasia measured 3.5 mm^2. At b, the stent CSA measured 7.9 mm^2, the lumen CSA measured 3.6 mm^2, and the intimal hyperplasia measured 4.4 mm^2. At c, the stent CSA measured 8.0 mm^2, the lumen CSA measured 2.5 mm^2, and the intimal hyperplasia measured 5.5 mm^2

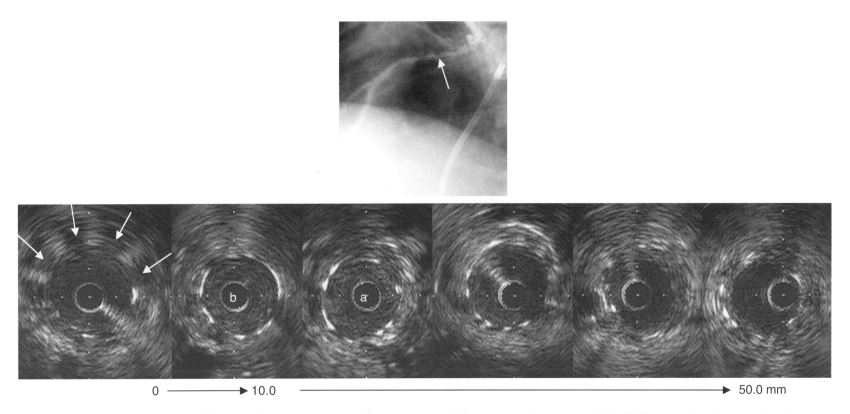

0 ⟶ 10.0 ⟶ 50.0 mm

Figure 8.9 This example shows a case of diffuse ostial right coronary artery in-stent restenosis (white arrow on the angiogram). The IVUS image shows the typical axial variation in intimal hyperplasia and lumen compromise. The maximum amount of intimal hyperplasia at a and b is associated with near-obliteration of the lumen. Note the malapposition (white arrows) proximally

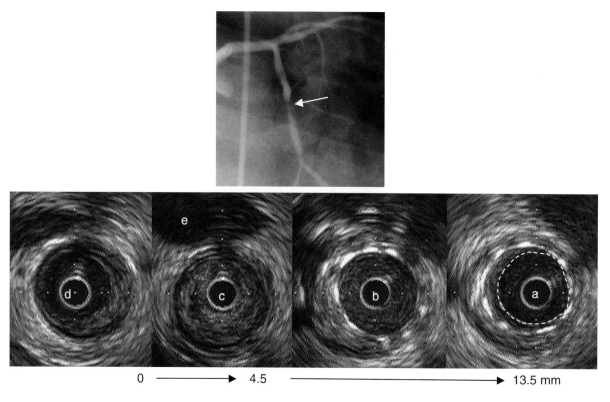

0 ⟶ 4.5 ⟶ 13.5 mm

Figure 8.10 There are two mechanisms of stent edge restenosis: intimal hyperplasia and a decrease in EEM CSA (or the combination). This example shows restenosis involving the proximal edge of a stent in the left circumflex coronary artery (white arrow on the angiogram) secondary to intimal hyperplasia. At the distal part of the stent (a), there is little intimal hyperplasia or lumen compromise; stent CSA measured 8.0 mm^2, the lumen CSA (dashed white line) measured 5.7 mm^2, and the intimal hyperplasia measured 2.3 mm^2. At the more proximal part of the stent (b), the stent CSA measured 7.5 mm^2, the lumen CSA measured 1.0 mm^2 (the size of the IVUS catheter), and the intimal hyperplasia CSA measured 6.5 mm^2. The intimal hyperplasia and lumen compromise extended into the proximal edge segment (c), where the EEM CSA measured 10.1 mm^2; this was similar to the proximal reference (d), whose EEM CSA measured 10.3 mm^2. Note the great cardiac vein (e). Contrast this with the distal edge restenosis shown in Figure 8.11

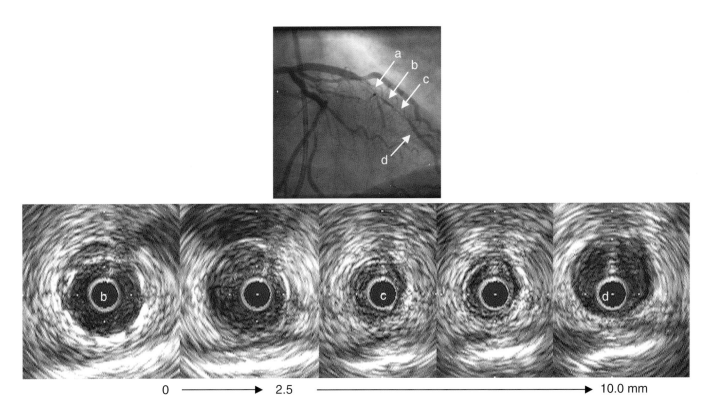

Figure 8.11 There are two mechanisms of stent edge restenosis: intimal hyperplasia and a decrease in EEM CSA (or the combination). This example shows restenosis involving the distal edge of the stent in the anterior descending artery secondary to a decrease in EEM CSA. In the angiogram, the white arrow a corresponds to the intra-stent restenosis, the white arrow b corresponds to a non-restenotic part of the distal end of the stent, the white arrow c indicates the distal edge restenosis, and the white arrow d shows the distal reference. Individual IVUS image slices (b–d) correspond to the similarly labeled arrows on the angiogram. The non-restenotic distal end of the stent (b) had a stent and lumen CSA of 6.3 mm^2. The distal edge restenosis (c) had an EEM of 3.7 mm^2 and a lumen CSA of 1.0 mm^2, both significantly smaller than the distal reference d whose EEM CSA and lumen CSA measured 7.2 mm^2 and 4.5 mm^2, respectively. Contrast this with the proximal edge restenosis in Figure 8.10

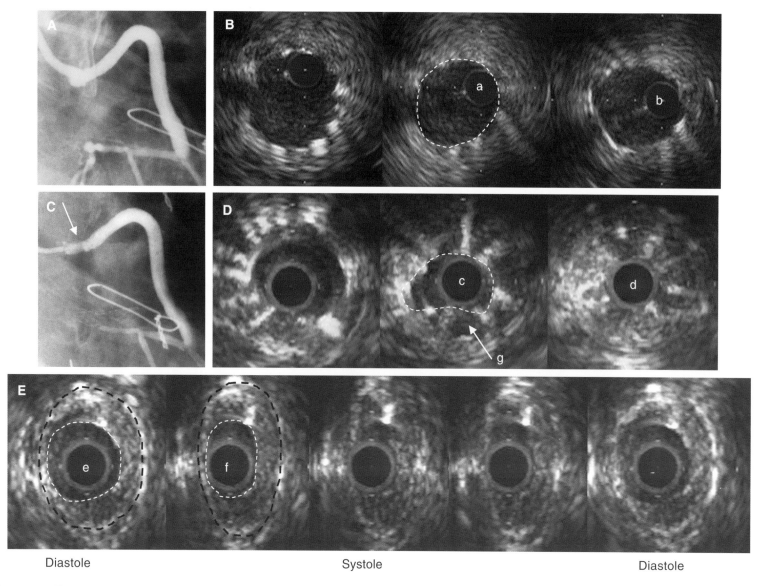

Diastole   Systole   Diastole

Figure 8.12   This is a rare example of chronic stent recoil of an ostial vein-graft Palmaz–Schatz stent. Panel A is the stent implantation angiogram, and Panel B is the stent implantation IVUS. The stent CSA measured 8.0 mm^2 at a and 7.8 mm^2 at b. Panel C is the angiogram 3 months later (note the ostial vein-graft restenosis lesion – white arrow); and Panel D is the corresponding IVUS imaging run. There has been a decrease in stent CSA from 8.0 mm^2 (dashed white line at a) to 5.4 mm^2 (dashed white line at c). Although the actual stent CSA at d is hard to measure, it is obviously deformed smaller than at implantation (b). Panel E shows systolic and diastolic eccentric compression and deformation of the vein graft at the central articulation of the Palmaz–Schatz stent; this deformation had the appearance of a "hinge point". Compare the EEM CSA (dashed black line) and lumen CSA (dashed white line) at e and f. Presumably, the eccentric vein-graft compression/deformation resulted in stent recoil and deformation that caused malapposition of the stent (g). In this case, malapposition resulted not from an increase in EEM CSA, but from a decrease in stent CSA. Panel A was recorded using a mechanical sector scanner; Panels D and E were recorded using an electronic-array instrument

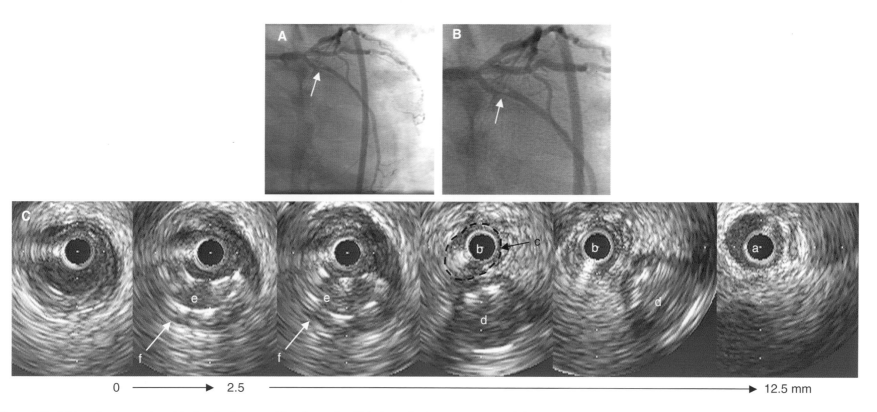

Figure 8.13   This patient was referred for brachytherapy with a diagnosis of left circumflex in-stent restenosis (white arrow in Panel A and in its magnified version, Panel B). IVUS imaging (Panel C) showed a small distal reference (a); an occlusive lumen (b) caused by shrinkage of the EEM CSA to 3.1 mm^2 (dashed black line, c); and a stent (d) in an angiographically non-visualized marginal branch. This stent extended into the proximal left circumflex, where it was partially crushed (e) against the arterial wall (f). The stent had been implanted to treat an ostial marginal branch stenosis; it had been placed from the proximal now-occluded marginal branch back to the main circumflex. Adjunct balloon angioplasty within the left circumflex crushed the proximal part of the stent against the wall. At follow-up, the marginal branch was totally occluded at its ostium, and there was no stent at the site of the angiographic "in-stent restenosis lesion". Brachytherapy was not performed

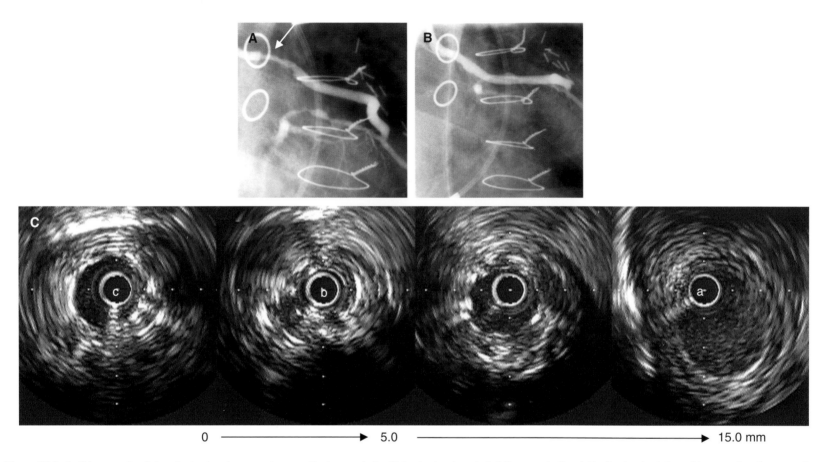

Figure 8.14 In this example of chronic stent underexpansion, a patient presented with in-stent restenosis (white arrow in Panel A) after implantation of two overlapping stents into an ostial vein-graft stenosis. IVUS imaging (Panel C) showed a distal reference lumen CSA (a) of 9.9 mm^2; a minimum stent CSA (b) of 3.3 mm^2; and a proximal stent CSA (c) of 5.3 mm^2. The vein-graft in-stent restenosis lesion was treated with high-pressure balloon inflations (22 atm), with the final angiographic result shown in Panel B

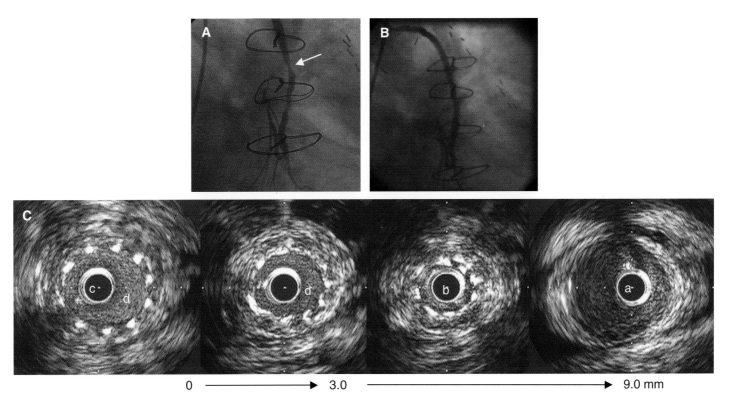

Figure 8.15 In this example of chronic stent underexpansion, a patient presented with in-stent restenosis (white arrow in Panel A) after stent implantation into a mid vein-graft stenosis. IVUS imaging (Panel C) showed a distal reference lumen CSA (a) of 8.0 mm^2; a minimum stent CSA (b) of 3.1 mm^2, and a proximal stent CSA (c) of 7.0 mm^2. There is intense blood speckle (d). The vein-graft in-stent restenosis lesion was treated with high-pressure balloon inflations (20 atm), with the final angiographic result shown in Panel B

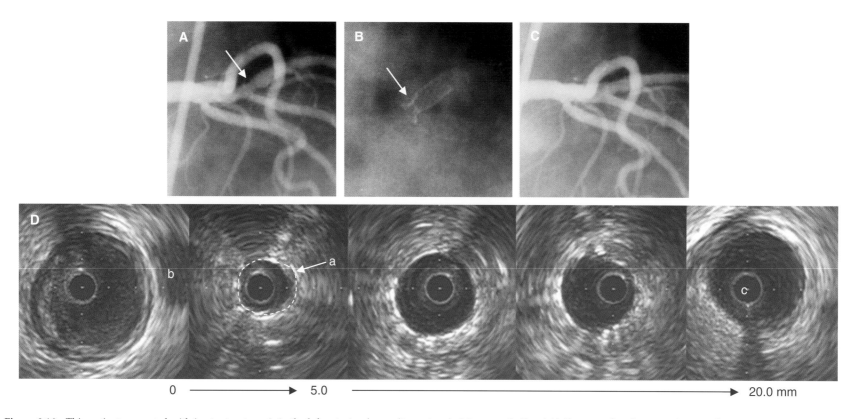

Figure 8.16   This patient presented with in-stent restenosis in the left anterior descending artery (white arrow in Panel A). Because of underexpansion, cinefluoroscopy (Panel B) showed focal, proximal stent under-expansion (white arrow). IVUS imaging (Panel D) showed a minimum stent CSA of 3.5 mm² (dashed white line a) just distal to the major diagonal branch (b), while the distal reference lumen CSA (c) measured 7.7 mm². The stent was aggressively expanded at 22 atm, with the final angiographic result shown in Panel C

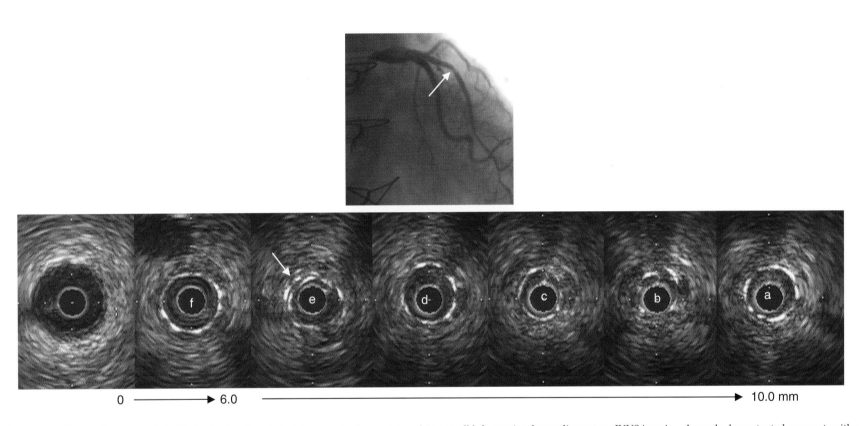

Figure 8.17 This patient presented with in-stent restenosis (white arrow in the angiogram) in a small left anterior descending artery. IVUS imaging showed a long stented segment, with a small stent CSA ranging from 2.5 mm² at a, to 1.8 mm² at b, to 2.0 mm² at c, to 3.2 mm² at d, to 2.7 mm² at e, and to 3.4 mm² at f. Note the overlapping stents (white arrow)

Figure 8.18 (opposite)   This patient presented with in-stent restenosis of an ostial right coronary lesion 2 months after implantation. The pre-intervention angiogram is showed in Panel A (with the lesion indicated by a white arrow), the post-stent implantation angiogram is shown in Panel B, and the in-stent restenosis angiogram 2 months later is shown in Panel C (with the restenosis lesion indicated by a white arrow). The IVUS imaging (Panel E) shows that the proximal edge of the previously placed stent (a) just missed the true ostial lesion (b). Note the transition to the aorta (c) and a small amount of intimal hyperplasia (d). The minimum lumen CSA (dashed white line) measured 3.8 mm^2. The patient was treated with additional stent implantation. The final angiogram is shown in Panel D. Panel F shows the final IVUS; the true ostium (e) is now covered by a stent. Note, again, the transition to the aorta (f)

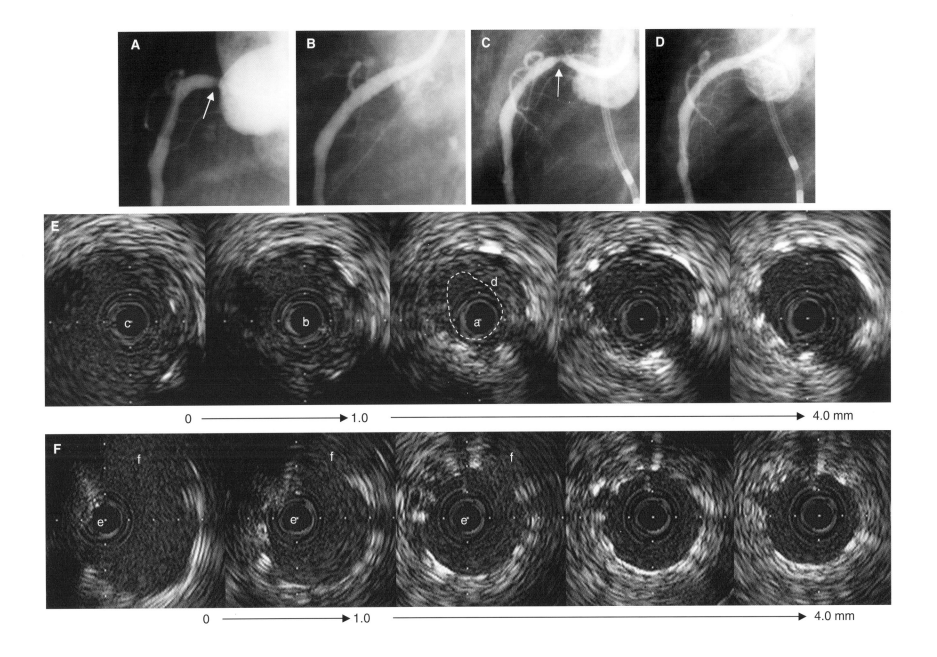

Figure 8.19 (opposite) This patient presented with a second episode of proximal right coronary artery in-stent restenosis (white arrow in Panel A) within 5 months of stent implantation. The pre-intervention IVUS (Panel C) shows a well-expanded distal part of the stent (a) with a stent CSA of $12.0\ mm^2$; a midportion of the stent (b) that is crushed against one side of the vessel wall (note that there are no stent struts against the opposite wall, c); and a proximal portion of the stent (d) that is asymmetric because of opposing arcs of calcium (e). During the intervention immediately after deploying the stent, the operator lost wire position. In rewiring the stent in order to post-dilate the stent, the guidewire exited through one of the proximal cells of the stent, coursed parallel to the midportion of the stent, and re-entered the distal portion of the stent through another one of its cells. When the stent was post-dilated, the midportion of the stent was crushed against one side of the artery. The dashed white line at f indicates the cell where the guidewire exited the stent, and the IVUS catheter at g is in the center of the cell where the guidewire re-entered the stent. These two cells have been stretched nearly circular by the original post-dilating balloon; the minimum inter-strut distance measured 2.5 mm in each distorted cell. The stent was then aggressively dilated, and the lumen restented; the final angiogram is shown in Panel B, and the final IVUS is shown in Panel D. Note the residual crushed stent (h) outside of the newly placed stent (dashed white line) and the transition to the aorta (i)

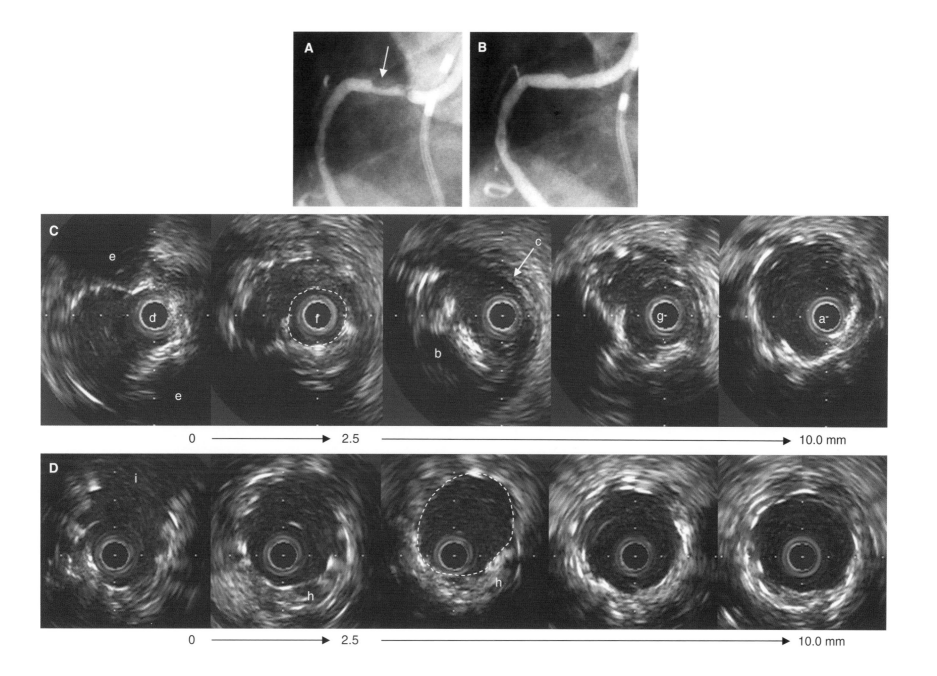

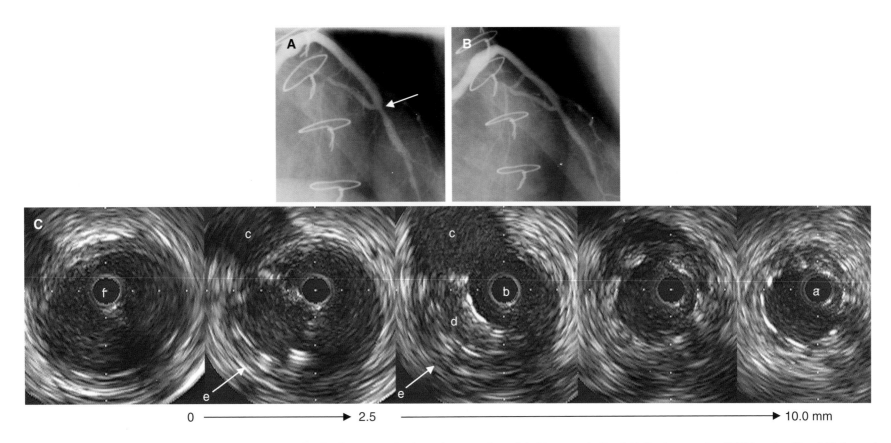

Figure 8.20 This patient presented with in-stent restenosis at the distal anastamosis of a saphenous vein graft (white arrow in Panel A). Pre-intervention IVUS imaging (Panel C) shows the stent in the native artery (a); the site of the distal anastamosis (b) – note the proximal native artery (c) – where the stent (d) was expanded and then crushed against one side of the vein-graft wall (e); and the vein graft proximal to the anastamosis (f). The patient was treated with balloon angioplasty, with the final angiogram shown in Panel B

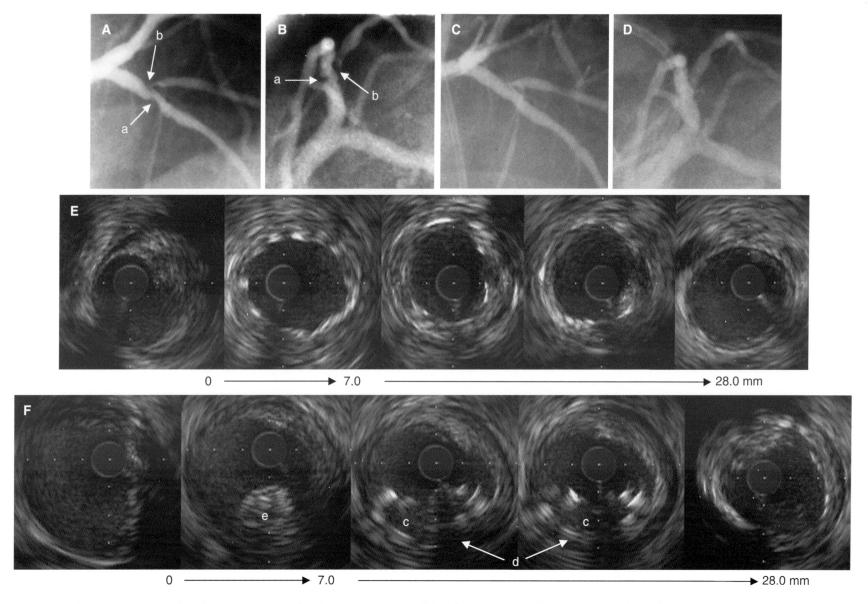

Figure 8.21 As shown in Panels A and B, this patient presented with in-stent restenosis of the left anterior descending artery (a) involving the major diagonal branch (b) 2 months after implantation of two tubular slotted stents. IVUS of the distal stent is shown in Panel E; the minimum stent CSA measured 8.9 mm^2, with little intimal hyperplasia. The IVUS of the proximal stent is shown in Panel F. Note that part of the stent had been expanded and then crushed (c) against the arterial wall (d), while part appears to have been stripped off the balloon and never expanded (e). The left anterior descending was restented, with the final angiograms shown in Panels C and D

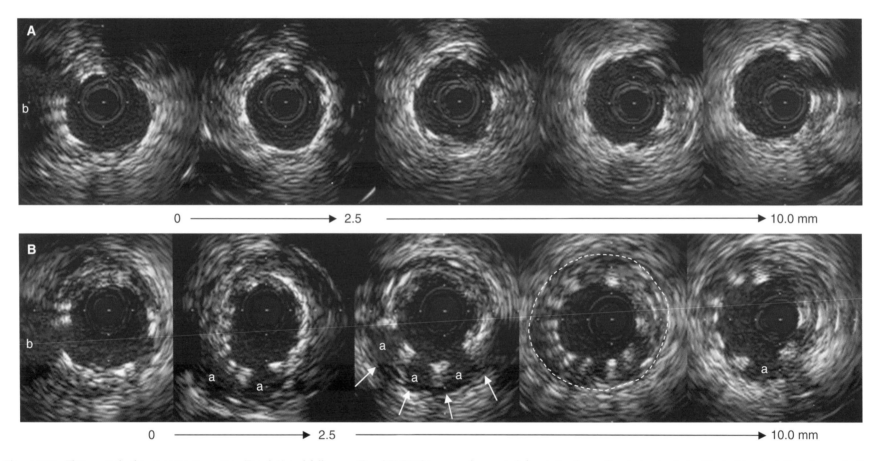

Figure 8.22 This example shows post-intervention (Panel A) and follow-up (Panel B) IVUS images of an acute left anterior descending lesion treated with stent implantation, demonstrating late stent malapposition after acute infarct intervention. In Panel A, it is difficult to determine the EEM CSA; this is seen with some thrombus-containing lesions, particularly after stent implantation. In Panel B, there is extensive late stent malapposition (a), particularly where the arterial wall is disease-free (white arrows). Unlike in the post-intervention study, the EEM (dashed white line) can be easily identified. These findings suggest that late stent malapposition in this patient was secondary to thrombus dissolution. Note where the stents cross the major diagonal branch (b); this should not be confused with stent-vessel wall malapposition

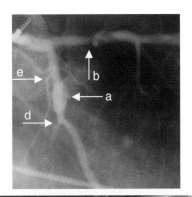

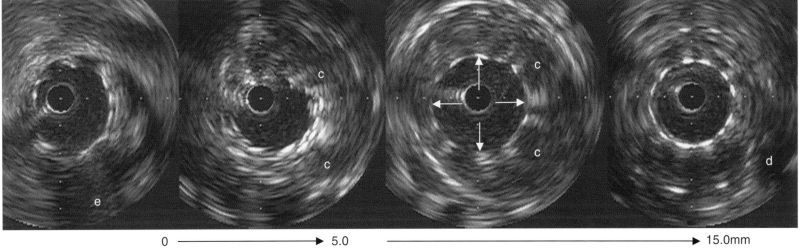

0 ⟶ 5.0 ⟶ 15.0mm

Figure 8.23 Two overlapping stents (white arrow a in the angiogram) were previously placed into this left circumflex artery; they were imaged at follow-up prior to treating the proximal left anterior descending stenosis (b). IVUS showed extensive stent malapposition (c). Because IVUS was not performed at implantation, it is not clear whether this malapposition is newly acquired or persistent from implantation. Note the lack of intimal hyperplasia at the site of late malapposition (white arrows) and the two branches (d and e), on both the angiogram and the IVUS, which are useful when comparing the two studies

Aorto-ostial lesions

Stent CSAs in aorto-ostial lesions are larger but restenosis rates are higher compared with non-ostial lesions. This is only possible if intimal hyperplasia is greater in aorto-ostial lesions compared with non-ostial lesions (Figure 8.24). Diabetes and aorto-ostial lesion location may have an additive effect in increasing intimal hyperplasia (see Figure 7.16).

Bifurcation stenting

Bifurcation stenoses are at high risk of restenosis, particularly when both the main artery and the side branch are stented. Frequently, when performing bifurcation stenting, one or both stents are not adequately expanded (see Figures 7.36 and 7.37), and this may contribute to restenosis. However, there have been no systematic studies of bifurcation stents – regardless of the technique ("T", "Y", "Culotte", or "crush") – in which both branches are imaged post-intervention and at follow-up to prove that chronic stent recoil is not a feature of bifurcation in-stent restenosis. Examples of IVUS follow-up after bifurcation stenting are shown in Figures 8.25–8.29. As these examples show, even when imaging both branches, it may be difficult to determine the presence of ostial "restenosis" of the contralateral branch. The size of the lumen of the contralateral ostium that is not covered by the stent can be measured, and intimal hyperplasia can be detected; however, flow into the artery (through the porous stent) is difficult to determine.

Other stent designs and stent grafts

There are few or no IVUS data on coiled stents. In particular, there are no serial IVUS data on Gianturco–Roubin stents to indicate whether chronic stent recoil, inadequate intial stent dimensions, or exaggerated intimal hyperplasia contributed to increased restenosis with this stent design (Figure 8.30).

Analysis of self-expanding stents showed late stent expansion with increased intimal hyperplasia, resulting in similar long-term lumen dimensions compared with balloon-expandable stents. The distribution of intra-stent intimal hyperplasia and the edge or reference-segment effects were similar to those with balloon-expandable stents.[78–86]

In two reports of small numbers of patients treated with ePTFE stent grafts, restenosis secondary to intimal hyperplasia occurred at the edges, not within the body of the stent graft.[87,88]

Serial IVUS studies of the bioabsorbable Igaki–Tamai, poly-L-lactic acid (PLLA) stent showed a stent CSA of 7.42 ± 1.51 mm^2 at implantation, 7.37 ± 1.44 mm^2 at day 1, 8.18 ± 2.42 mm^2 at 3 months, and 8.13 ± 2.52 mm^2 at 6 months, with intimal hyperplasia CSA at 3 and 6 months of 2.51 ± 0.94 mm^2 and 2.50 ± 0.65 mm^2, respectively.[89] IVUS studies revealed stent signatures at 6 months (PLLA and metal have a very similar IVUS appearance), but the struts were difficult to see at 3 years.

Predictors of in-stent restenosis in bare-metal stents

The single major IVUS predictor of clinical, angiographic, or IVUS in-stent restenosis is the final stent CSA.[35–42,90–96] This is true even when the stent is "overexpanded" compared with the reference (overexpansion does not increase restenosis).[97,98] The data in Figure 7.16 are supported by other studies, including the results of the CRUISE trial, in which the 9-month target-lesion revascularization rate was 27% for a final stent CSA 4.0–5.9 mm^2, 19% for a final stent CSA 6.0–6.9 mm^2, 12% for a final stent CSA 7.0–8.9 mm^2, and 4% for a final stent CSA > 9.0 mm^2. The final stent CSA is even a predictor of restenosis after stenting chronic total occlusions.[99]

The power of the final stent CSA to predict clinical or angiographic restenosis is explained by the finding that intimal hyperplasia thickness is independent of the final stent CSA. The same intimal hyperplasia thickness, when superimposed on a smaller final stent CSA, results in a smaller follow-up lumen CSA, and ischemia is related, at least in part, to the absolute lumen area. However, in bare-metal stents, the predictive value of the minimum stent CSA is only 50–60%, indicating that 40–50% of restenosis is explained by biologic factors (such as diabetes) or underlying lesion morphology that increase intimal hyperplasia.[100]

De Feyter *et al.* reported the interaction between stent length and minimum stent CSA (see Figure 7.17). For the same final stent CSA, a longer stent was more likely to restenose than a shorter stent, and this interaction was greater in smaller than in larger final stent CSAs. More stent metal increases the heterogeneity and variability of the neointimal response and the probability that there will be an exaggerated focal accumulation of neointima within a particular segment.[101] In addition, one study showed that the final minimum stent CSA was less optimal in long lesions compared with short lesions.[102] Thus, it was not surprising that the TULIP trial indicated that IVUS guidance can mitigate against this interaction by optimizing the final stent area in longer lesions.[103]

There have been other weaker, less consistent, or less well-studied IVUS predictors of bare-metal in-stent restenosis. Five studies compared restenosis with pre-intervention remodeling. Three studies showed that positive remodeling was associated with more clinical restenosis or neointimal hyperplasia;[104–106] one study showed no difference between lesions with positive versus intermediate/negative remodeling;[107] and one study showed that negative remodeling was associated with more neointimal hyperplasia or restenosis.[99,108] Two studies showed that the amount and spatial orientation of the intimal hyperplasia was related to the amount and distribution of the pre-intervention plaque burden.[109,110] Three studies showed that the residual plaque burden predicted restenosis or neointimal hyperplasia,[96,111,112] and two did not.[113,114] Three reports showed no impact of residual edge dissections – described as minor or non-obstructive – on subsequent clinical, angiographic, or IVUS restenosis.[115–117] In one of these studies with serial IVUS, 75% of the edge dissections had healed by 6 months.[117] In one study, asymmetric stent expansion was associated with more intimal hyperplasia.[118] However, stent asymmetry is difficult to "control", and more aggressive post-dilation may only make it worse (see Figure 7.24).[119] In one study of patients with acute myocardial infarction, the presence of a ruptured plaque was predictive of in-stent restenosis.[120]

PREVENTION OF BARE METAL IN-STENT RESTENOSIS

IVUS guidance

This is discussed in detail in Chapter 7. However, a recent meta-analysis of nine studies enrolling 2972 patients showed that IVUS-guided stenting was associated with less target-vessel revascularization (odds ratio = 0.62, $p < 0.0001$), major adverse cardiac events (odds ratio = 0.79, $p = 0.03$), and binary angiographic restenosis (odds ratio = 0.75, $p = 0.01$), while it had a neutral effect on death or non-fatal myocardial infarction.[121]

Local drug delivery

HIPS randomized 179 patients to intraluminal or intramural delivery of unfractionated heparin prior to stent implantation. At 6 months, there was no difference in IVUS measures of intimal hyperplasia.[122] IMPRESS (Intravascular Ultrasound Makes Possible Reliable Assessment of Neointima After Stenting) randomized 250 patients to intramural delivery of nadroparin versus control (no local delivery) and showed no difference in intimal hyperplasia at 6 months between the two groups.[123] ITALICS (Investigation by the Thoraxcentre of Antisense DNA Using Local Delivery and IVUS After Coronary Stenting) randomized 85 patients to intracoronary delivery of *c-myc* antisense versus saline; 6-month intimal hyperplasia was almost identical in the two groups.[124]

Systemic drug therapies

ERASER (Evaluation of ReoPro And Stenting to Eliminate Restenosis) was a trial of abciximab versus placebo in patients treated with the Palmaz–Schatz stents.[125] DANTE was a trial of abciximab versus placebo in diabetic patients treated with various stents.[126] TRAPIST (TRApidil versus placebo to Prevent In-STent intimal hyperplasia) was a trial of trapidil versus controls in patients treated with the self-expanding Wallstent.[80] PRESTO (Prevention of REStenosis with Tranilast and its Outcomes) compared four dose regimens of tranilast versus placebo in patients treated with a variety of interventions, but mostly (84%) stent implantation.[127] All of these studies showed no differences in IVUS measurements of intimal hyperplasia in the treatment group compared with controls.

CART-1, a study of AGI-1067 and probucol (beginning 14 days pre-intervention) versus placebo in patients treated mostly with stent implantation also showed no difference in intimal hyperplasia compared with placebo.[128] However, despite the lack of an impact of these drugs on in-stent neointima, there was a curious dose-responsive increase in lesion and reference-segment lumen volume with AGI-1067 compared with placebo, as well as with probucol compared with placebo; this benefit was detected immediately post-stent implantation and persisted at follow-up.

Recently, the success of sirolimus-eluting stents in reducing in-stent restenosis has prompted studies of oral rapamycin for preventing in-stent restenosis. Most of these studies include IVUS analyses. The results are pending, but have shown no benefit to date.

Finally, six smaller IVUS studies have shown benefits of various systemic drug therapies in reducing in-stent intimal hyperplasia: (1) troglitazone in non-insulin-dependent diabetics,[129] (2) pioglitazone in non-insulin-dependent diabetics,[130] (3) quinapril,[131] (4) candesartan plus probucol,[132] (5) amlodipine,[133] and (6) pemirolast.[134]

Stent implantation technique modifications

One study randomized 249 patients to direct stenting (without pre-dilation) versus conventional stenting following pre-dilation. At 6 months, there was no difference in IVUS measures of intimal hyperplasia.[135] These same investigators randomized 120 Multi-Link HP stents to implantation at either low (8–10 atm) or high (16–20 atm) inflation pressures. At 6 months, there was also no difference in IVUS measures of intimal hyperplasia.[136] Thus, it is the final result that is important, not how this result is obtained.

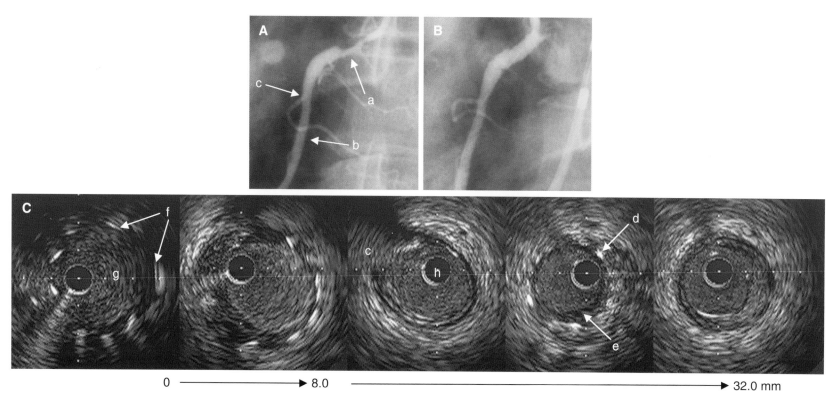

Figure 8.24 Two stents had previously been placed in this right coronary artery; the ostial stent restenosed (white arrow a on the angiogram), while the proximal stent did not (white arrow b on the angiogram). Note the branch (c), on both the angiogram and the IVUS (Panel C), which was useful when comparing the two studies. IVUS showed that the proximal stent (d, 7.5 mm^2) had only mild intimal hyperplasia (e, 2.8 mm^2), while the ostial stent CSA (f) (which measured 13.2 mm^2) had extensive intimal hyperplasia (12.2 mm^2, g). Note the intervening segment (h) between the two stents; it was nearly normal. The ostial lesion was restented, with the angiographic result shown in Panel B

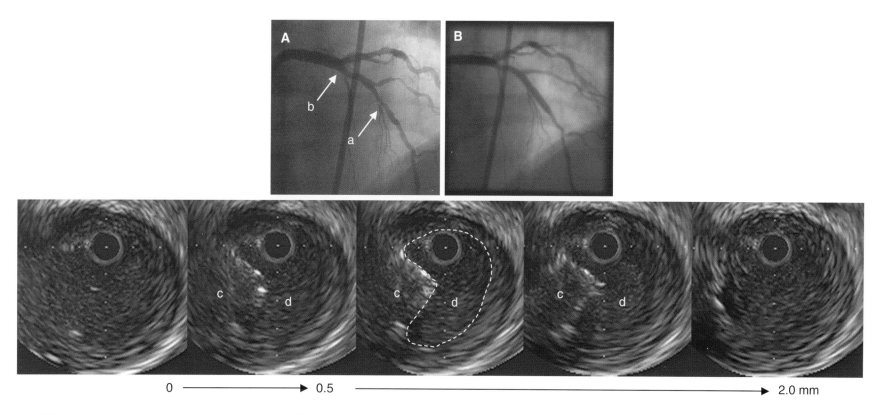

Figure 8.25 A stent had previously been placed in the ostium of the left circumflex; the patient presented for intervention of a mid left anterior descending stenosis (white arrow a on Panel A). The IVUS imaging run (Panel C) began in the left circumflex (right-hand images), continued proximally alongside the left anterior descending stent, and terminated in the left main (left-hand images). The IVUS images showed the ostium of the left anterior descending, corresponding to the white arrow b on the angiogram in Panel A. Note the ostial left circumflex stent (c), which protruded into the lumen of the left anterior descending (d); however, the uncovered lumen CSA of the left anterior descending at this point (dashed white line) measured 10.2 mm^2. The guidewire and the IVUS catheter entered the left anterior descending proximal to the proximal edge of the stent, not through a cell in the stent (see Figure 8.29 for comparison). Panel B shows the mid left anterior descending stenosis after stent implantation

Figure 8.26 (opposite)   This patient underwent stent implantation into a proximal left anterior descending stenosis (white arrow in Panel A), with the result shown in Panel B. At that time, the IVUS images (Panel C) showed a minimum stent CSA that measured 6.0 mm^2, and the stent covered most, but not all, of the left circumflex ostium (a). The patient presented 1 month later with recurrent symptoms and the angiogram shown in Panel D; note the linear density across the ostium of the left circumflex (white arrow in Panel D). The ostia of the left anterior descending and left circumflex were dilated with kissing-balloon inflations, with the angiographic result shown in Panel E. The IVUS sequences that corresponded to Panels D and E are shown in Figure 8.27

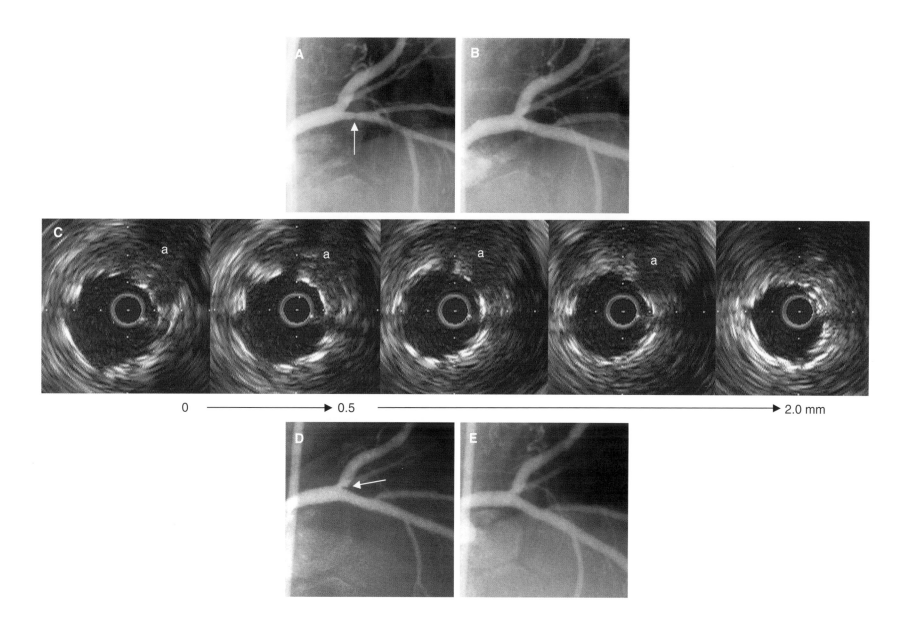

Figure 8.27 (opposite)   The sequences of IVUS images that correspond to Panels D and E in Figure 8.26 are shown. The IVUS imaging runs in Panels A and B began in the left circumflex (right-hand images), continued proximally alongside (but not through) a cell in the left anterior descending stent, and terminated in the left main (left-hand images). Panel A shows the pre-intervention IVUS images of the left circumflex ostium. Note that the IVUS catheter entered the left circumflex proximal to the proximal edge of the left anterior descending stent (a, similar to Figure 8.25, but different from Figure 8.29). The area of the left circumflex ostium (dashed white line) not covered by the stent (b) measured 4.2 mm^2. Kissing-balloon inflations were performed using a 3.0 mm balloon in each artery (see Panel E in Figure 8.26). Panel B shows the final imaging of the left anterior descending. The area of the ostium of the left circumflex not covered by the stent (dashed white line) increased to 5.2 mm^2; note the flattening of the arc of the proximal edge of the stent (white arrows), which formed the new carina between the left anterior descending and the left circumflex (c). Panel C shows the final imaging of the left circumflex. There was an increase in minimum stent CSA to 7.2 mm^2, and flattening of the arc of the proximal edge of the facing stent (d) formed the carina with the left anterior descending (e). While it is possible to assess the extent to which a stent covers the ostium of a contralateral artery in a bifurcation, it is not possible to assess flow since the stent is porous, and blood will flow through the cells into the vessel

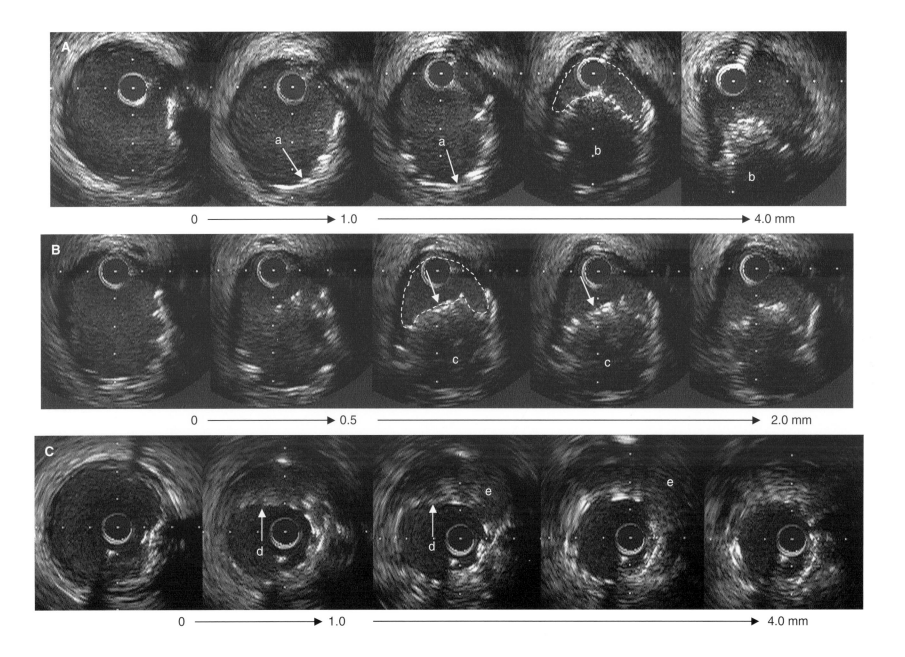

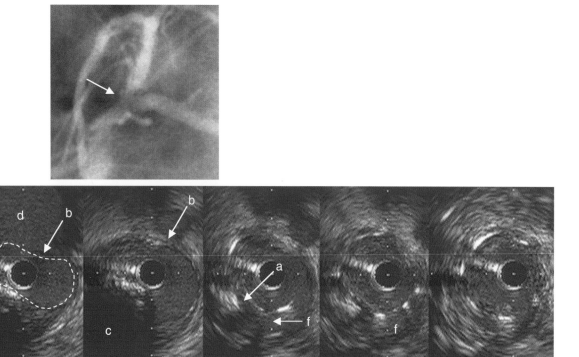

Figure 8.28 A stent had previously been placed into the proximal left anterior descending artery. At angiographic follow-up, there was concern about the ostium of the left anterior descending. The IVUS sequence showed that the proximal edge of the stent (a) stopped just short of the proximal edge of the carina (b). The ostium of the left anterior descending (dashed white line) measured 5.1 mm^2 and was partially narrowed by an eccentric calcific plaque (c), which was opposite the left circumflex (d) and which extended proximally into the distal left main (e). This calcific plaque corresponded to the white arrow in the angiogram; it caused distortion and malapposition of the proximal edge of the stent (e) and should not be confused with another stent

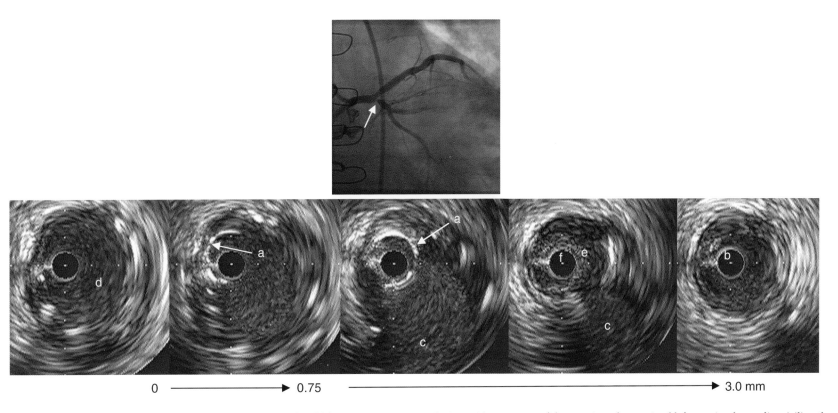

0 ⟶ 0.75 ⟶ 3.0 mm

Figure 8.29   This patient had a stent implanted into a protected distal left main coronary artery lesion, with cross-over of the stent into the proximal left anterior descending, jailing the origin of the left circumflex; the patient subsequently presented with a stenosis of the ostium of the left circumflex (white arrow on the angiogram). In order to assess this lesion, the IVUS catheter was advanced over the guidewire through one of the cells in the stent (a) into the left circumflex (b). The IVUS imaging run began in the left circumflex (right-hand images), continued proximally to enter the stent through a middle cell (middle images), and terminated in the left main (left-hand images). This has a distinctly different appearance from Figures 8.25 and 8.27, in which the IVUS catheter entered the left circumflex proximal to the proximal edge of the stent (i.e. alongside the stent). Note the left anterior descending (c) and the stent in the distal left main artery (d). Also, note the focal intimal hyperplasia (e) at the ostium of the left circumflex (f). There is negative remodeling at the ostium of the left circumflex, with an EEM CSA that measured 9.3 mm^2 compared with the EEM CSA at a, which measured 10.9 mm^2

Figure 8.30 (opposite)   This patient presented with restenosis (white arrows in Panel A) of a Gianturco–Roubin II stent implanted into the right coronary artery. IVUS imaging (Panel C) showed marked axial variation in metallic arcs of the stent (a) with reverberations (b) and the central spine (c) – typical of this stent design. While there was some intimal hyperplasia (d), the minimum stent CSA measured only 2.1 mm^2. Because there are no serial IVUS studies of Gianturco–Roubin stents, it is not clear whether this most likely represented inadequate initial stent expansion, acute recoil (plastic deformation), or chronic recoil

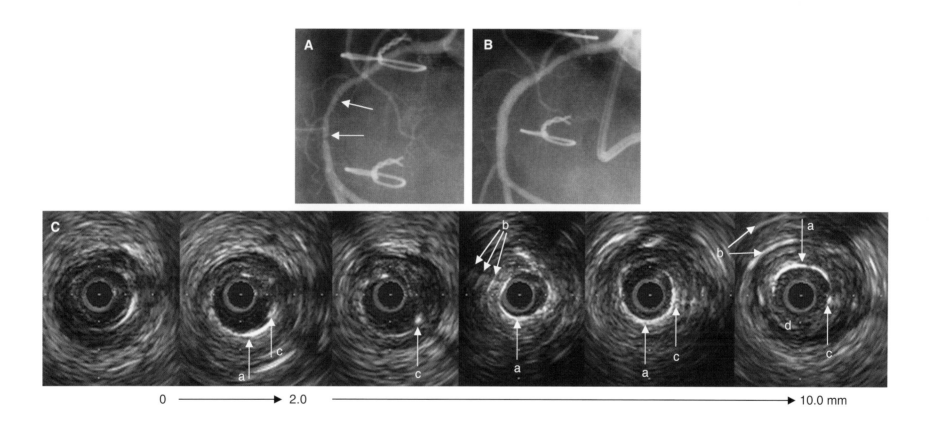

Atherectomy before stenting

IVUS studies have shown the following: (1) a relationship exists between restenosis versus pre-intervention remodeling and/or pre- and post-intervention plaque burden; (2) restenosis after atherectomy is mostly arterial shrinkage, while stent implantation resists arterial shrinkage; (3) a large plaque burden often prevents optimal stent expansion even with the use of high inflation pressures. These findings lead to the intuitive assumption that pre-stent atherectomy would reduce in-stent restenosis. Preliminary registry data and single-center experiences supported this concept. However, multicenter studies (AMIGO (Atherectomy before Multi-Link Improves lumen Gain and clinical Outcomes) and DESIRE) that randomized patients to directional coronary atherectomy prior to stenting versus stenting alone were negative. This is discussed in detail in Chapter 7.

Radiation-emitting stents

The Isostent (^{32}P-emitting stent) experience illustrated the importance of detailed IVUS analysis mm-by-mm within the stent and 5 mm-long proximal and distal edges (Figure 8.31). Dose-finding studies from Milan, core lab analysis of the global Isostent experience, and analyses from the Thoraxcenter showed that radioactive stents decreased intra-stent intimal hyperplasia CSA assessed at 6 months. However, there were three limitations to this technology.[137–142] The first limitation has been called the "candy-wrapper" effect. When analyzed mm-by-mm, there was a profound, focal, and sharply demarcated lumen loss peaking approximately 1 mm outside the edge of the beta-radiation emitting stent resulting from a focal increase in neointimal tissue.[143,144] (Conversely, when 5 mm-long segments proximal and distal to the stent edges were analyzed as a volume, the conclusions were quite different.[137,144] This highlights the importance of mm-by-mm analysis.) Two modifications to the Isostent were tried in an attempt to eliminate the "candy-wrapper" effect. Creating cold ends (25 mm-long stents with 15 mm-long beta-emitting centers and 5 mm-long non-emitting ends) broadened the peak of the "edge" effect, shifted the peak intimal hyperplasia within the body of the stents, and caused more in-stent neointima.[145] Conversely, creating hot ends appeared to attenuate the edge effect, but was associated with marked late stent malapposition in 20% of cases – higher than in the original Isostents (5.9%). This was consistent with a dose-responsive effect.[144] As with other causes of late stent malapposition, the cause was an increase in EEM CSA that was greater than the peri-stent increase in P&M CSA.[146] Late catch-up was the third main limitation of beta-radiation emitting stents. In one serial IVUS study, there was a 50% increase in intimal hyperplasia volume between 6 and 12 months.[147] An example of restenosis after radioactive stent implantation is shown in Figure 8.32.

Echolucent neointimal tissue (the so-called black hole or black wall) has been reported after implantation of radioactive stents.[148] It was tissue rich in proteoglycans, but poor in mature collagen and elastin.

Radiation following *de novo* stent implantation

Data on the use of beta-irradiation prior to *de novo* stenting come from two sources. In BERT, cross-over to stent implantation was permitted in clinically significant dissections or residual stenosis > 30%. At follow-up, the in-stent intimal hyperplasia volume was less than in historic controls and similar to other brachytherapy trials. The edge effect in stent cross-over lesions was similar to the edge effect in non-stented lesions in BERT.

PREVENT randomized patients with in-stent restenosis ($n = 25$), restenosis after balloon angioplasty ($n = 7$), and *de novo* lesions treated with stents ($n = 64$) or balloon angioplasty ($n = 9$) to one of three dose schedules of intracoronary radiation with ^{32}P or placebo.[149] The IVUS analysis was limited primarily to patients who received stents. Within the stented segment, the intimal hyperplasia volume in irradiated patients was less than in placebo patients. An analysis of 40 stent edges in 23 patients showed that the decrease in edge lumen dimensions resulted from a decrease in EEM CSA, but there was no change in P&M CSA.[150,151] There was geographic miss in 30 of 40 edges; in 77% of these 30 edges, the decrease in EEM CSA was the dominant etiology for edge lumen loss. Conversely, in the 10 edges with adequate radiation coverage, a decrease in EEM CSA was seen in only 20%, and the main mechanism of edge lumen loss was intimal hyperplasia. In BetaCath, the largest trial of beta-irradiation following *de novo* stenting, there were not enough IVUS data for meaningful analysis.

Most cases of late stent malapposition after beta-irradiation occurred in newly stented segments with little plaque burden.[152] In these patients, late stent malapposition depended on the dose delivered to the adventitia and was associated with a late event in only one patient.

Inert stent designs

In one study, all patients with allergies to nickel or molybdenum developed in-stent restenosis – enough to suggest that the overall restenosis rate after bare-metal stenting was, at least in part, related to the high restenosis rate in the subgroup of patients with metal allergies.[153] Therefore, coated, inert (non-drug-eluting) stents were developed with the hope of reducing the overall bare-metal in-stent restenosis rate. Figure 8.33 includes the IVUS findings in patients treated with inert titanium nitride oxide-, silicon carbide-, or carbon ion-coated stents; these modifications did not reduce intimal hyperplasia in unselected patients.

DRUG-COATED AND DRUG-ELUTING STENTS

Almost all drug-eluting stent studies – particularly the first-in-man initial reports – have included IVUS analysis. Initially, it was assumed that almost any combination of stent, coating, and drug would reduce restenosis compared with controls. This has not been the case. A summary of the IVUS results is shown in Figure 8.33.

Substantial data are available for only three devices: the sirolimus-eluting Cypher stent (RAVEL, Randomized Study with the Sirolimus-eluting Velocity Balloon-expandable Stent in the Treatment of Patients with De Novo Native Coronary Artery Lesions, and SIRIUS, Sirolimus-coated Bx Velocity Balloon-expandable stent in the Treatment of Patients with De Novo Native Coronary Artery Lesions); the non-polymeric paclitaxel-coated Supra-G stent (ASPECT); and the polymeric-based paclitaxel-eluting Taxus stent (TAXUS-II and TAXUS-IV). Both the mean and standard deviation of intimal hyperplasia volume obstruction are important. In successful drug-eluting stents, the mean percentage of intimal hyperplasia is less, and the standard deviation is narrower compared with bare-metal stents. Therefore, even patients with relatively more intimal hyperplasia are below the threshold of a neointimal response needed to cause symptoms.

Sirolimus

The Cypher (sirolimus-eluting) stent reduced intimal hyperplasia compared with control Bx Velocity stents.[62] In RAVEL, intimal hyperplasia averaged 1.3% and in SIRIUS, intimal hyperplasia averaged 3.1% of stent volume.[60,62] Diabetic patients in SIRIUS treated with the Cypher stents also had a significantly lower percentage volume obstruction compared with bare-metal stents (1.8% vs. 35.3%); the IVUS findings from insulin-treated and non-insulin-dependent patients were not reported separately. There was less intimal hyperplasia in the middle of the Cypher stent than at the edges; in other words, there was a greater suppression of neointima in the middle of the stent compared with the edges.

In the 4-year follow-up from the first-in-man experience, in 14 patients treated with the fast-release formulation, intimal hyperplasia was 2.3% at 1 year, 9.2% at 2 years, and 9.1% at 4 years; in the 14 patients treated with the slow-release formulation, intimal hyperplasia was 2.2% at 1 year, 3.3% at 2 years, and 5.7% at 4 years.[154–156]

In SIRIUS, a minimum stent CSA of 5.0 mm^2 was shown to have a 90% predictive value versus the IVUS minimum lumen CSA at follow-up.[100] Therefore, most cases of Cypher stent failure were due to inadequate stent expansion. In support of this, a recent presentation showed that the majority of Cypher intra-stent restenoses were in lesions with a minimum stent CSA of < 5.0 mm^2.[157] Recently, Cypher stent failure has also been attributed to either stent strut fractures or gaps between adjacent stents; the authors suggested that strut fractures or gaps between stents caused local under-dosing as well as local "irritation", leading to very focal intimal hyperplasia (while there was complete abolition of intimal hyperplasia within the rest of the stent).[158,159] The diagnosis of stent strut fracture requires a post-intervention study showing stent struts that were not present at follow-up. In fact, ideally, there should be an absence of stent struts at follow-up, since transducer angulation can affect the number and distribution of the struts seen on a single frame. Examples of Cypher stent failure are shown in Figures 8.34 and 8.35. In bare-metal stents, frank mechanical complications (crushed stent, etc.) account for 4–5% of in-stent restenosis; because Cypher stents suppress neointima, it is probable that these mechanical complications will account for a larger percentage of Cypher stent failure (Figure 8.36).

Of 31 patients with Cypher stent failure in SIRIUS, 27 restenoses were focal, and 19 of the focal restenoses were at the stent edges. In SIRIUS, volumetric analysis of 5 mm-long stent edges did not show a difference compared with controls; but, to date, mm-by-mm analysis has not been presented, and few patients with angiographic edge restenosis had complete serial (baseline and follow-up) IVUS studies. Therefore, the mechanism of Cypher stent edge effects cannot be explained by currently reported IVUS analysis. An example of Cypher stent edge restenosis is shown in Figure 8.37.

A recent randomized trial of Cypher stent implantation for bifurcation stenoses reported a restenosis rate of 25.7% that was not significantly different from double stenting (28.0%) and provisional side-branch stenting (18.7%).[160] Four cases of main-branch restenosis and four cases of side-branch restenosis were imaged at follow-up, often showing stent underexpansion. An example is shown in Figure 8.38.

Cypher stents may have more late stent malapposition compared with controls. In the RAVEL trial, only follow-up IVUS was performed; therefore, the higher Cypher stent follow-up malapposition rate (21% vs. 4% in controls) could not be separated into late stent malapposition versus persistent stent malapposition.[60] A subsequent analysis indicated that malapposition discovered at follow-up did not progress over the subsequent 12 months.[161] The serial IVUS analysis from SIRIUS suggested that, indeed, late stent malapposition was more common after sirolimus-eluting stent implantation. An example is shown in Figure 8.39.

There are no data available on the impact of sirolimus on the healing of dissections and other complications, although it would not be surprising if healing was affected (Figure 8.40).

Figure 8.31 (opposite) The Isostent experience illustrates the importance of the analysis plan in understanding edge effects. As shown in the upper left-hand panel, when analyzed mm-by-mm throughout the stent and contiguous 5 mm-long proximal and distal edges, there was a profound, focal, and sharply demarcated lumen loss, peaking approximately 1 mm outside the edge of the beta-radiation emitting stent resulting from a focal increase in intimal hyperplasia (IH) tissue. (Conversely, when 5 mm-long segments proximal and distal to the stent edges were analyzed as a volume, the conclusion was different: (1) a decrease in lumen volume and (2) a decrease in EEM volume, but (3) no significant change in P&M volume.)

Thereafter, as shown in the upper right-hand panel, between 6 and 12 months, there was a significant increase in intimal hyperplasia in the regular Isostents, mainly in the mid and distal portions of the stent, with no change in edge lumen CSA.

Two modifications were tried. Creating "cold ends" (25 mm stent length with 15 mm-long beta-emitting centers and 5 mm-long non-emitting ends) broadened the peak of the edge effect, shifted the peak intimal hyperplasia response within the body of the stents, and caused more in-stent neointima within the body of the stent. This is shown in the bottom left-hand panel.

Conversely, creating "hot ends" – approximately 8 mCi within the 14 mm body (0.57 mCi/mm) and approximately 10 mCi at the two 2 mm long "hot" ends combined (2.6 mCi/mm) for a total activity of approximately 18 mCi – appeared to attenuate the edge effect. This is shown in the bottom right-hand panel. (The data used in the upper left, lower left, and lower right panels are courtesy of Neil Weissman. The upper right-hand panel was adapted from Kay IP *et al*.[147])

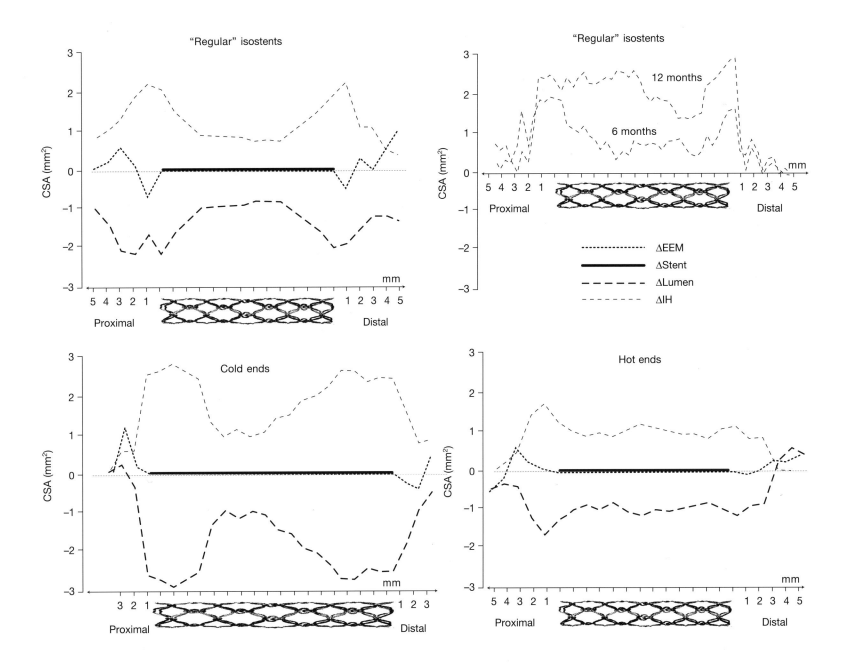

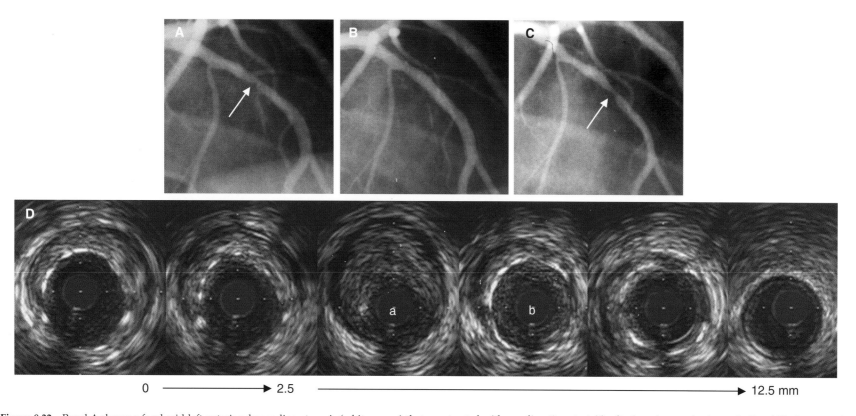

Figure 8.32 Panel A shows a focal mid left anterior descending stenosis (white arrow) that was treated with a radioactive stent (the final angiogram is shown in Panel B). At 6 months follow-up (Panel C), there was focal restenosis (white arrow). IVUS imaging at 6 months (Panel D) showed that the focal restenosis was located at (a) and just distal (b) to the central articulation

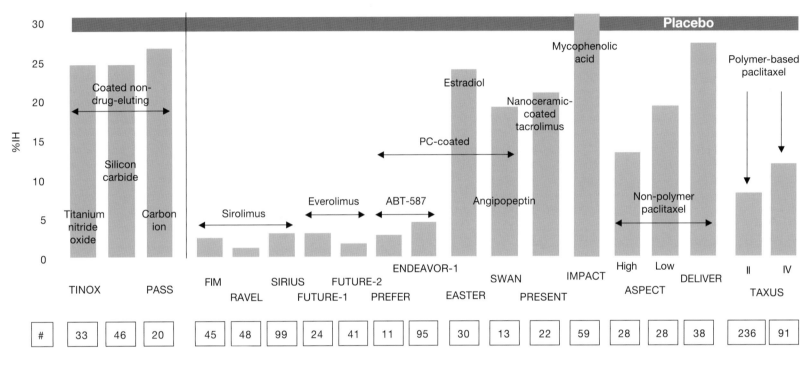

Figure 8.33 This illustration shows the percentage of intimal hyperplasia (%IH or percentage of stent volume obstruction) from trials of inert, coated non-drug-eluting stents as well as drug-coated and drug-eluting stents. The inert stent covering or the drug and its carrier vehicle (polymeric or non-polymeric), the name of the trial, and the number of patients (#) in the active arm of each analysis, when known, are shown. The time point of the IVUS analysis ranged from 4 to 9 months post-implantation, depending on the trial. As shown by the horizontal bar, meta-analysis of bare-metal stent studies shows that intimal hyperplasia averages 29% in placebo controls

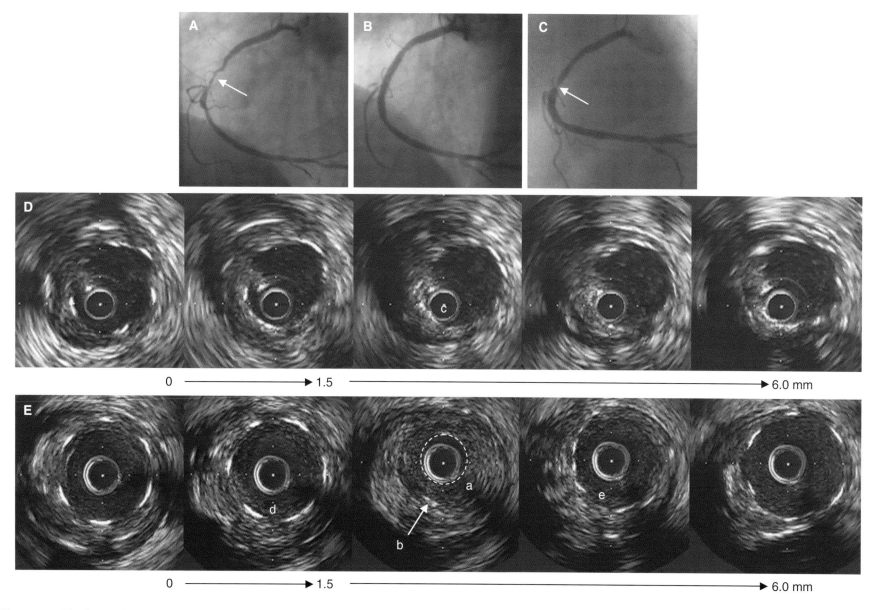

Figure 8.34 This long right coronary artery stenosis (white arrow in Panel A) was treated with two overlapping Cypher stents (33 and 15 mm in length), with the final result shown in Panel B. At 7-month follow-up, there was focal in-stent restenosis (white arrow in Panel C). Panel D shows the final (post-stent implantation) IVUS, and Panel E shows the follow-up IVUS. The two imaging sequences show identical image slices. Note the superior resolution (sharpness) of Panel E, which was recorded using a 40-MHz transducer, compared with Panel D, which was recorded using a 30-MHz transducer. At the site of focal intimal hyperplasia (a), the minimum lumen CSA (dashed white line) measured 2.0 mm², and there was a paucity of stent struts (actually, only one stent strut, b) compared with the same image slice (c) on the post-intervention study. The intimal hyperplasia was very focal and extended for less than 2 mm proximally (d) and distally (e). This is an example of focal intra-sirolimus-eluting stent restenosis, possibly from strut fracture (struts were apparent at implantation that were not seen at follow-up)

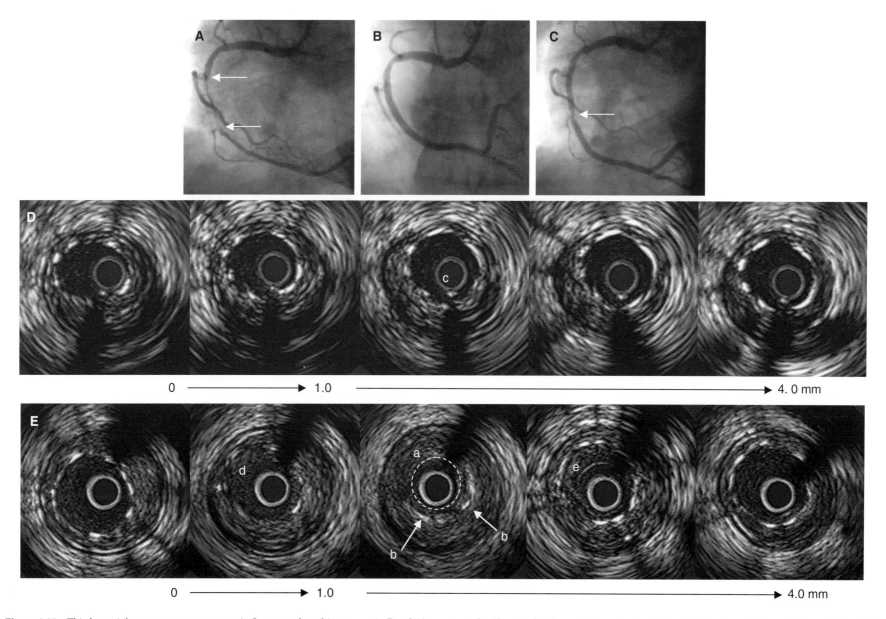

Figure 8.35 This long right coronary artery stenosis (between the white arrows in Panel A) was treated with a single 33 mm Cypher stent, with the final angiographic result shown in Panel B. The 8-month follow-up angiogram is shown in Panel C; note the focal in-stent restenosis (white arrow). Panel D shows the final (post-stent implantation) IVUS, and Panel E shows the follow-up IVUS. Note the superior resolution (sharpness) of Panel E, which was recorded using a 40-MHz transducer, compared with Panel D, which was recorded using a 30-MHz transducer. As in Figure 8.34, the two imaging sequences show identical image slices. At the site of focal intimal hyperplasia (a), the minimum lumen CSA (dashed white line) measured 2.9 mm², and there were fewer stent struts (b) compared with the same image slice (c) on the post-intervention study. The intimal hyperplasia was very focal and extended for only approximately 1 mm proximally (d) and distally (e). This is an example of focal intra-sirolimus-eluting stent restenosis, possibly from strut fracture (struts were apparent at implantation that were not seen at follow-up). (This example was courtesy of Alexandre Abizaid.)

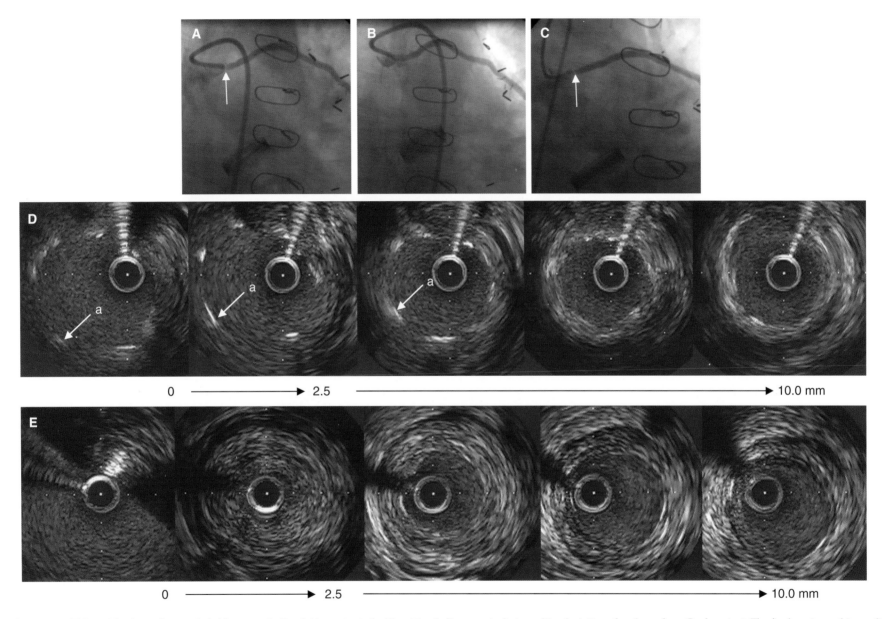

Figure 8.36 This ostial vein-graft stenosis (white arrow in Panel A) was treated with cutting-balloon angioplasty and implantation of an 8 mm-long Cypher stent. The final angiographic result is shown in Panel B. At 7-month follow-up, there was focal restenosis (white arrow in Panel C). Panel D shows the final (post-stent implantation) IVUS; note that approximately half of the length of the stent (a) protrudes into the aorta. No stent is seen at follow-up (Panel E); presumably, removal of the guiding catheter dislodged the stent

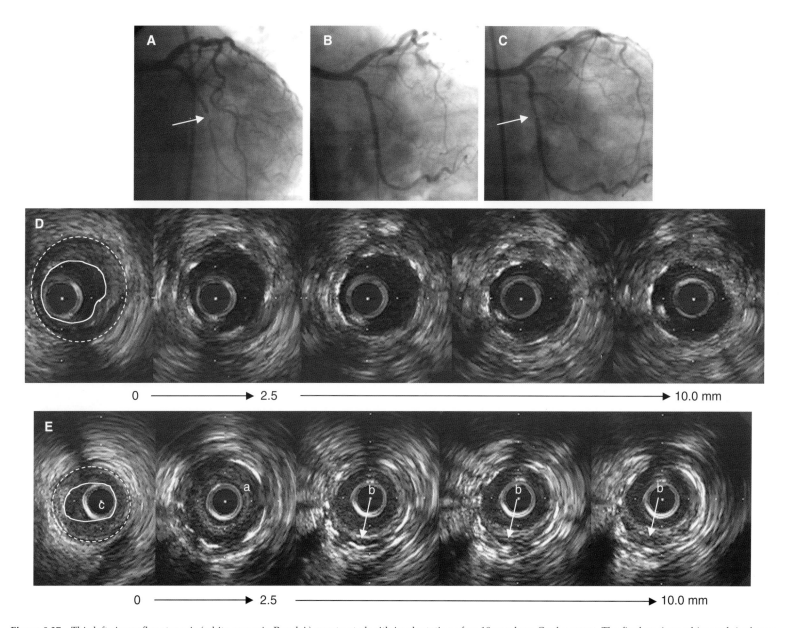

Figure 8.37   This left circumflex stenosis (white arrow in Panel A) was treated with implantation of an 18 mm-long Cypher stent. The final angiographic result is shown in Panel B. At 9-month follow-up, there was focal restenosis (white arrow in Panel C). Panel D shows the final (post-stent implantation) IVUS, and Panel E shows the follow-up IVUS. Note the focal proximal-edge intimal hyperplasia (a), which extends distally (b). In addition, there is a decrease in proximal-edge EEM CSA from 10.5 mm^2 (dashed white line in Panel D) to 6.9 mm^2 (dashed white line at c in Panel E), as well as a decrease in lumen CSA from 4.6 mm^2 (solid white line in Panel D) to 2.4 mm^2 (solid white line at c in Panel E). This is an example of focal proximal-edge sirolimus-eluting stent restenosis from a combination of intimal hyperplasia precisely at the edge of the stent (a) and a decrease in EEM CSA more proximally (c)

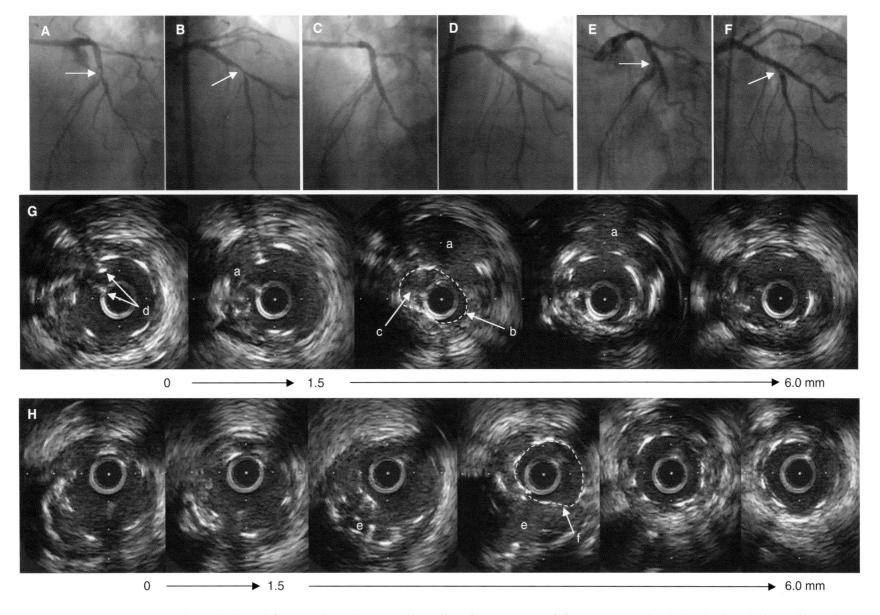

Figure 8.38 The white arrows in Panels A and B show a left anterior descending artery diagonal branch stenosis prior to bifurcation stenting. Panels C and D show the lesion after implantation of a Cypher stent into each branch. The white arrows in Panels E and F show restenosis in the left anterior descending just distal to the diagonal branch. Panel G is the IVUS imaging of the left anterior descending; note the relationship to the diagonal branch stent (a). The minimum stent CSA (dashed white line b) within the left anterior descending measured 3.0 mm^2, the minimum lumen CSA measured 2.0 mm^2, and the intimal hyperplasia CSA (c) measured 1.0 mm^2. Also note the two guidewires (d) in the left anterior descending proximal to the diagonal branch. Panel H is the imaging of the diagonal branch; note the relationship to the left anterior descending stent (e). The minimum stent CSA (dashed white line f) within the diagonal branch measured 5.0 mm^2, with a lack of intimal hyperplasia. Thus, the left anterior descending restenosis was the result of Cypher stent underexpansion

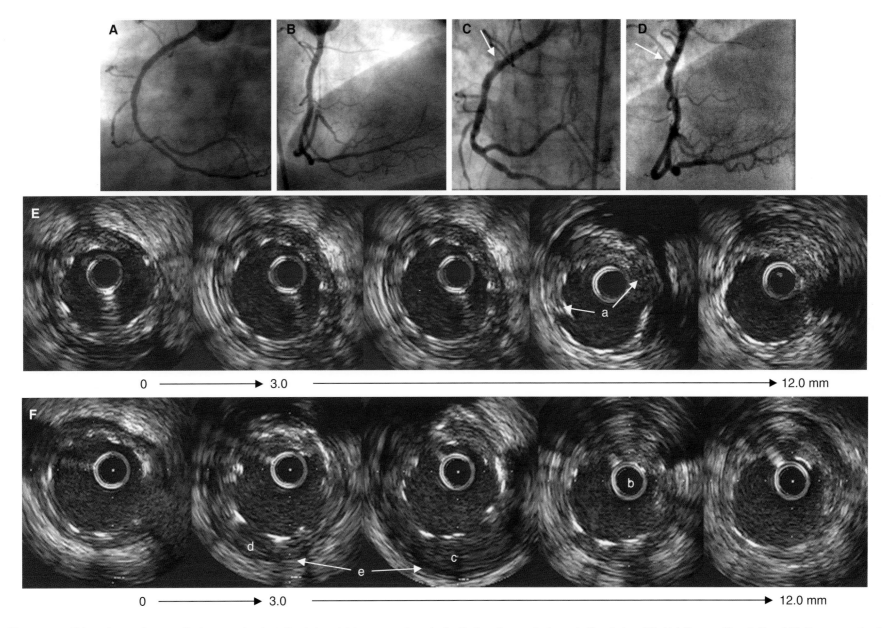

Figure 8.39 This patient underwent Cypher-stent implantation into a right coronary stenosis; the final angiogram is shown in Panels A and B. At follow-up (Panels C and D), there was a focal angiographic aneurysm in the proximal right coronary (white arrows). The final (post-stent implantation) IVUS is shown in Panel E, and the follow-up IVUS is shown in Panel F. Note the plaque prolapse (a), which is not present on the same image slice at follow-up (b). Also note the late stent malapposition (c and d), which involves the arc of normal vessel wall (e). At the site of maximum late stent malapposition (c), there has been an increase in EEM CSA from 17.8 to 28.9 mm^2, together with an increase in effective lumen CSA (intra-stent lumen CSA plus area of malapposition) from 8.8 to 16.8 mm^2. The stent CSA (8.8 mm^2) and the peri-stent P&M CSA (8.9 mm^2) have not changed

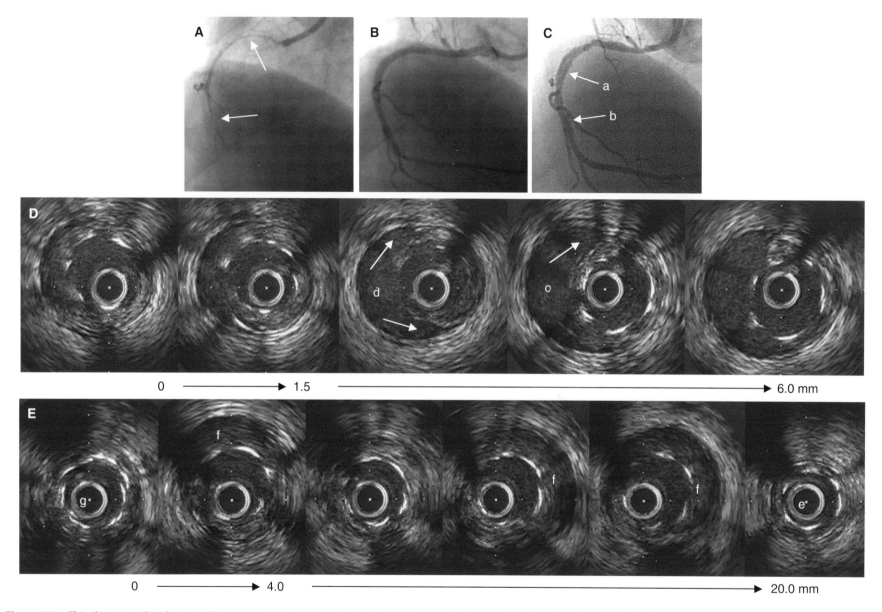

Figure 8.40 This chronic total occlusion (white arrows in Panel A) was treated with balloon angioplasty and implantation of multiple Cypher stents (Panel B). At follow-up (Panel C), there was a proximal double lumen (a) and a beaded appearance (b) in the midportion. Panel D shows the follow-up IVUS, which corresponds to the double lumen (a) in Panel C. The stent and the IVUS catheter are in the true lumen, and there is a large, unhealed false lumen (c and d) from a dissection down to the media. Note how the plaque has separated from the media, shown best by the white arrows at c and d. (For a complete discussion of dissections and their description, see Chapter 7.) In Panel E (which corresponds to the "beaded" appearance, b, in the follow-up angiogram), there is complete apposition distally (e), skip areas of late malapposition (f), and overlapping stents (g) proximally. The "beaded" appearance in the angiogram is caused by the skip areas of late stent malapposition

Non-polymeric paclitaxel

Non-polymeric paclitaxel-coated stents were tested in two trials. ASPECT (using the Supra-G stent platform) showed a significant step-wise reduction in intra-stent intimal hyperplasia volume from control (30% of stent volume) to low dose (1.28 mg/mm^2 stent surface area, 19% of stent volume) to high dose (3.10 mg/mm^2 stent surface area, 13% of stent volume).[61,162] The axial distribution of intimal hyperplasia tended to be similar to controls, and there was no increase in the rate of late stent malapposition compared with controls. In addition, at high-dose stent edges, there was an increase in EEM CSA resulting in no decrease in lumen CSA despite an increase in P&M CSA (presumably IH CSA) that was similar to control stents; this was particularly notable in the first millimeter from the stent edge (Figure 8.41). Subsequent analyses showed that, like bare-metal stents, positive pre-intervention remodeling was associated with more neointimal hyperplasia compared with negative/intermediate remodeling and that intimal hyperplasia thickness was independent of stent size.[163,164]

The results of ASPECT were not confirmed in the larger DELIVER trial that used the MultiLink Penta stent platform, suggesting that non-polymeric delivery of paclitaxel may be less controllable and reproducible than polymeric delivery of this drug.

Polymeric paclitaxel

The slow- and moderate-release formulations of paclitaxel were studied in TAXUS-II; there was a reduction in intimal hyperplasia compared with the control stent with identical amounts of intimal hyperplasia (7.8% stent volume obstruction) at 6 months in both the slow- and moderate-release formulations.[165] The distribution of intimal hyperplasia over the length of the stent was uniform and similar to controls.[166] There was no increase in late stent malapposition compared with controls, although there was a greater increase in peri-stent EEM CSA in the moderate-release formulation compared with controls (but not in the slow-release formulation compared with controls), suggesting a possible release-dependent effect of the drug on EEM dimensions.

When analyzed mm-by-mm, there was an increase in EEM CSA and a reduction in lumen loss at the edges of both slow- and moderate-release polymeric paclitaxel-eluting stents compared with controls.[167] This was most notable closest to the edge of the stent (within the first 1 mm from the proximal edge and within the first 3 mm from the distal edge), where the dose of paclitaxel was presumably greatest (Figure 8.41). Conversely, this edge effect was less obvious when the proximal and distal 5 mm-long edge segments were analyzed as a volume.

The findings of TAXUS-II are supported by preliminary analyses from TAXUS-IV that compared the slow-release formulation with controls. In TAXUS-IV, intimal hyperplasia averaged 12.2% of the stent volume, and the beneficial effects of paclitaxel were seen at the distal, but not the proximal, edges.

There are no data available on the impact of paclitaxel on the healing of dissections and other complications, although it would not be surprising if healing was affected. In bare-metal stents, frank mechanical complications account for 4–5% of in-stent restenosis; because paclitaxel-eluting stents suppress neointima, it is probable that these complications and stent under-expansion will account for a larger percentage of Taxus stent failure.

CONVENTIONAL TREATMENT OF IN-STENT RESTENOSIS

Pre-intervention assessment

Does in-stent restenosis always require treatment? Nishioka *et al.*[168] presented an analysis of 142 patients with 150 intermediate in-stent restenosis lesions (angiographic diameter stenosis of 40–75%, with 34% having a diameter stenosis > 50% and 17% having a positive exercise thallium). Repeat intervention was deferred if the IVUS minimum lumen CSA measured > 3.5 mm^2 regardless of symptoms, non-invasive testing, or angiographic findings. At follow-up that averaged 32 months, only 10% of patients had events; and the 2-year event-free survival rate was 96.5%. Therefore, not all in-stent restenosis lesions need to be treated – if they have reached the plateau of intimal hyperplasia growth that tends to occur at 6 months.[63,64] An example of an intermediate in-stent restenosis lesion in which re-intervention was deferred is shown in Figure 8.42. When measuring lumen dimensions, particularly within a restenotic stent, it is important not to misuse machine settings. As discussed in Chapter 1 (see Figure 1.21), excessive reduction in near-field intensity (in an attempt to reduce blood speckle, ring-down, or other near-field artifacts) can blank out echolucent neointimal tissue and artificially increase lumen dimensions.

Although it is uncommon, chronic prolapse of tissue through stent struts (or prolapse of tissue between adjacent stents) can occur after the patient leaves the catheterization laboratory. Prolapsed tissue tends to be more complex and often contains echodense plaque elements (typical of atherosclerosis), while intimal hyperplasia is hypoechoic and uniform in appearance. Prolapsed tissue tends to be localized, eccentric, and protruding into the lumen, while intimal hyperplasia tends to involve the entire stent circumference even though it may vary in thickness. It is difficult to see stent struts at the site of plaque prolapse, while intimal hyperplasia rarely obscures stent struts.

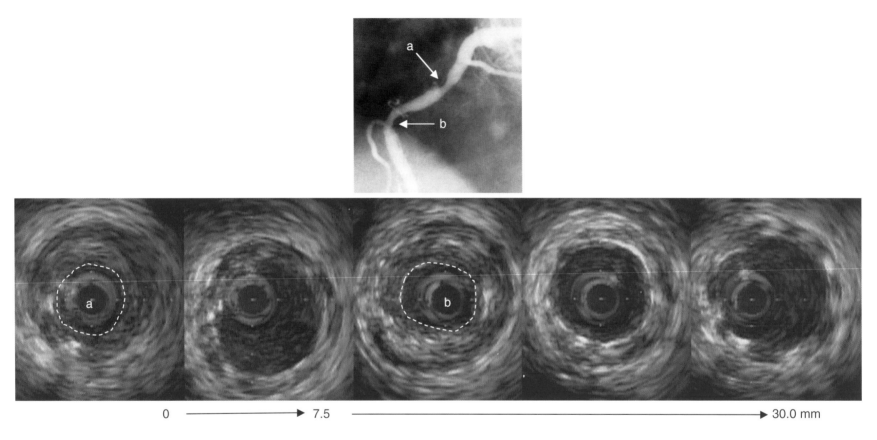

Figure 8.42 This patient underwent routine follow-up angiography after implantation of two stents into the right coronary artery; each was associated with an angiographic intermediate lesion (white arrows a and b). The IVUS study showed a lumen CSA of 5.5 mm^2 at the site of each stent (dashed white lines a and b, which corresponded to the white arrows on the angiogram). No intervention was performed

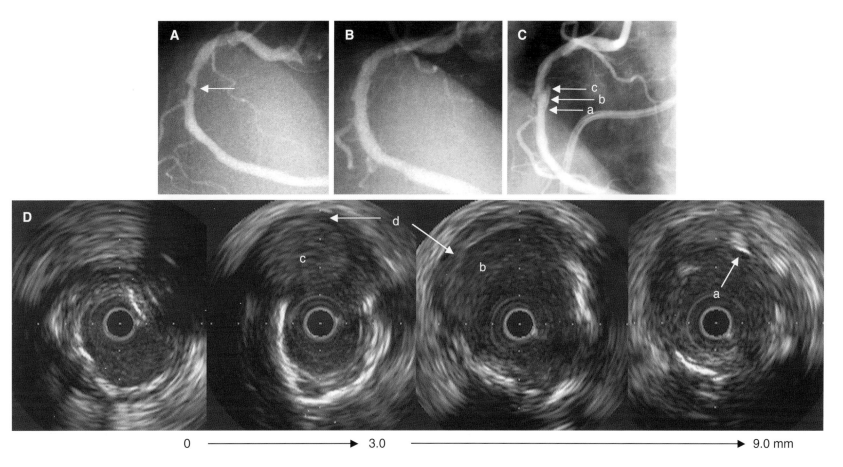

Figure 8.43   Panel A is the pre-intervention angiogram, with the lesion shown by the white arrow; Panel B is the post-intervention angiogram; and Panel C is the 5-month follow-up angiogram, with an aneurysm shown by the white arrows a, b, and c; these arrows correspond to the individual image slices on the IVUS study. On the IVUS image (Panel D), note the proximal edge of the stent (a), the body of the aneurysm (b), and the blood-stasis-filled proximal end of the aneurysm (c). The intact vessel wall (d) is consistent with a true aneurysm

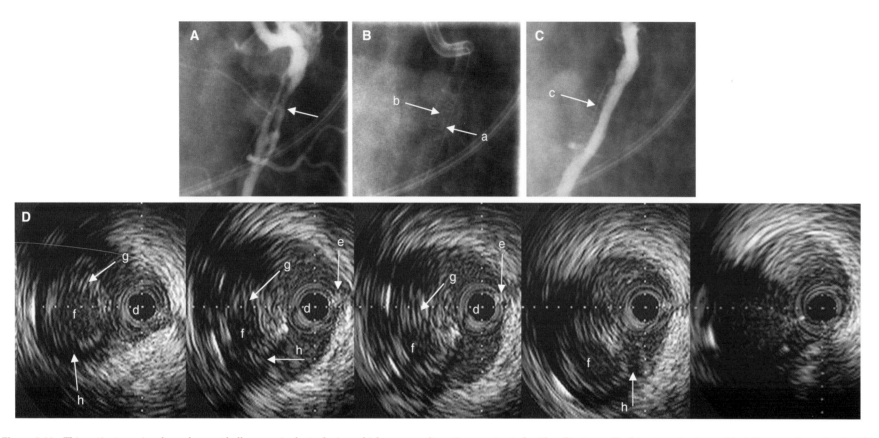

Figure 8.44   This patient previously underwent balloon angioplasty during which a severe dissection was treated with a Gianturco–Roubin stent. Angiographic follow-up showed a double-lumen appearance (white arrow in Panel A). Cinefluoroscopy (Panel B) showed that the guidewire (a) was outside the stent (b). IVUS imaging (Panel D) showed that the IVUS catheter (d) and guidewire (e) were in the false lumen. The true lumen (f) was surrounded by plaque (g) and echolucent media (h). The false lumen was stented with a tubular-slotted stent (Panel C); note that the Gianturco–Roubin stent (c) remained outside the newly stented lumen

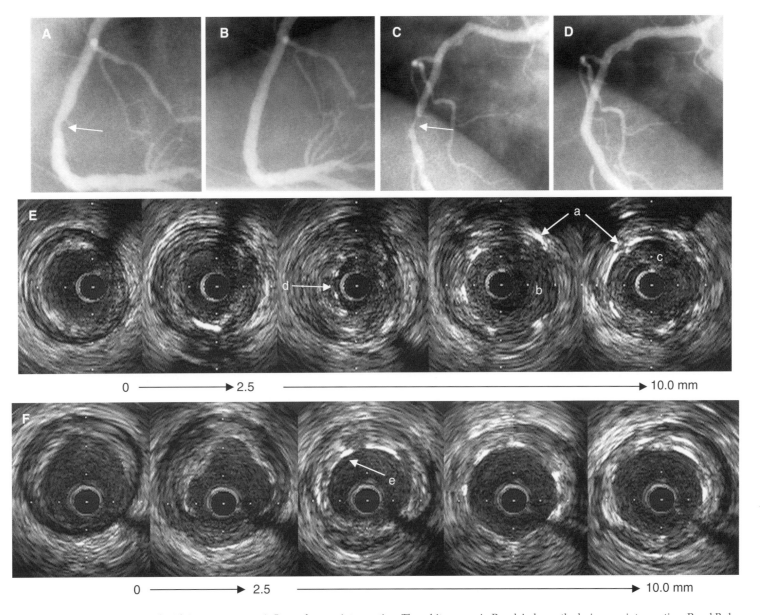

Figure 8.45 This patient presented with in-stent restenosis 5 months post-intervention. The white arrow in Panel A shows the lesion pre-intervention; Panel B shows the lesion post-stent implantation; and the white arrow on Panel C shows the restenotic lesion. IVUS imaging (Panel E) showed that the body of the stent (a) was well expanded, measured 9.6 mm^2, and contained 7.6 mm^2 (b) and 6.5 mm^2 (c) of intimal hyperplasia. Conversely, IVUS imaging showed that the proximal edge of the stent (d) measured 3.6 mm^2, with 1.5 mm^2 of intimal hyperplasia. After balloon angioplasty (Panel D), IVUS imaging (Panel F) showed additional stent expansion, particularly at the proximal edge (e), which then measured 7.5 mm^2

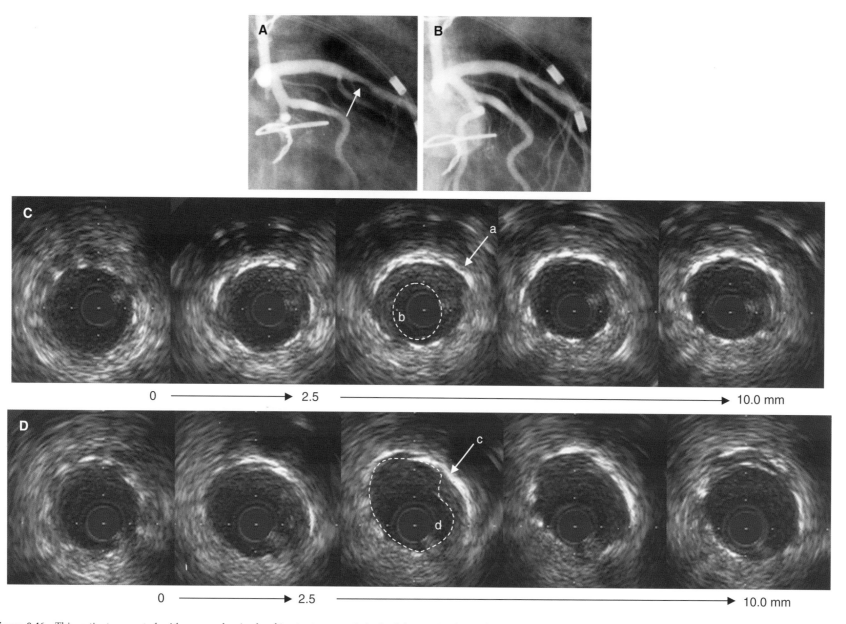

Figure 8.46 This patient presented with a second episode of in-stent restenosis in the left anterior descending (white arrow in Panel A). The pre-intervention IVUS (Panel C) showed a minimum stent CSA (a) of 8.5 mm^2 and a minimum lumen CSA (dashed white line b) of 3.2 mm^2. After balloon angioplasty (Panel B), the IVUS imaging (Panel D) showed additional stent expansion to 10.5 mm^2 (c), with a residual lumen CSA of 7.6 mm^2 (dashed white line d). Lumen improvement of 4.4 mm^2 was 45% from additional stent expansion and 55% from tissue extrusion. Because this was the second episode of in-stent restenosis, stent CSA in Panel C no longer reflected the lumen CSA at the time of the original stent-implantation procedure

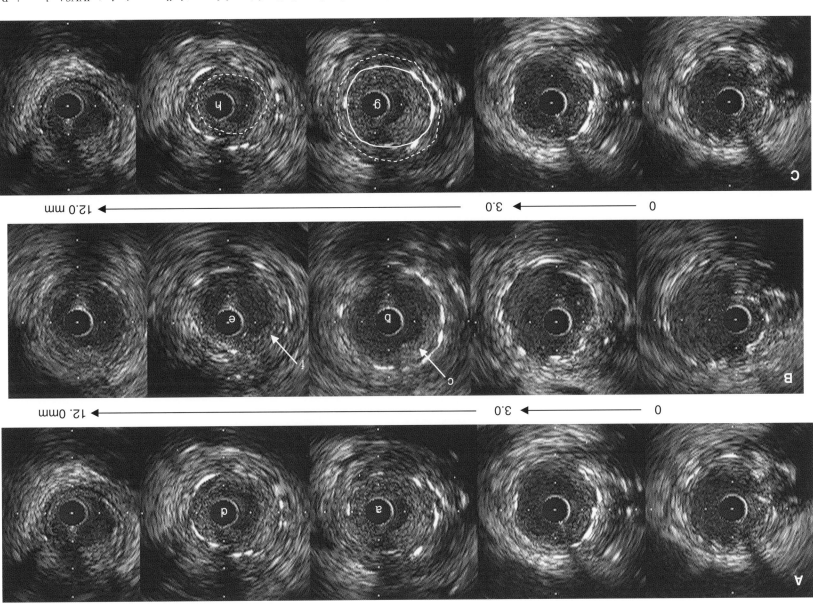

Figure 8.47 This in-stent restenosis lesion was treated with balloon angioplasty. The pre-angioplasty IVUS is shown in Panel A, and the post-balloon angioplasty IVUS is shown in Panel B. Two image slices are analyzed. The pre-angioplasty lumen CSA of 1.7 mm² (a) increased to 6.2 mm² (b), with a residual intimal hyperplasia CSA of 45%; the pre-angioplasty lumen CSA of 2.0 mm² (d) increased to 5.0 mm² (e), with a residual intimal hyperplasia burden (f) of 48%. In Panel C, the post-angioplasty IVUS contours are superimposed on a copy of the pre-angioplasty IVUS. As shown at g, stent CSA increased from 8.0 mm² pre-angioplasty (solid white line) to 11.4 mm² post-angioplasty (dashed white line). Therefore 72% of lumen improvement was the result of additional stent expansion. Because chronic stent recoil is rare, the pre-angioplasty stent CSA accurately reflects the final lumen CSA after stent implantation. As shown at h, the post-angioplasty lumen CSA of 5.0 mm² (dotted white line) is less than the pre-angioplasty stent CSA of 7.9 mm²; therefore, treatment of in-stent restenosis recovered only 63% of the lumen CSA of the original stent implantation procedure

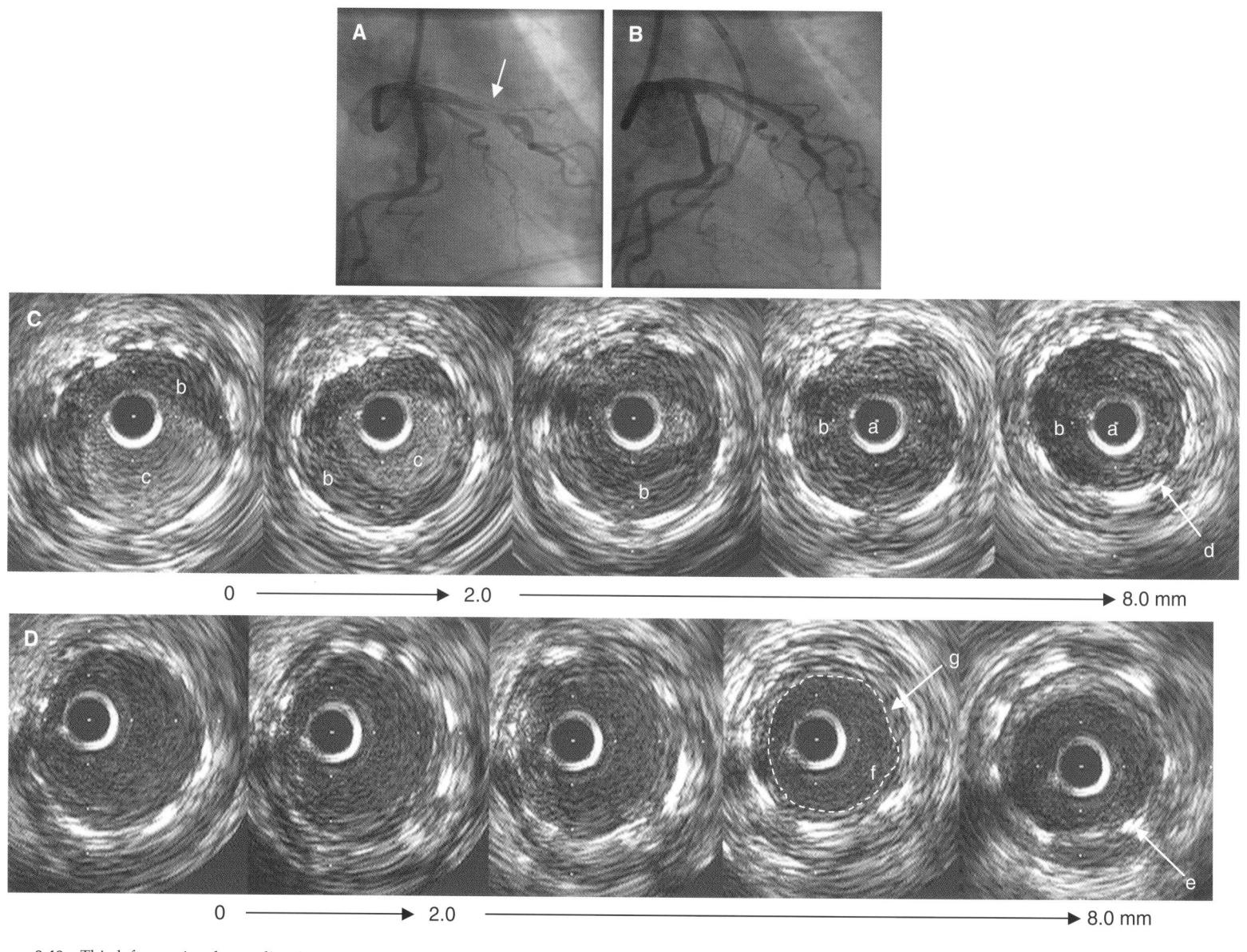

Figure 8.48 This left anterior descending in-stent restenosis lesion (white arrow in Panel A) was treated with a cutting balloon; the angiographic result is shown in Panel B. Panel C shows the pre-cutting balloon IVUS; the minimum lumen CSA was the size of the IVUS catheter (a). Note that the intimal hyperplasia (b) was less echoreflective than the blood stasis (c) proximal to the site of the minimum lumen CSA. Panel D shows the post-cutting balloon IVUS. The stent CSA increased from 10.0 mm^2 (d) to 12.1 mm^2 (e). Because chronic stent recoil is rare, the pre-cutting balloon stent CSA accurately reflects the final lumen CSA at the time of stent implantation. The residual minimum lumen CSA (dashed white line, f) measured 7.4 mm^2, i.e. 74% of the pre-cutting balloon stent CSA, indicating that treatment of this in-stent restenosis lesion recovered only 74% of the lumen of the original stent implantation procedure. The residual intimal hyperplasia burden (g) measured 35%

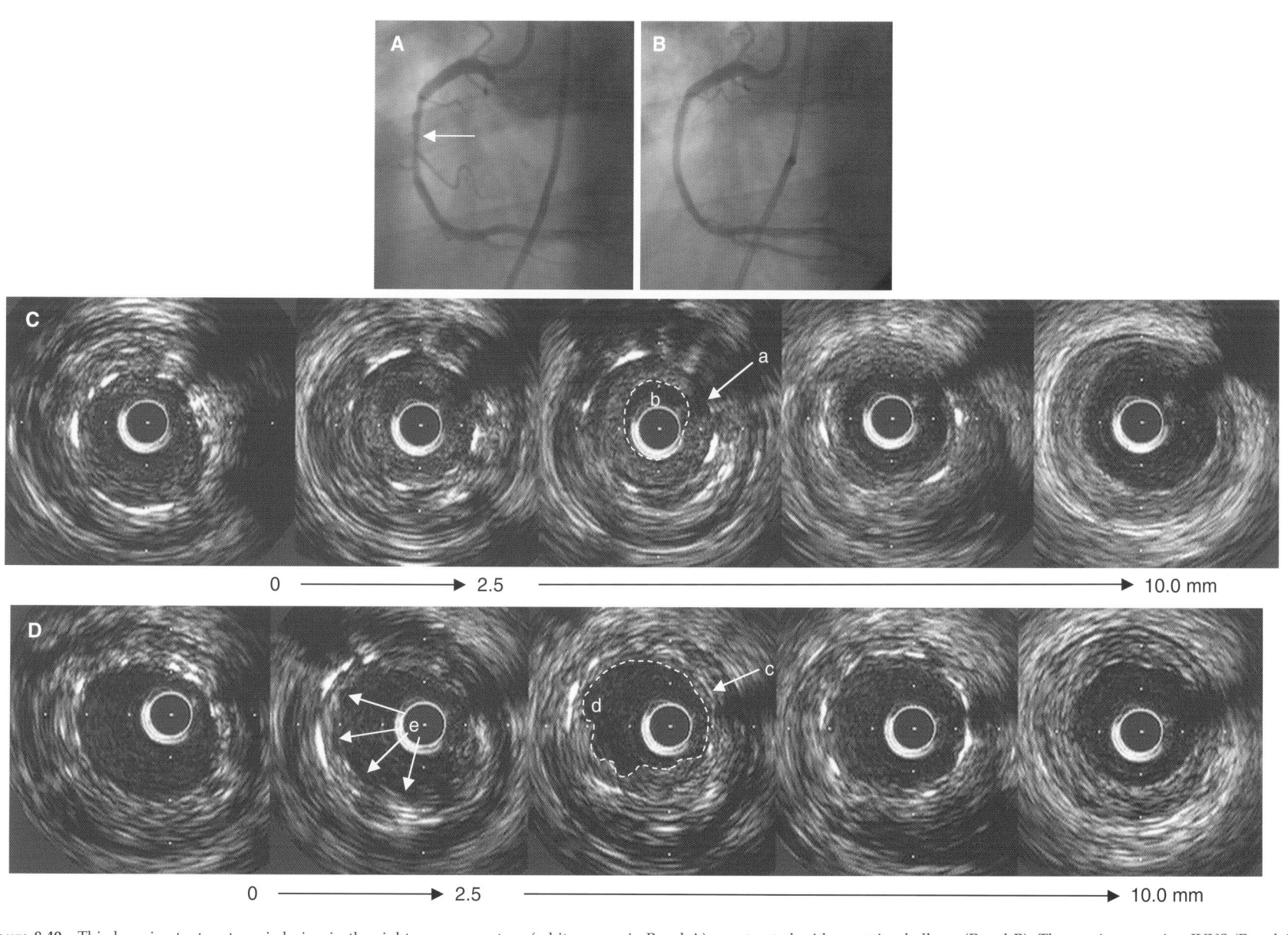

Figure 8.49   This long in-stent restenosis lesion in the right coronary artery (white arrow in Panel A) was treated with a cutting balloon (Panel B). The pre-intervention IVUS (Panel C) showed a minimum stent CSA (a) of 7.6 mm^2 and a minimum lumen CSA (dashed white line b) of 2.3 mm^2. After the cutting balloon, the IVUS imaging (Panel D) showed additional stent expansion to 9.9 mm^2 (c), with a residual lumen CSA of 6.0 mm^2 (dashed white line d). Lumen improvement of 3.7 mm^2 was 62% from additional stent expansion and 38% from tissue extrusion. Note the scalloped contour of the residual lumen (e)

Figure 8.50 (opposite)   This in-stent restenosis lesion (white arrow in Panel A, with the pre-intervention IVUS shown in Panel B) was treated with excimer laser angioplasty (Panel C, with the post-laser angioplasty IVUS shown in Panel D) followed by adjunct balloon angioplasty (Panel E, with the final IVUS shown in Panel F). The sequential IVUS studies show the same three anatomic image slices. Despite the angiographic lumen improvement, there was no increase in IVUS minimum lumen CSA from pre-intervention (dashed white line a, 1.0 mm^2) to post-laser angioplasty (dashed white line b, 1.0 mm^2); however, adjunct balloon angioplasty increased the lumen CSA to 7.5 mm^2 (dashed white line c), although this represented only 73% of the pre-intervention stent CSA (d). Because chronic stent recoil is rare, the pre-laser angioplasty stent CSA accurately reflected the final lumen CSA at the time of stent implantation. During adjunct balloon angioplasty, the mean stent CSA increased from 10.2 mm^2 (f) to 12.4 mm^2 (g), with a residual intimal hyperplasia burden (h) that averaged 40%

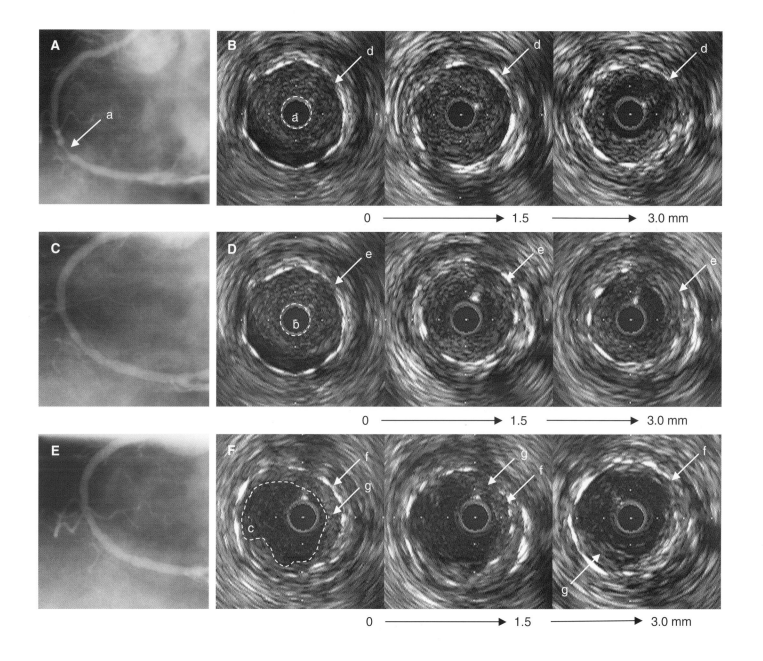

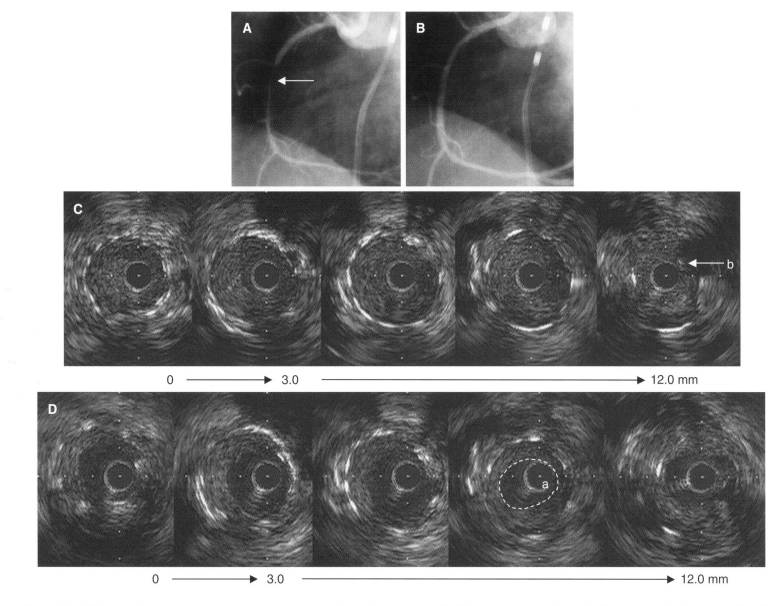

Figure 8.51 This long right coronary artery in-stent restenosis lesion (white arrow in Panel A) was treated with stand-alone rotational atherectomy. The final angiographic result is shown in Panel B. The pre-rotational atherectomy IVUS study is shown in Panel C, with the final IVUS study shown in Panel D. The residual lumen CSA (dashed white line a) measured 3.4 mm², with a residual neointimal hyperplasia burden of 63%. There was no increase in stent CSA; it measured 8.6 mm², both pre- and post-intervention. Because chronic stent recoil is rare, the pre-rotational atherectomy stent CSA accurately reflected the final lumen CSA after stent implantation; thus, treatment of this in-stent restenosis lesion recovered only 37% of the pre-intervention stent CSA (or the final lumen CSA immediately after stent implantation). Note the single unexpanded stent strut (b), which was not seen on the post-intervention study, indicating that it was ablated by the rotational atherectomy burr

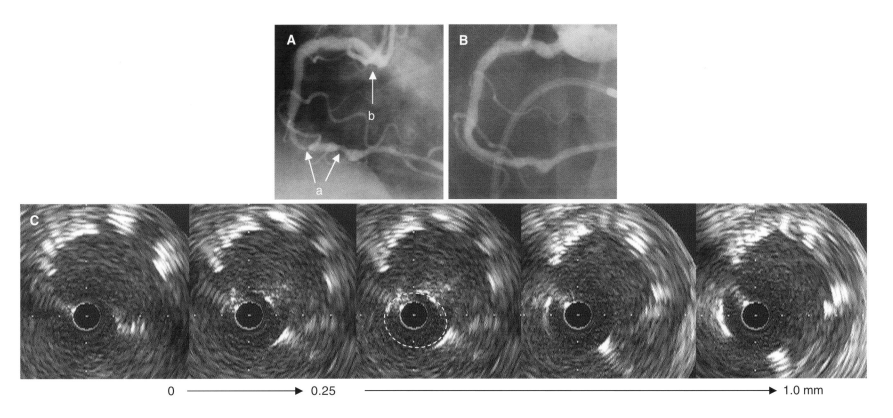

Figure 8.52 These distal right coronary artery in-stent restenosis lesions (white arrows a in Panel A) were treated with 2.0 mm rotational atherectomy burr plus adjunct balloon angioplasty; the final result is shown in Panel B. However, there was another, non-restenotic stent in the ostium of the right coronary artery (white arrow b). In wiring the artery, the guidewire entered the ostial stent through the side of one of the cells. Activating the rotational atherectomy burr to enter the right coronary ablated the ostial stent metal, creating an elliptical cell with a lumen area of 3.3 mm^2 and an inter-strut distance of 2.0 mm (dashed white line in Panel C)

Figure 8.53 (opposite)   This distal left main in-stent restenosis lesion (white arrow in Panel A) was treated with directional coronary atherectomy (Panel B). The pre-intervention IVUS (Panel C) showed a minimum stent CSA (a) of 11.1 mm^2 and a minimum lumen CSA (dashed white line b) of 3.4 mm^2. Note the ostium of the left circumflex (c) and the fact that the struts that cover the left circumflex are free of neointima; note also the calcium (d), which deformed the stent. After directional atherectomy, the IVUS imaging (Panel D) showed additional stent expansion to 13.3 mm^2, with a residual lumen CSA of 6.3 mm^2 (dashed white line e). Despite the angiographic appearance, there was only modest lumen improvement, which was almost entirely from additional stent expansion, with significant residual neointima (f)

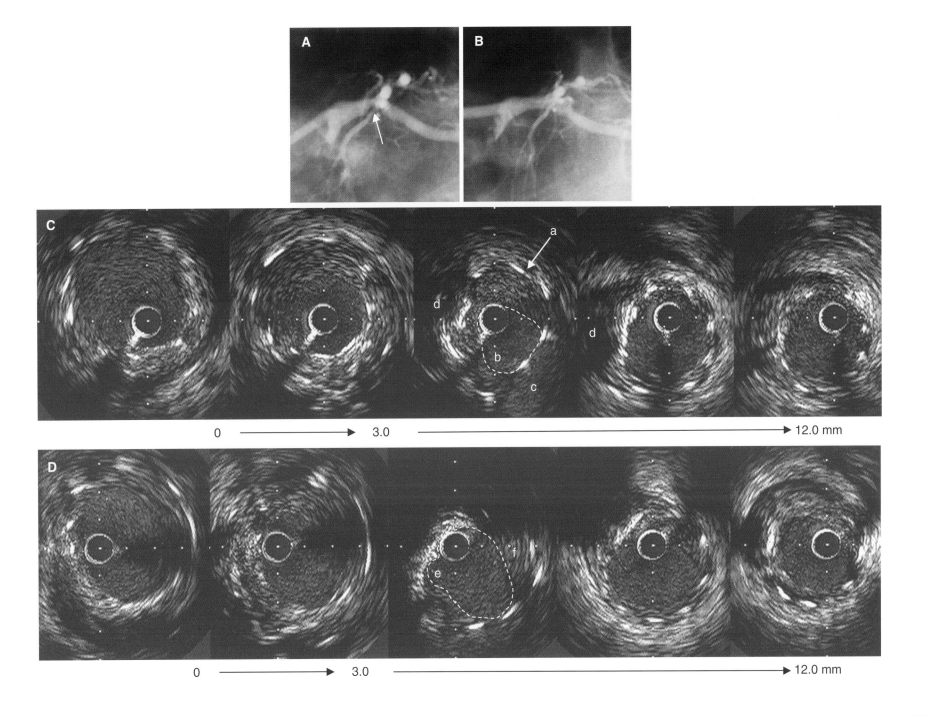

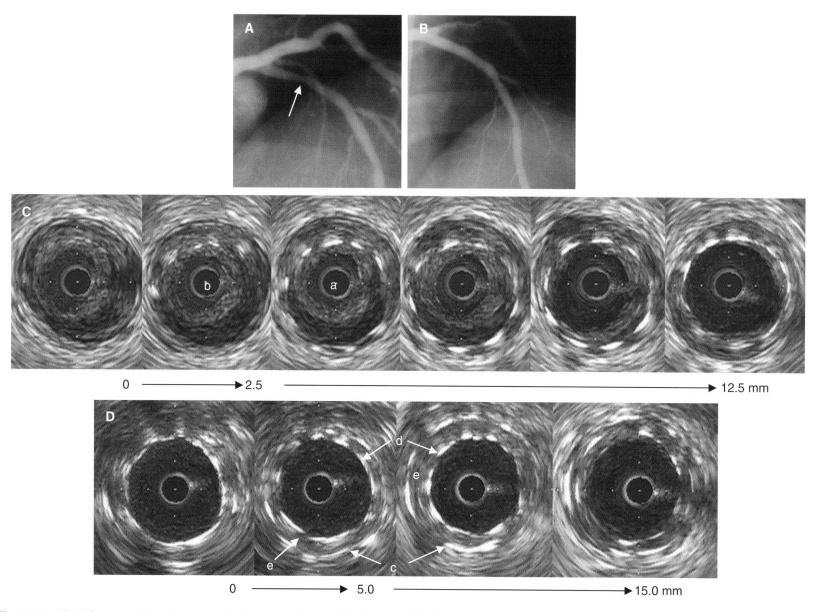

Figure 8.54 This left anterior descending artery in-stent restenosis lesion (white arrow in Panel A) was treated with additional stent implantation (Panel B). The pre-intervention IVUS (Panel C) showed this to be a proximal edge in-stent restenosis lesion; the maximum intimal hyperplasia CSA measured 8.3 mm^2 at the proximal edge (a) and extended more proximally (b). At the proximal edge, the minimum lumen CSA measured 2.9 mm^2, and the minimum stent CSA measured 11.2 mm^2. The post-intervention IVUS (Panel D) showed the double-stent layer typical of restenting an in-stent restenosis lesion: c represents the original stent, d represents the new stent, and e indicates the intimal hyperplasia that was sandwiched between them. The final lumen CSA measured 9.2 mm^2. Note that the new stent overlapped the original stent and then extended proximally. Note also the lack of residual intimal hyperplasia within the newly placed stent

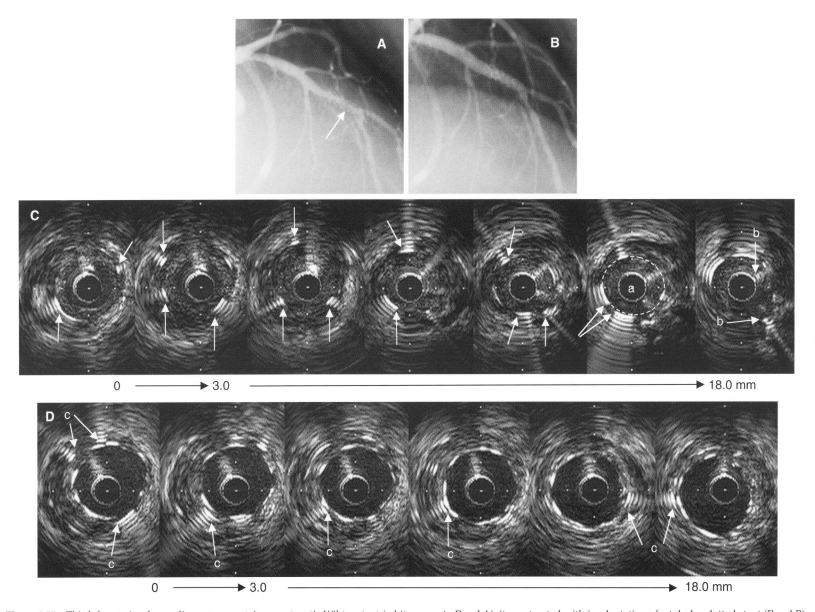

Figure 8.55 This left anterior descending artery contains a restenotic Wiktor stent (white arrow in Panel A); it was treated with implantation of a tubular slotted stent (Panel B). The pre-intervention IVUS (Panel C) shows the features of the Wiktor stent: marked variation in pattern of the coiled stent wire – sometimes many and sometimes few, some narrow and some wide, and many with intense reverberations or shadowing (most, but not all of these wire coils are shown by unlabeled white arrows). Although it was difficult to measure with confidence, the minimum stent CSA (dashed white line at a) was estimated to be 3.7 mm^2. Note the two guidewire artifacts (b), since the diagonal branch was also wired. Panel D shows the IVUS after implantation of a tubular slotted stent. Note the lack of residual intimal hyperplasia tissue within the newly placed stent and the Wiktor stent coils (c) outside the new stent

Figure 8.56 (opposite) This patient had a stent implanted into a protected distal left main coronary artery lesion, with cross-over of the stent into the proximal left anterior descending, jailing the origin of the left circumflex; the patient subsequently presented with involvement of the ostium of the left circumflex (the angiogram is shown in Figure 8.29). The IVUS catheter entered the left circumflex through one of the cells in the stent. Each IVUS imaging run began in the left circumflex (right-hand images), continued proximally to enter the stent through a middle cell (middle images), and terminated in the left main (left-hand images). Panel A is the pre-intervention IVUS. Note the left circumflex (a), the stent cell (b) through which the IVUS catheter entered the left circumflex, the left anterior descending (c), the stent in the distal left main artery (d), and the focal intimal hyperplasia (e) at the ostium of the left circumflex (dashed white line f), whose lumen CSA measured 1.8 mm^2. The ostial lesion was treated first with balloon angioplasty and then with additional stent implatation. Panel B shows the IVUS after balloon angioplasty. There has been a minimal increase in the area of the stent cell from 2.1 mm^2 (b) to 2.9 mm^2 (g), with an increase in minimum lumen CSA only to 2.3 mm^2 (dashed white line h). Implantation of a stent (Panel C) did not increase the size of the stent cell (i), although just distal to the stent cell, the ostial left circumflex lumen CSA improved to 4.9 mm^2 (j). Note that the stent protruded proximally (k), with a gap (l) with the previous stent

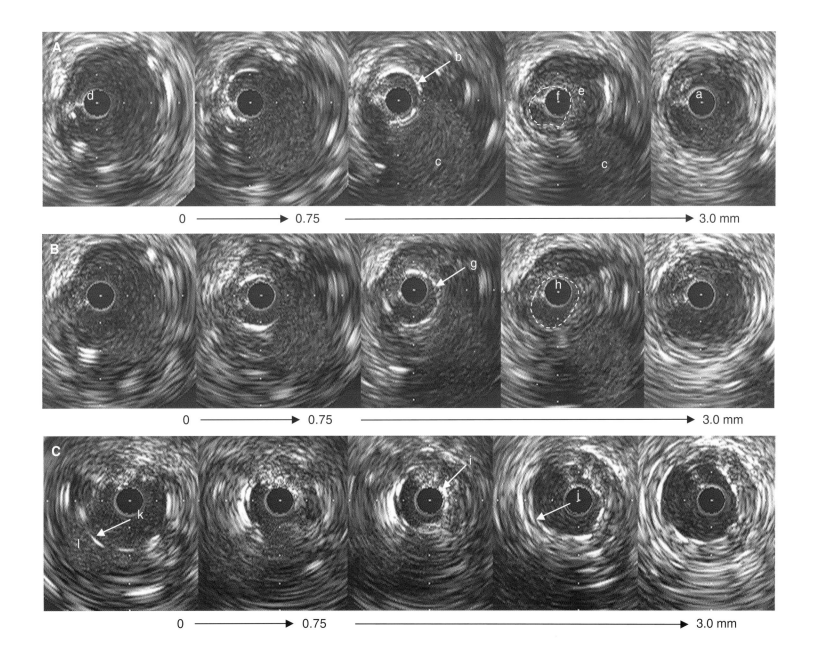

There have been no consistent studies showing the superiority of one device over another, although two studies indicated that the final lumen CSA as assessed by IVUS was predictive of recurrence.[190,191] Mehran proposed an angiographic and IVUS classification of in-stent restenosis: (1) focal in-stent restenosis (≤ 10 mm in length to include intra-stent, stent edge, and multifocal patterns); (2) diffuse intra-stent restenosis (> 10 mm within the stent), (3) proliferative in-stent restenosis (> 10 mm extending outside the stent); and (4) total occlusions. Target-lesion revascularization at 1 year was 19% in focal, 35% in diffuse intra-stent, 50% in proliferative, and 83% in totally occluded in-stent restenosis lesions. Multivariate analysis showed that diabetes (odds ratio = 2.8, $p = 0.0003$), previously treated in-stent restenosis (odds ratio = 2.7, $p = 0.0006$), and the in-stent restenosis classification (odds ratio = 1.7, $p = 0.038$) were independent predictors of recurrence.[192] These predictors are all markers of biological activity. The actual device used did not affect recurrence, suggesting that in-stent restenosis is a biological process that does respond to a mechanical approach.

Complications during treatment of in-stent restenosis are less common than with *de novo* interventions, except, perhaps, when the restenosis process involves the edges and adjacent reference segments. IVUS findings are similar to complications during *de novo* interventions (see Chapter 7). Examples are shown in Figures 8.58 and 8.59. Furthermore, additional stent expansion (which occurs during most procedures to treat in-stent restenosis) can cause the neointima to peel away from the stent metal, resulting in an intra-stent dissection. An example is shown in Figure 8.60.

Mechanisms and assessment of recurrent in-stent restenosis

There have not been any specific studies addressing the mechanisms of in-stent restenosis recurrence after traditional catheter-based intervention. However, information can be extracted from the placebo arms of various brachytherapy trials.[101,189,193–196] Recurrent in-stent restenosis is the result of intimal hyperplasia reaccumulation; chronic stent recoil is not a factor. Reference-segment effects appear to be similar to *de novo* stenting. Recurrent vein-graft lesions have similar amounts of intimal hyperplasia reaccumulation compared with native artery in-stent restenosis lesions. Longer lesions are associated with a more heterogeneous neointimal response that may contribute to their higher recurrence rate.[197]

Larger final lumen dimensions are associated with both a larger follow-up lumen and with a greater neointimal hyperplasia response.[191] However, the largest acute lumen dimensions are achieved by restenting; therefore, it is difficult to separate the effect of restenting from the larger post-treatment lumen *per se*.

There are, however, differences in IVUS findings compared with *de novo* stenting. With the exception of restenting an in-stent restenosis lesion, most procedures are associated with a significant residual neointimal hyperplasia response. Therefore, %intimal hyperplasia at follow-up is a problematic end-point since it reflects both the residual intimal hyperplasia and the amount of tissue reaccumulation. Figure 8.61 includes the placebo arms of various brachytherapy trials, indicating that there is a wide variation in the increase in mean intimal hyperplasia CSA (the most commonly reported end-point) after conventional treatment strategies.

Late stent malapposition is much less common after treatment of in-stent restenosis compared with *de novo* stent implantation. However, when it does occur, it is usually in the setting of new stent implantation.

BRACHYTHERAPY TREATMENT OF IN-STENT RESTENOSIS

Gamma-irradiation

There are extensive IVUS randomized clinical trial data showing that brachytherapy using gamma sources reduces recurrent in-stent restenosis. The first report was the SCRIPPS (Scripps Coronary Radiation to Inhibit Intimal Proliferation Post Stenting) trial, in which most of the lesions were in-stent restenosis lesions.[193] The distance from the center of the IVUS catheter (assumed to be the position of the radiation source) to the leading edge of the adventitia (the target) was used to determine the dose prescription. At follow-up, the increase in intimal hyperplasia volume was less in iridium-192 (^{192}Ir)-treated patients than in placebo patients (Figure 8.61). There was no edge analysis in SCRIPPS because edge effects were under-recognized at that time, and the edges were not imaged.

The WRIST and Gamma-1 trials specifically addressed treatment of in-stent restenosis.[194,198] In both studies, there was a smaller increase in intimal hyperplasia volume and mean CSA in the ^{192}Ir group compared with placebo (Figure 8.61). Of note, in over half of the lesions in WRIST, there was a reduction in intimal hyperplasia between radiation and follow-up (Figure 8.62).

Although uncommon, distal edge recurrence was noted in eight gamma-irradiated patients from WRIST. Compared with irradiated patients with no recurrence, distal edge recurrence lesions had (1) a greater decrease in distal lumen CSA; (2) no change in distal EEM CSA versus an increase in distal EEM CSA in non-recurrence lesions; (3) a greater increase in distal P&M CSA; and (4) a significant increase in intra-stent intimal hyperplasia, particularly closer to the distal edge of the stent.[199] These findings suggested that edge recurrence after gamma-irradiation was part of diffuse treatment failure. One proposed solution to edge effects was to irradiate longer segments. To determine the short-term safety of this approach, since it would involve radiating angiographically normal arterial segments, the effect of brachytherapy on irradiated, but uninjured, reference segments more than 5 mm from the stent edge was analyzed. There was an increase in P&M CSA in both ^{192}Ir and placebo patients.[200] However, in the ^{192}Ir group, there was an increase in EEM CSA, while in the placebo group there was a decrease in EEM CSA. As a result, there was no change in lumen CSA in the ^{192}Ir group, while in the placebo group there was a decrease in lumen CSA.

In-stent restenosis lesion length was an independent predictor of radiation failure in these studies. In an attempt to understand the impact of lesion length on treatment of in-stent restenosis, irradiated long WRIST lesions (length 36–80 mm) were compared with irradiated native artery WRIST lesions (10–47 mm in length).[201] Post-intervention lumen areas were smaller in longer lesions. Combining both groups, the maximum source-to-target distance could be correlated directly with in-stent restenosis length; and the decrease in minimum lumen CSA, the increase in intimal hyperplasia CSA, and the ratio of maximum/minimum follow-up intimal hyperplasia CSA could all be correlated with the maximum source-to-target distance. This indicated that more recurrence in longer in-stent restenosis lesions was related to a greater heterogeneity in the neointimal response, which was superimposed on smaller post-intervention lumen dimensions; a more heterogeneous neointimal response was, in turn, related to a greater variability in lesion geometry and source eccentricity. Two parameters determine source eccentricity: (1) centering the source within the lumen and (2) P&M eccentricity. These two factors may be additive (to exaggerate dose heterogeneity), or they may cancel each other. There appeared to be a greater possibility that these two factors were additive in longer lesions. To test the hypothesis that increasing the dose prescription would overcome this geometric problem, a group of patients with long, diffuse in-stent restenosis lesions were treated with a higher dose, with improved results (Figure 8.61).[195]

Other studies showed that gamma-irradiation treatment of saphenous vein-graft in-stent restenosis lesions was superior to placebo (Figure 8.61) and similar to native artery lesions.[202]

Restenting the in-stent restenosis lesion prior to brachytherapy caused more recurrent neointimal hyperplasia. This was similar to non-irradiated lesions.[188,189,203]

Beta-irradiation

Beta WRIST was a registry; there was no actual control group. The source was a centered yttrium-90 (^{90}Y) wire, and the results were comparable to those of the gamma-irradiated patients in WRIST.[204] START (Stents and Radiation

Therapy) was a randomized trial assessing the same brachytherapy system used in BERT. The findings were similar to gamma-emitter studies.[205] Hong *et al.*[206] evaluated a beta-emitting, liquid rhenium-188 ([188]Re)-MAG[3] filled balloon in patients with diffuse in-stent restenosis with similar results. However, these and other investigators have recently reported late catch-up 12–24 months after beta-irradiation treatment of in-stent restenosis similar to *de novo* implantation of radioactive stents.[207] Results from beta-irradiation studies are also shown in Figure 8.61.

IVUS dosimetry

There have been numerous reports suggesting the advantage of IVUS-based treatment planning for intracoronary brachytheraphy as well as the advantage of centering versus non-centering.[208–214] Two gamma-irradiation studies (SCRIPPS and Gamma-1) used IVUS dosimetry; WRIST did not. None of the beta-irradiation studies used IVUS dosimetry. The results of fixed dosimetry were similar to those of IVUS dosimetry, questioning the need for IVUS dosimetric calculations. In addition, accurate identification of the EEM (the target) can be difficult in stented arteries. Furthermore, dose–volume histogram analysis from both gamma- and beta-irradiation trials showed no relationship between calculated dose delivered to the adventitia and efficacy.[215,216]

Geographic miss

In six of the distal edge recurrence lesions from WRIST, there was evidence of geographic miss. Lesions with geographic miss had a greater decrease in lumen CSA because there was no change in EEM CSA (compared with an increase in EEM CSA in lesions with adequate coverage) to counteract the increase in P&M CSA in the two groups. Hong *et al.*[217] showed similar results in lesions treated with liquid [188]Re-MAG[3] filled balloons. As in BERT and PREVENT, edge lumen loss in the setting of inadequate radiation coverage of injured segments appeared to be related to either a decrease or no change in EEM CSA in the face of an increase in P&M CSA.

IVUS "complications" of brachytherapy

The most important complication of brachytherapy is stent thrombosis or late total occlusion. There are no IVUS studies of patients who have presented with stent thrombosis post-irradiation. However, clinical studies have shown that restenting an in-stent restenosis lesion is associated with an increased rate of late thrombosis; and IVUS analysis has shown that this practice leads to more intimal hyperplasia compared with non-restented segments.[188,189,203]

Late stent-vessel wall malapposition is the result of exaggerated positive remodeling in the absence of neointimal hyperplasia. It is more common in newly stented segments than in segments with in-stent restenosis.[152] An example is shown in Figure 8.62. Pregowski and Kalinczuk analyzed 133 radiated patients with in-stent restenosis from several brachytherapy trials. Dose–volume histograms showed that the adventitia in segments that developed late stent malapposition received a higher dose than the opposite wall with complete stent-vessel wall apposition or control segments with complete circumferential apposition. Positive remodeling and neointima inhibition – the combination that appears to lead to late stent malapposition – were dose-related.[152,218]

IVUS studies have assessed the impact of brachytherapy on the healing of post-angioplasty dissections in *de novo* lesions, but not after treatment of in-stent restenosis. While post-angioplasty dissections are common, dissections after treatment of in-stent restenosis are usually not seen. However, in all probability, the effect on healing is the same as with treatment of *de novo*, non-stented lesions (Figure 8.63).

Echolucent neointimal tissue – the "black hole" phenomenon that should be renamed the "black wall" – has been seen after both gamma- and beta-emitters (Figure 8.64).[148] Histologic analysis of directional coronary atherectomy-retrieved "black hole" tissue revealed large myxoid areas rich in proteoglycans, but poor in mature collagen and elastin.[148] However, the clinical implications of this finding are not known.

Mechanisms of recurrence after brachytherapy

The reported studies cited above all showed that recurrence late lumen loss after either gamma- or beta-irradiation was the result of intimal hyperplasia reaccumulation, not chronic stent recoil. This was true whether or not an additional stent was placed.

DRUG-ELUTING STENTS AND TREATMENT OF IN-STENT RESTENOSIS

There are only preliminary data available on the use of drug-eluting stents to treat bare-metal stent restenosis. Acute IVUS findings are similar to those for bare-metal restenting, including complications (Figure 8.65). IVUS images of patients who developed recurrence have shown: (1) incomplete in-stent restenosis lesion coverage (either gaps between multiple stents or uncovered edges) and (2) poor drug-eluting stent expansion (Figure 8.66).[219–222] While the frequency of recurrent restenosis is not known and may depend on the complexity of the underlying in-stent restenosis lesion, a recent report from Dante Pazzanese suggests that drug-eluting stents may be more efficacious than brachytherapy.[223]

In an analysis of sirolimus-eluting stent implantation to treat brachytherapy failures, neointimal hyperplasia averaged 11.8% of stent volume at follow-up.[224] Of 11 patients with significant neointimal hyperplasia reaccumulation, 6 patients showed echolucent neointima ("black hole" or "black wall" phenomenon), similar to some patients after brachytherapy (Figure 8.64).[225]

Trials assessing drug-eluting stent treatment of bare-metal in-stent restenosis as well as post-drug-eluting stent restenosis are in progress.

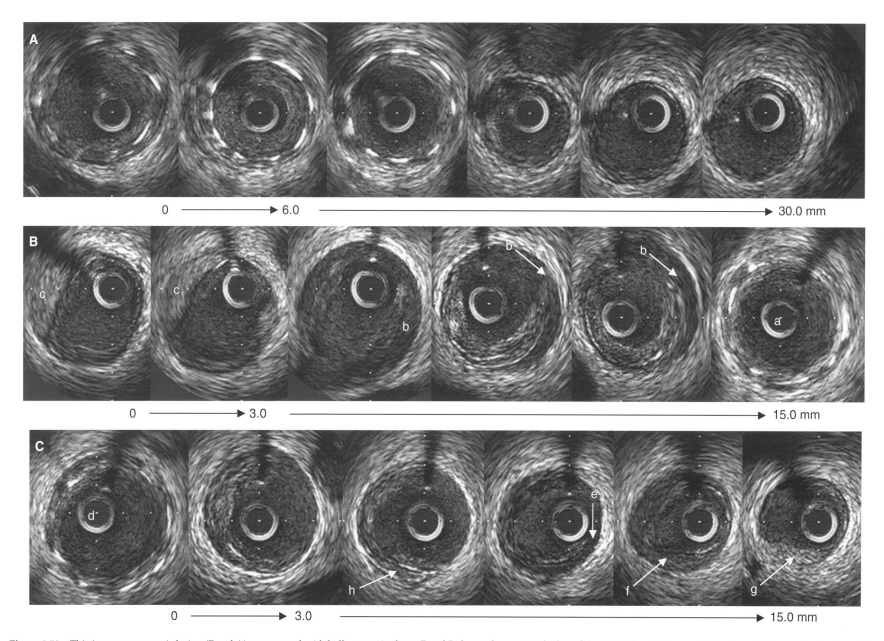

Figure 8.58 This in-stent restenosis lesion (Panel A) was treated with balloon angioplasty. Panel B shows the proximal edge of the stent after balloon angioplasty; note the proximal edge of the stent (a) and a dissection down to the media (b), which ends proximally to form an intramural hematoma (c). Panel C shows the distal edge of the stent after balloon angioplasty; note the distal edge of the stent (d), and the dissection down to the media (e), which becomes circumferential (f) and ends distally as an intramural hematoma (g). Note also the small extramural hematoma (h). For a more complete discussion and description of the IVUS findings of intramural hematoma, see Chapter 7

Figure 8.59 (opposite) The white arrow in Panel A shows a proximal edge in-stent restenosis lesion in the right coronary artery that was treated with balloon angioplasty, resulting in a large dissection (white arrow in Panel B) that required stent implantation (Panel C). Panel D shows the pre-intervention IVUS study. Note that the minimum lumen CSA of 1.5 mm^2 (dashed white line a) is proximal to the proximal edge of the stent (b) and that the proximal edge appears underexpanded (5.9 mm^2) compared with the proximal reference (c). Panel E shows the proximal edge after balloon angioplasty. Note the nearly circumferential dissection (d) which tracked distally behind the stent (e), with evidence of perforation and contrast or saline extravasation (f). For a more complete discussion and description of the IVUS findings of perforation, see Chapter 7

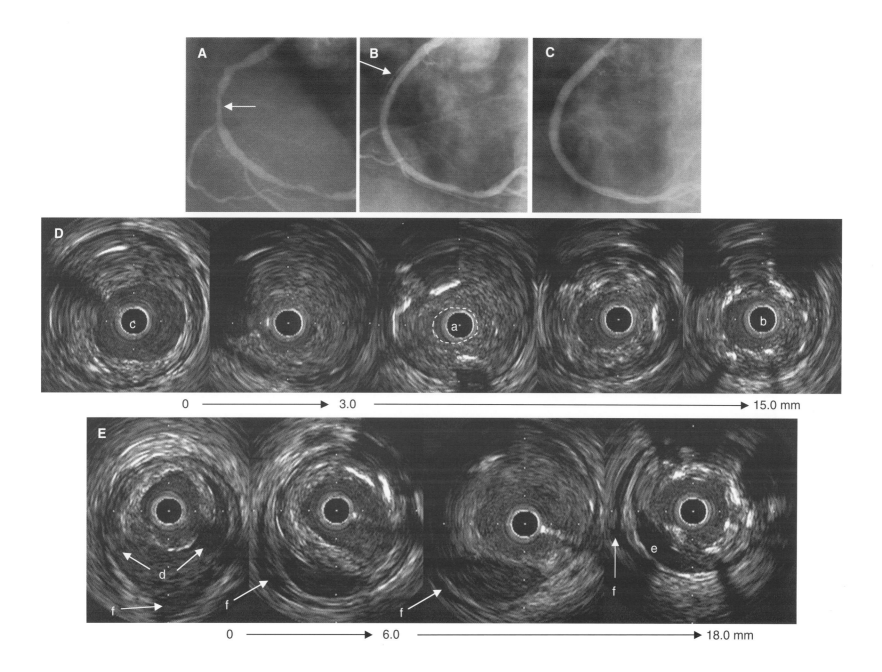

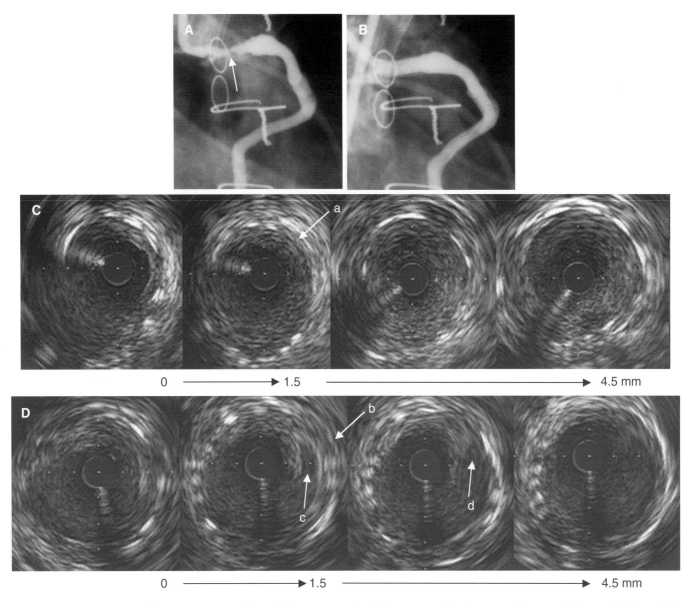

Figure 8.60   This ostial vein-graft in-stent restenosis lesion (white arrow in Panel A) was treated with excimer laser angioplasty and adjunct balloon angioplasty (Panel B). The pre-intervention IVUS is shown in Panel C. Post-laser angioplasty, the minimum lumen CSA increased to only 2.3 mm² (not shown). The post-balloon angioplasty IVUS is shown in Panel D. Note that the stent CSA has increased from 15.1 mm² (a) to 19.8 mm² (b). Expansion of the stent was associated with disruption within the neointima (c) and peeling of the neointimal hyperplasia away from the underlying stent (d)

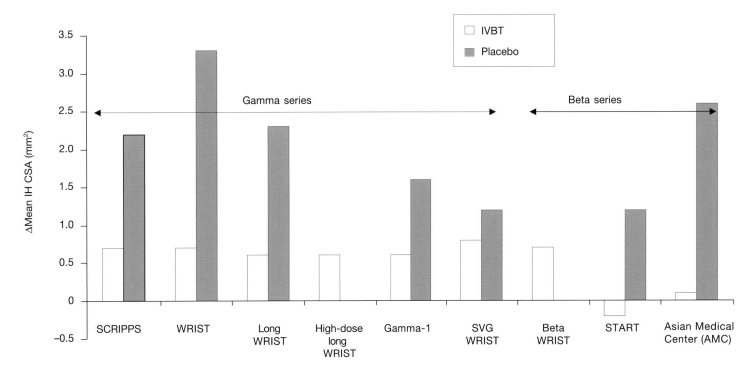

Figure 8.61   This illustration summarizes the results of the published series of intravascular brachytherapy treatment (IVBT) of in-stent restenosis in which IVUS was performed at treatment and follow-up. Note the heterogeneity of the mean recurrent intimal hyperplasia (IH) cross-sectional area (CSA) in the placebo groups, the fact that there are scant IVUS data with beta-irradiation, and the relatively consisted mean recurrent IH CSA with IVBT

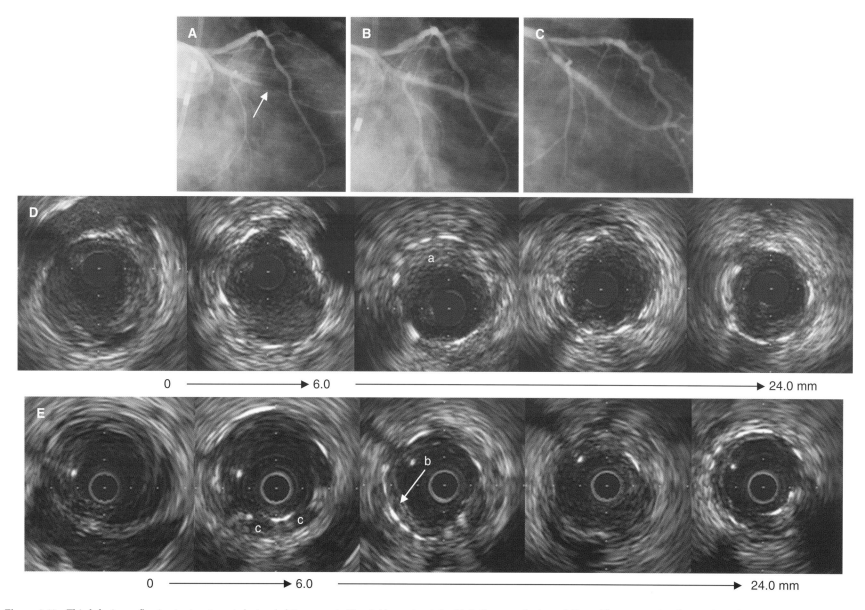

Figure 8.62 This left circumflex in-stent restenosis lesion (white arrow in Panel A) was treated with balloon angioplasty followed by gamma-irradiation (Panel B). At follow-up (Panel C), there has been an improvement in lumen dimensions. Panel D shows the post-irradiation IVUS, and Panel E shows the follow-up IVUS. Note the decrease in intimal hyperplasia area from 5.6 mm^2 (a) to 3.4 mm^2 (b), together with late stent malapposition (c)

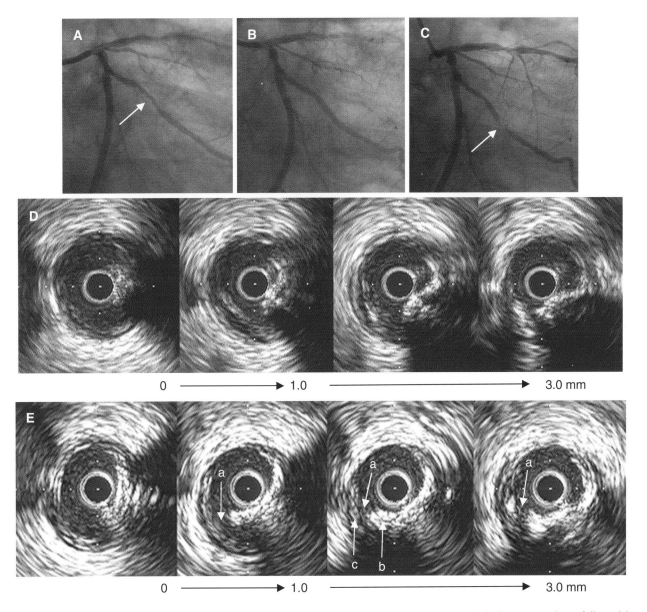

Figure 8.63 This left circumflex in-stent restenosis lesion (white arrow in Panel A) was treated with balloon angioplasty followed by gamma-irradiation (Panel B). At follow-up, there was edge recurrence (white arrow in Panel C). Panel C shows the post-irradiation IVUS, and Panel E shows the follow-up IVUS. Note the persistent and unhealed dissection (white arrows, a, in Panel E) at the junction of calcium (b) and relatively normal vessel wall (c)

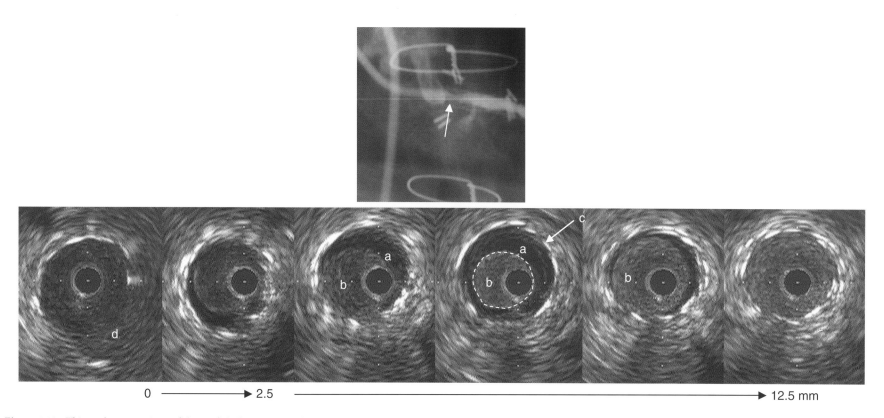

0 ——→ 2.5 ——————————————————————→ 12.5 mm

Figure 8.64 This saphenous vein-graft lesion failed gamma-irradiation (white arrow in the angiogram). The IVUS imaging run showed echolucent intimal hyperplasia (a), which was less dense than the blood speckle (b). The stent CSA (c) measured 10.6 mm^2, and the minimum lumen CSA (dashed white line) measured 3.4 mm^2. Note the transition to the aorta (d) proximally

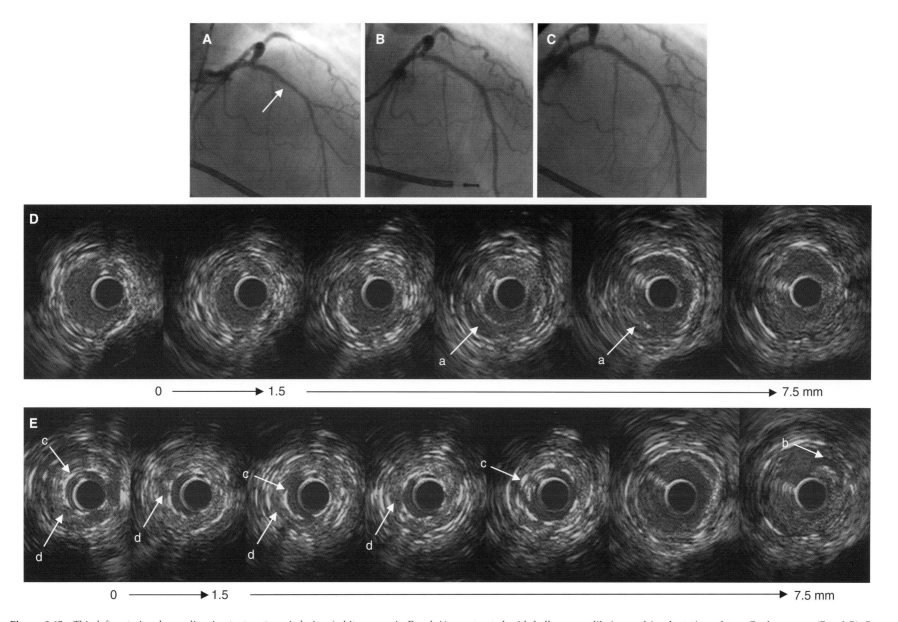

Figure 8.65 This left anterior descending in-stent restenosis lesion (white arrow in Panel A) was treated with balloon pre-dilation and implantation of two Cypher stents (Panel B). Pre-intervention IVUS (Panel D) showed disruption of the neointima (a). The IVUS after pre-dilation and implantation of two Cypher stents (Panel E) showed a separation (b) of the intimal hyperplasia from the underlying stent caused by additional stent expansion. More importantly, in the proximal left anterior descending, there was a new, unexpanded stent (c). During delivery of the second Cypher stent, it was stripped from the delivery balloon and became lodged proximally; this is the stent shown by the arrow c. Note the gap (d) between the original restenotic stent and the Cypher stent. This stripped, unexpanded stent was then expanded, and a third Cypher stent was implanted to cover the entire in-stent restenosis lesion. The final angiogram is shown in Panel C

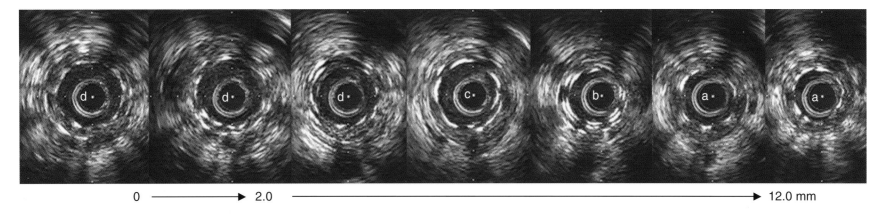

0 ———————▶ 2.0 ————————————————————————————▶ 12.0 mm

Figure 8.66 This IVUS example shows a 12 mm-long segment of a bare-metal in-stent restenosis lesion after placement of multiple Cypher stents. Note that the distal edge of the in-stent restenosis lesion (beyond the margin of the restenotic stent) is covered with a newly placed Cypher stent (a). Within the length of the restenotic stent, there are three stent layers (b), representing both the restenotic stents and the new Cypher stent, a gap between the two Cypher stents (c), where only the original restenotic stents are seen, and multiple stent layers proximally (d), representing the both the restenotic and Cypher stents. When restenting an in-stent restenosis lesion, multiple stent layers should be seen throughout, with the newly implanted stent visualized uninterrupted. The newly placed Cypher stent should fully cover the restenotic stents, extending proximally and distally if necessary. The minimum stent CSA measured only 2.8 mm^2

REFERENCES

1. O'Brien ER, Alpres CE, Stewart DK, et al. Proliferation in primary and restenotic coronary atherectomy specimens: implications for antiproliferative therapy. Circ Res 1993; 73: 223–31

2. Currier JW, Faxon DP, Restenosis after percutaneous transluminal coronary angioplasty: Have we been aiming at the wrong target? J Am Coll Cardiol 1995; 25: 516–20

3. Kakuta T, Currier JW, Haudenschild CC, et al. Differences in compensatory vessel enlargement, not intimal proliferation, account for restenosis after angioplasty in the hypercholesterolemic rabbit. Circulation 1994; 89: 2809–15

4. Lafont A, Guzman L, Whitlow P, et al. Restenosis after experimental angioplasty: intimal, medial, and adventitial changes associated with constrictive remodeling. Circ Res 1995; 76: 996–1002

5. Guzman LA, Mick MJ, Arnold AM, et al. Role of intimal hyperplasia and arterial remodeling after balloon angioplasty. An experimental study in the atherosclerotic rabbit model. Arterioscler Thromb Vasc Biol 1996; 16: 1–19

6. Andersen HR, Maeng M, Thorwest M, et al. Remodeling rather than neointimal formation explains luminal narrowing after deep vessel wall injury. Insights from a porcine coronary restenosis model. Circulation 1996; 93: 1716–24

7. Post MJ, Borst C, Kuntz RE, The relative importance of arterial remodeling compared with intimal hyperplasia in lumen renarrowing after balloon angioplasty. Circulation 1994; 89: 2816–21

8. de Smet BJ, van der Zande J, van der Helm YJ, et al. The atherosclerotic Yucatan animal model to study the arterial response after balloon angioplasty: the natural history of remodeling. Cardiovasc Res 1998; 39: 224–32

9. Labinaz M, Pels K, Hoffert C, et al. Time course and importance of neoadventitial formation in arterial remodeling following balloon angioplasty of porcine coronary arteries. Cardiovasc Res 1999; 41: 255–64

10. Pels K, Labinaz M, Hoffert C, et al. Adventitial angiogenesis early after coronary angioplasty: correlation with arterial remodeling. Arterioscler Thromb Vasc Biol 1999; 19: 229–38

11. Kakuta T, Usui M, Coats WD Jr, et al. Arterial remodeling at the reference site after angioplasty in the atherosclerotic rabbit model. Arterioscler Thromb Vasc Biol 1998; 18: 47–51

12. Nakamura Y, Zhao H, Yutani C, et al. Morphometric and histologic assessment of remodeling associated with restenosis after percutaneous transluminal coronary angioplasty. Cardiology 1998; 90: 115–21

13. Sangiorgi G, Taylor AJ, Carter AJ, et al. Histopathology of postpercutaneous transluminal coronary angioplasty remodeling in human coronary arteries. Am Heart J 1999; 138: 681–7

14. Maeng M, Olesen PG, Emmertsen NC, et al. Time course of vascular remodeling, formation of neointima and formation of neoadventitia after angioplasty in a porcine model. Coron Artery Dis 2001; 12: 285–93

15. Lansky AJ, Mintz GS, Popma JJ, et al. Remodeling after directional coronary atherectomy (with and without adjunct percutaneous transluminal coronary angioplasty): a serial angiographic and intravascular ultrasound analysis from the Optimal Atherectomy Restenosis Study. J Am Coll Cardiol 1998; 32: 329–37

16. Mintz GS, Popma JJ, Pichard AD, et al. Arterial remodeling after coronary angioplasty. A serial intravascular ultrasound study. Circulation 1996; 94: 35–43

17. Kornowski R, Mintz GS, Kent KM, et al. Increased restenosis in diabetes mellitus after coronary interventions is due to exaggerated intimal hyperplasia: a serial intravascular ultrasound study. Circulation 1997; 95: 1366–9

18. Di Mario C, Gil R, Camenzind E, et al. Quantitative assessment with intracoronary ultrasound of the mechanisms of restenosis after percutaneous transluminal coronary angioplasty and directional coronary atherectomy. Am J Cardiol 1995; 75: 772–7

19. Meine TJ, Bauman RP, Yock PG, et al. Coronary artery restenosis after atherectory is primarily due to negative remodeling. Am J Cardiol 1999; 84: 141–6

20. Kawamura A, Asakura Y, Okabe T, et al. Predictors of vessel remodeling following directional coronary atherectomy. Catheter Cardiovasc Interv 2004; 61: 44–51

21. Okura H, Hayase M, Shimodozono S, et al. Impact of pre-intervention arterial remodeling on subsequent vessel behavior after balloon angioplasty: a serial intravascular ultrasound study. J Am Coll Cardiol 2001; 38: 2001–5

22. Okura H, Shimodozono S, Hayase M, et al. Impact of deep vessel wall injury and vessel stretching on subsequent arterial remodeling after balloon angioplasty: a serial intravascular ultrasound study. Am Heart J 2002; 144: 323–8

23. Suzumura H, Hosokawa H, Suzuki T, et al. Comparison of dilatation mechanism and long-term vessel remodeling between directional coronary atherectomy and balloon angioplasty assessed by volumetric intravascular ultrasound. J Invasive Cardiol 2002; 14: 315–20

24. Sumitsuji S, Katoh O, Tsuchikane E, et al. Role of plaque proliferation in late lumen loss after directional coronary atherectomy. Circ J 2002; 66: 362–6

25. Oikawa Y, Kirigaya H, Aizawa T, et al. Mechanisms of acute gain and late lumen loss after atherectomy in different preintervention arterial remodeling patterns. Am J Cardiol 2002; 89: 505–10

26. Costa MA, Kozuma K, Gaster AL, et al. Three dimensional intravascular ultrasonic assessment of the local mechanism of restenosis after balloon angioplasty. Heart 2001; 85: 73–9

27. Tsuchikane E, Sumitsuji S, Awata N, et al. Final results of the STent versus directional coronary Atherectomy Randomized Trial (START). J Am Coll Cardiol 1999; 34: 1050–7

28. Meine TJ, Bauman RP, Yock PG, et al. Coronary artery restenosis after atherectomy is primarily due to negative remodeling. Am J Cardiol 1999; 84: 141–6

29. Cote G, Tardif JC, Lesperance J, et al. Effects of probucol on vascular remodeling after coronary angioplasty. Multivitamins and Protocol Study Group. Circulation 1999; 99: 30–5

30. Luo H, Nishioka T, Eigler NL, et al. Coronary artery restenosis after balloon angioplasty in humans is associated with circumferential coronary constriction. Arterioscler Thromb Vasc Biol 1996; 16: 1393–8

31. Lansky AJ, Mintz GS, Popma JJ, et al. Remodeling after directional coronary atherectomy (with and without adjunctive percutaneous coronary angioplasty): a serial angiographic and intravascular ultrasound analysis from the Optimal Atherectomy Restenosis Study. J Am Coll Cardiol 1998; 32: 329–37

32. Kimura T, Kaburagi S, Tamura T, et al. Remodeling of human coronary arteries undergoing coronary angioplasty or atherectomy. Circulation 1997; 96: 475–83

33. Schoenhagen P, Ziada KM, Vince DG, et al. Arterial remodeling and coronary artery disease: the concept of "dilated" versus "obstructive" coronary atherosclerosis. J Am Coll Cardiol 2001; 38: 297–306

34. de Vrey E, Mintz GS, Kimura T, et al. Arterial remodeling after directional coronary atherectomy: a volumetric analysis from the Serial Ultrasound REstenosis (SURE) trial. J Am Coll Cardiol 1997; 29: 280A (abstract)

35. Meerkin D, Tardif JC, Bertrand OF, et al. The effects of intracoronary brachytherapy on the natural history of postangioplasty dissections. J Am Coll Cardiol 2000; 36: 59–64

36. Mintz GS, Popma JJ, Pichard AD, et al. Intravascular ultrasound predictors of restenosis following percutaneous transcatheter coronary revascularization. J Am Coll Cardiol 1996; 27: 1678–87

37. The GUIDE Trial Inventigators. IVUS-determined predictors of restenosis in PTCA and DCA: final report from the GUIDE trial. J Am Coll Cardiol 1996; 27: 156A

38. Tardif JC, Cote G, Lesperance J, et al. Impact of residual plaque burden after balloon angioplasty in the MultiVitamins and Probucol (MVP) trial. Can J Cardiol 2001; 17: 49–55

39. Jain SP, Jain A, Collins TJ, et al. Predictors of restenosis: a morphometric and quantitative evaluation by intravascular ultrasound. Am Heart J 1994; 128: 664–73

40. Honda Y, Yock PG, Fitzgerald PJ. Impact of residual plaque burden on clinical outcomes of coronary interventions. Catheter Cardiovasc Interv 1999; 46: 265–76

41. Peters RJG, Kok WEM, Di Mario C, et al. Prediction of restenosis after coronary angioplasty. Results of PICTURE (Post-IntraCoronary Treatment Ultrasound Result Evaluation), a prospective multicenter intracoronary ultrasound imaging study. Circulation 1997; 95: 2254–61

42. Kok WE, Peters RJ, Pasterkamp G, et al. Early lumen diameter loss after percutaneous transluminal coronary angioplasty is related to coronary plaque burden: a role for viscous plaque properties in early lumen diameter loss. Int J Cardiovasc Imaging 2001; 17: 111–21

43. Dangas G, Mintz GS, Mehran R, et al. Preintervention arterial remodeling as an independent predictor of target-lesion revascularization after nonstent coronary intervention: an analysis of 777 lesions with intravascular ultrasound imaging. Circulation 1999; 99: 3149–54

44. Wexberg P, Gyongyosi M, Sperker W, et al. Pre-existing arterial remodeling is associated with in-hospital and late adverse cardiac events after coronary interventions in patients with stable angina pectoris. J Am Coll Cardiol 2000; 36: 1860–9

45. Mintz GS, Kimura T, Nobuyoshi M, et al. Relation between preintervention remodeling and late arterial responses to coronary angioplasty or atherectomy. Am J Cardiol 2001; 87: 392–6

46. Schroeder S, Baumbach A, Mahrholdt H, et al. The impact of untreated coronary dissections on acute and long-term outcome after intravascular ultrasound guided PTCA. Eur Heart J 2000; 21: 137–45

47. Lee HS, Tardif JC, Harel F, et al. Effects of plaque composition on vascular remodelling after angioplasty in the MultiVitamins and Probucol (MVP) trial. Can J Cardiol 2002; 18: 271–5

48. Cote G, Tardif JC, Lesperance J, et al. Effects of probucol on vascular remodeling after coronary angioplasty. Multivitamins and Protocol Study Group. Circulation 1999; 99: 30–5

49. Meerkin D, Tardif J-C, Crocker IR, et al. Effects of intracoronary beta-radiation therapy after coronary angioplasty: an intravascular ultrasound study. Circulation 1999; 99: 1660–6

50. Sabate M, Serruys PW, van der Giessen WJ, et al. Geometric vascular remodeling after balloon angioplasty and beta-radiation therapy: a three-dimensional intravascular ultrasound study. Circulation 1999; 100: 1182–8

51. Sabate M, Marijnissen JP, Carlier SG, et al. Residual plaque burden, delivered dose, and tissue composition predict 6-month outcome after balloon angioplasty and beta-radiation therapy. Circulation 2000; 101: 2472–7

52. Kay IP, Sabate M, Van Langenhove G, et al. Outcome from balloon induced coronary artery dissection after intracoronary beta radiation. Heart 2000; 83: 332–7

53. Mintz GS, Popma JJ, Hong MK, et al. Intravascular ultrasound to discern device-specific effects and mechanisms of restenosis. Am J Cardiol 1996; 78: 18–22

54. Suzuki T, Hosakawa H, Katoh O, et al. Effects of adjunctive balloon angioplasty after intravascular ultrasound-guided directional coronary atherectomy: the results of Adjunctive Balloon Angioplasty After Coronary Atherectomy Study (ABACAS). J Am Coll Cardiol 1999; 343: 1028–35

55. Hoffmann R, Mintz GS, Dussaillant GR, et al. Patterns and mechanisms of in-stent restenosis: a serial intravascular ultrasound study. Circulation 1996; 94: 1247–54

56. Mudra H, Blasini R, Regar E, et al. Intravascular ultrasound assessment of the balloon-expandable Palmaz-Schatz coronary stent. Coron Artery Dis 1993; 4: 791–9

57. Hong MK, Park SW, Lee CW, et al. Intravascular ultrasound comparison of chronic recoil among different stent designs. Am J Cardiol 1999; 84: 1247–50

58. Costa MA, Sabate M, Kay IP, et al. Three-dimensional intravascular ultrasonic volumetric quantification of stent recoil and neointimal formation of two new generation tubular stents. Am J Cardiol 2000; 85: 135–9

59. Weissman NJ, Wilensky RL, Tanguay JF, et al. Extent and distribution of in-stent intimal hyperplasia and edge effect in a non-radiation stent population. Am J Cardiol 2001; 88: 248–52

60. Serruys PW, Degertekin M, Tanabe K, et al. Intravascular ultrasound findings in the multicenter, randomized, double-blind RAVEL (RAndomized study with the sirolimus-eluting VElocity balloon-expandable stent in the treatment of patients with de novo native coronary artery Lesions) trial. Circulation 2002; 106: 798–803

61. Hong MK, Mintz GS, Lee CW, et al. Paclitaxel coating reduces in-stent intimal hyperplasia in human coronary arteries: a serial volumetric intravascular ultrasound analysis from the Asian Paclitaxel-Eluting Stent Clinical Trial (ASPECT). Circulation 2003; 107: 517–20

62. Moses JW, Leon MB, Popma JJ, et al. Sirolimus-eluting stents versus standard stents in patients with stenosis in a native coronary artery. N Engl J Med 2003; 349: 1315–23

63. Kuroda N, Kobayashi Y, Nameki M, et al. Intimal hyperplasia regression from 6 to 12 months after stenting. Am J Cardiol 2002; 89: 869–72

64. Suzumura H, Suzuki T, Hosokawa H, et al. Neointima in coronary stent does not increase during over 1-year in non-restenosed lesion at 6 months follow-up: serial volumetric intravascular ultrasound study. Jpn Heart J 2002; 43: 581–91

65. Hoffmann R, Jansen C, Konig A, et al. Stent design-related neointimal tissue proliferation in human coronary arteries; an intravascular ultrasound study. Eur Heart J 2001; 22: 2007–14

66. Hoffmann R, Mintz GS, Haager PK, et al. Relation of stent design and stent surface material to subsequent in-stent intimal hyperplasia in coronary arteries determined by intravascular ultrasound. Am J Cardiol 2002; 89: 1360–4

67. Hoffmann R, Mintz GS, Pichard AD, et al. Intimal hyperplasia thickness at follow-up is independent of stent size: a serial intravascular ultrasound study. Am J Cardiol 1998; 82: 1168–72

68. Castagna MT, Mintz GS, Leiboff BO, et al. The contribution of "mechanical" problems to in-stent restenosis: an intravascular ultrasonographic analysis of 1090 consecutive in-stent restenosis lesions. Am Heart J 2001; 142: 970–4

69. Hoffmann R, Mintz GS, Popma JJ, et al. Chronic arterial responses to stent implantation: a serial intravascular ultrasound analysis of Palmaz–Schatz stents in native coronary arteries. J Am Coll Cardiol 1996; 1134–9

70. Nakamura M, Yock PG, Bonneau HN, et al. Impact of peri-stent remodeling on restenosis: a volumetric intravascular ultrasound study. Circulation 2001; 103: 2130–2

71. Okabe T, Asakura Y, Asakura K, et al. Usefulness of residual percent plaque area after percutaneous coronary intervention in predicting peristent positive remodeling. Am J Cardiol 2003; 92: 1399–403

72. Shah VM, Mintz GS, Apple S, et al. "Background" incidence of late malapposition following bare metal stent implantation. Circulation 2002; 106: 1753–5

73. Hong MK, Mintz GS, Lee CW, et al. Incidence, mechanism, predictors, and long-term prognosis of late stent malapposition after bare-metal stent implantation. Circulation 2004; 109: 881–6

74. Nakamura N, Kataoka T, Honda Y, et al. Late incomplete stent apposition and focal vessel expansion after bare metal stenting. Am J Cardiol 2003; 92: 1217–9

75. Mintz GS, Shah VM, Weissman NJ. Regional remodeling as the cause of late stent malapposition. Circulation 2003; 107: 2660–3

76. Takagi T, Yoshida K, Akasaka T, et al. Hyperinsulinemia during oral glucose tolerance test is associated with increased neointimal tissue proliferation after coronary stent implantation in nondiabetic patients: a serial intravascular ultrasound study. J Am Coll Cardiol 2000; 34: 731–8

77. Abizaid A, Kornowski R, Mintz GS, et al. The influence of diabetes mellitus on acute and late clinical outcomes following coronary stent implantation. J Am Coll Cardiol 1998; 32: 584–9

78. Konig A, Schiele M, Rieber J, et al. Stent design-related coronary artery remodeling and patterns of neointima formation following self-expanding and balloon-expandable stent implantation. Catheter Cardiovasc Interv 2002; 56: 478–86

79. Han RO, Schwartz RS, Kobayashi Y, et al. Comparison of self-expanding and balloon-expandable stents for the reduction of restenosis. Am J Cardiol 2001; 88: 253–9

80. Serruys PW, Foley DP, Pieper M, et al. The TRAPIST study. A multicentre randomized placebo-controlled clinical trial of trapidil for prevention of restenosis after coronary stenting, measured by 3-D intravascular ultrasound. Eur Heart J 2001; 22: 1938–47

81. Nageh T, de Belder AJ, Thomas MR, et al. A randomised trial of endoluminal reconstruction comparing the NIR stent and the Wallstent in angioplasty of long segment coronary disease: results of the RENEWAL study. Am Heart J 2001; 141: 971–6

82. Konig A, Klauss V, Regar E, et al. Serial intravascular ultrasound and quantitative coronary angiography after self-expandable Wallstent coronary artery implantation. Am J Cardiol 2000; 86: 1015–8, A10

83. Kobayashi Y, Honda Y, Christie GL, et al. Long-term vessel response to a self-expanding coronary stent: a serial volumetric intravascular ultrasound analysis from the ASSURE trial. A stent vs. stent ultrasound remodeling evaluation. J Am Coll Cardiol 2001; 37: 1329–34

84. Oshima A, Ochiai M, Takeshita S, et al. Serial automated three-dimensional intravascular ultrasound analysis of the self-expanding Radius stent. Am J Cardiol 2000; 85: 388–91, A9

85. Kay IP, Sabate M, Van Langenhove G, et al. The ESSEX (European Scimed Stent Experience) study. Catheter Cardiovasc Interv 2000; 50: 419–25

86. Yu ZX, Tamai H, Kyo E, et al. Comparison of the self-expanding Radius stent and the balloon-expandable Multilink stent for elective treatment of coronary stenoses: a serial analysis by intravascular ultrasound. Catheter Cardiovasc Interv 2002; 56: 40–5

87. Gercken U, Lansky AJ, Buellesfeld L, et al. Results of the Jostent coronary stent graft implantation in various clinical settings: procedural and follow-up results. Catheter Cardiovasc Interv 2002; 56: 353–60

88. Lukito G, Vandergoten P, Jaspers L, et al. Six months clinical, angiographic, and IVUS follow-up after PTFE graft stent implantation in native coronary arteries. Acta Cardiol 2000; 55: 255–60

89. Tamai H, Igaki K, Kyo E, et al. Initial and 6-month results of biodegradable poly-*l*-lactic acid coronary stents in humans. Circulation 2000; 102: 399–404

90. Kasaoka S, Tobis JM, Akiyama T, et al. Angiographic and intravascular ultrasound predictors of in-stent restenosis. J Am Coll Cardiol 1998; 32: 1630–5

91. Ziada KM, Kapadia SR, Belli G, et al. Prognostic value of absolute versus relative measures of the procedural result after successful coronary stenting: importance of vessel size in predicting long-term freedom from target vessel revascularization. Am Heart J 2001; 141: 823–31

92. Morino Y, Honda Y, Okura H, et al. An optimal diagnostic threshold for minimal stent area to predict target lesion revascularization following stent implantation in native coronary lesions. Am J Cardiol 2001; 88: 301–3

93. Hong K, Lee CW, Kim JH, et al. Impact of various intravascular ultrasound criteria for stent optimization on the six-month angiographic restenosis. Catheter Cardiovasc Interv 2002; 56: 178–83

94. Hong MK, Park SW, Mintz GS, et al. Intravascular ultrasonic predictors of angiographic restenosis after long coronary stenting. Am J Cardiol 2000; 85: 441–5

95. de Feyter PJ, Kay P, Disco C, et al. Reference chart derived from post-stent-implantation intravascular ultrasound predictors of 6-month expected restenosis on quantitative coronary angiography. Circulation 1999; 100: 1777–83

96. Hoffmann R, Mintz GS, Mehran R, et al. Intravascular ultrasound predictors of angiographic restenosis in lesions treated with Palmaz–Schatz stents. J Am Coll Cardiol 1997; 31: 43–9

97. Kuriyama N, Kobayashi Y, Kuroda N, et al. Effect of coronary stent overexpansion on lumen size and intimal hyperplasia at follow-up. Am J Cardiol 2002; 89: 1297–9

98. Nakamura S, Di Francesco L, Finci L, et al. Focal wall overstretching after high-pressure coronary stent implantation does not influence restenosis. Catheter Cardiovasc Interv 1999; 48: 24–30

99. Werner GS, Gastmann O, Ferrari M, et al. Determinants of stent restenosis in chronic coronary occlusions assessed by intracoronary ultrasound. Am J Cardiol 1999; 83: 1164–9

100. Sonoda S, Morino Y, Ako Y, et al. Impact of final stent dimensions on long-term results following sirolimus-eluting stent implantation: Serial IVUS analysis from the SIRIUS trial. J Am Coll Cardiol 2004; 43: 1959–63

101. Ahmed JM, Mintz GS, Waksman R, et al. Comparison of native coronary artery in-stent recurrence rates with longer versus shorter narrowings. Am J Cardiol 2002; 90: 422–5

102. Nageh T, De Belder AJ, Thomas MR, et al. Intravascular ultrasound-guided stenting in long lesions: an insight into possible mechanisms of restenosis and comparison of angiographic and intravascular ultrasound data from the MUSIC and RENEWAL trials. J Interv Cardiol 2001; 14: 397–405

103. Oemrawsingh PV, Mintz GS, Schalij MJ, et al. Intravascular ultrasound guidance improves angiographic and clinical outcome of stent implantation for long coronary artery stenoses: final results of a randomized comparison with angiographic guidance (TULIP study). Circulation 2003; 107: 62–7

104. Okura H, Morino Y, Oshima A, et al. Preintervention arterial remodeling affects clinical outcome following stenting: an intravascular ultrasound study. J Am Coll Cardiol 2001; 37: 1031–5

105. Endo A, Hirayama H, Yoshida O, et al. Arterial remodeling influences the development of intimal hyperplasia after stent implantation. J Am Coll Cardiol 2001; 37: 70–5

106. Sahara M, Kirigaya H, Oikawa Y, et al. Arterial remodeling patterns before intervention predict diffuse in-stent restenosis: an intravascular ultrasound study. J Am Coll Cardiol 2003; 42: 1731–8

107. Dangas G, Mintz GS, Mehran R, et al. Stent implantation neutralizes the impact of pre-intervention arterial remodeling on subsequent target lesion revascularization. Am J Cardiol 2000; 86: 452–5

108. Hong MK, Park SW, Lee CW, et al. Preintervention arterial remodeling as a predictor of intimal hyperplasia after intracoronary stenting: a serial intravascular ultrasound study. Clin Cardiol 2002; 25: 11–15

109. Hibi K, Suzuki T, Honda Y, et al. Quantitative and spatial relation of baseline atherosclerotic plaque burden and subsequent in-stent neointimal proliferation as determined by intravascular ultrasound. Am J Cardiol 2002; 90: 1164–7

110. Shiran A, Wiessman NJ, Leiboff B, et al. Effect of pre-intervention plaque burden on subsequent intimal hyperplasia in stented coronary arteries. Am J Cardiol 2000; 86: 1318–21

111. Prati F, Di Mario C, Moussa I, et al. In-stent neointimal proliferation correlates with the amount of residual plaque burden outside the stent: an intravascular ultrasound study. Circulation 1999; 99: 1011–14

112. Alfonso F, Garcia P, Pimentel G, et al. Predictors and implications of residual plaque burden after coronary stenting: an intravascular ultrasound study. Am Heart J 2003; 145: 254–61

113. Hong MK, Park SW, Lee CW, et al. Relation between residual plaque burden after stenting and six-month angiographic restenosis. Am J Cardiol 2002; 89: 368–71

114. Casserly IP, Aronow HD, Schoenhagen P, et al. Relationship between residual atheroma burden and neointimal growth in patients undergoing stenting: analysis of the atherectomy before MultiLink improves lumen gain and clinical outcomes trial intravascular ultrasound substudy. J Am Coll Cardiol 2002; 40: 1573–8

115. Nishida T, Colombo A, Briguori C, et al. Outcome of nonobstructive residual dissections detected by intravascular ultrasound following percutaneous coronary intervention. Am J Cardiol 2002; 89: 1257–62

116. Hong MK, Park SW, Lee NH, et al. Long-term outcomes of minor dissection at the edge of stents detected with intravascular ultrasound. Am J Cardiol 2000; 86: 791–5

117. Sheris SJ, Canos MR, Weissman NJ, Natural history of intravascular ultrasound-detected edge dissections from coronary stent deployment. Am Heart J 2000; 139: 59–63

118. Murata T, Hiro T, Fujii T, et al. Impact of the cross-sectional geometry of the post-deployment coronary stent on in-stent neointimal hyperplasia: an intravascular ultrasound study. Circ J 2002; 66: 489–93

119. Vavuranakis M, Toutouzas K, Stefanidis C, et al. Stent deployment in calcified lesions: can we overcome calcific restraint with high-pressure balloon inflations? Catheter Cardiovasc Interv 2001; 52: 164–72

120. Tanaka A, Kawarabayashi T, Nishibori Y, et al. In-stent restenosis and lesion morphology in patients with acute myocardial infarction. Am J Cardiol 2003; 92: 1208–11

121. Casella G, Klauss V, Ottani F, et al. Impact of intravascular ultrasound-guided stenting on long-term clinical outcome: a meta-analysis of available studies comparing intravascular ultrasound-guided and angiographically guided stenting. Catheter Cardiovasc Interv 2003; 59: 314–21

122. Wilensky RL, Tanguay JF, Ito S, et al. Heparin infusion prior to stenting (HIPS) trial: final results of a prospective, randomized, controlled trial evaluating the effects of local vascular delivery on intimal hyperplasia. Am Heart J 2000; 139: 1061–70

123. Meneveau N, Schiele F, Grollier G, et al. Local delivery of nadroparin for the prevention of neointimal hyperplasia following stent implantation: results of the IMPRESS trial. A multicentre, randomized, clinical, angiographic and intravascular ultrasound study. Eur Heart J 2000; 21: 1767–75

124. Kutryk MJ, Foley DP, van den Brand M, et al. Local intracoronary administration of antisense oligonucleotide against c-*myc* for the prevention of in-stent restenosis: results of the randomized investigation by the Thoraxcenter of antisense DNA using local delivery and IVUS after coronary stenting (ITALICS) trial. J Am Coll Cardiol 2002; 39: 281–7

125. The ERASER Investigators. Acute platelet inhibition with abciximab does not reduce in-stent restenosis (ERASER study). Circulation 1999; 100: 799–806

126. Chaves AJ, Sousa AG, Mattos LA, et al. Volumetric analysis of in-stent intimal hyperplasia in diabetic patients treated with or without abciximab: results of the Diabetes Abciximab steNT Evaluation (DANTE) randomized trial. Circulation 2004; 109: 861–6

127. Holmes DR Jr, Savage M, LaBlanche JM, et al. Results of Prevention of REStenosis with Tranilast and its Outcomes (PRESTO) trial. Circulation 2002; 106: 1243–50

128. Tardif JC, Gregoire J, Schwartz L, et al. Effects of AGI-1067 and probucol after percutaneous coronary interventions. Circulation 2003; 107: 552–8

129. Takagi T, Akasaka T, Yamamuro A, et al. Troglitazone reduces neointimal tissue proliferation after coronary stent implantation in patients with non-insulin dependent diabetes mellitus: a serial intravascular ultrasound study. J Am Coll Cardiol 2000; 36: 1529–35

130. Takagi T, Yamamuro A, Tamita K, et al. Pioglitazone reduces neointimal tissue proliferation after coronary stent implantation in patients with type 2 diabetes mellitus: an intravascular ultrasound scanning study. Am Heart J 2003; 146: E5

131. Kondo J, Sone T, Tsuboi H, et al. Effect of quinapril on intimal hyperplasia after coronary stenting as assessed by intravascular ultrasound. Am J Cardiol 2001; 87: 443–5, A6

132. Wakeyama T, Ogawa H, Iida H, et al. Effects of candesartan and probucol on restenosis after coronary stenting: results of insight of stent intimal hyperplasia inhibition by new angiotensin II receptor antagonist (ISHIN) trial. Circ J 2003; 67: 519–24

133. Yamazaki T, Taniguchi I, Kurusu T, et al. Effect of amlodipine on vascular responses after coronary stenting compared with an angiotensin-converting enzyme inhibitor. Circ J 2004; 68: 328–33

134. Ohsawa H, Noike H, Kanai M, et al. Preventive effect of an antiallergic drug, pemirolast potassium, on restenosis after stent placement: quantitative coronary angiography and intravascular ultrasound studies. J Cardiol 2003; 42: 13–22

135. Hoffmann R, Takimoglu-Boerekci M, Langenberg R, et al. Randomized comparison of direct stenting with predilatation followed by stenting on vessel trauma and restenosis. Am Heart J 2004; 147: E13

136. Hoffmann R, Haager P, Mintz GS, et al. The impact of high pressure vs low pressure stent implantation on intimal hyperplasia and follow-up lumen dimensions; results of a randomized trial. Eur Heart J 2001; 22: 2015–24

137. Kay IP, Sabate M, Costa MA, et al. Positive geometric vascular remodeling is seen after catheter-based radiation followed by conventional stent implantation but not after radioactive stent implantation. Circulation 2000; 102: 1434–9

138. Albiero R, Adamian M, Kobayashi Y, et al. Short- and intermediate-term results of 32P radioactive beta-emitting stent implantation in patients with coronary artery disease: the Milan Dose–Response Study. Circulation 2001; 101: 16–26

139. Weissman NJ, Tinana A, Canos DA, et al. Comparison of IVUS findings of the beta-emitting Isostent versus a non-radiation control group from the HIPS trial. Circulation 2000; 102: II-691

140. Weissman NJ, Albiero R, Di Mario C, et al. Final IVUS results from the Isostent BXI multicenter dose response study. Circulation 2000; 102: II-567

141. Albiero R, Nishida T, Adamian M, et al. Edge restenosis after implantation of high activity 32P radioactive beta-emitting stents. Circulation 2000; 101: 2454–7

142. Weissman NJ, Albiero R, De Bruyne B, et al. Final IVUS results from the multicenter "cold ends" Isostent study. Circulation 2000; 102: II-568

143. Hansen A, Hehrlein C, Hardt S, et al. Is the "candy-wrapper" effect of 32P radioactive beta-emitting stents due to remodeling or neointimal hyperplasia? Insights from intravascular ultrasound. Catheter Cardiovasc Interv 2001; 54: 41–8

144. Wexberg P, Kirisits C, Gyongyosi M, et al. Vascular morphometric changes after radioactive stent implantation: a dose-response analysis. J Am Coll Cardiol 2002; 39: 400–7

145. Kay IP, Wardeh AJ, Kozuma K, et al. The pattern of restenosis and vascular remodelling after cold-end radioactive stent implantation. Eur Heart J 2001; 22: 1311–17

146. Kalinczuk L, Pregowski J, Mintz GS, et al. Incidence and mechanism of late stent malapposition after phosphorus-32 radioactive stent implantation. Am J Cardiol 2003; 92: 970–2

147. Kay IP, Wardeh AJ, Kozuma K, et al. Radioactive stents delay but do not prevent in-stent neointimal hyperplasia. Circulation 2001; 103: 14–17

148. Kay IP, Ligthart JM, Virmani R, et al. The black hole: echolucent tissue observed following intracoronary radiation. Int J Cardiovasc Intervent 2003; 5: 137–42

149. Raizner AE, Oesterle SN, Waksman R, et al. Inhibition of restenosis with beta-emitting radiotherapy: Report of the Proliferation Reduction with Vascular Energy Trial (PREVENT). Circulation 2000; 102: 951–8

150. Okura H, Lee DP, Handen CE, et al. Contribution of vessel remodeling to "edge effect" following intracoronary beta-irradiation: a serial volumetric intravascular ultrasound study. Circulation 1999; 100: I-511

151. Lee DP, Okura H, Handen CE, et al. Reference segment and target lesion effects of 32P radiation: intravascular ultrasound results of the PREVENT trial. Circulation 1999; 100: I-517

152. Okura H, Lee DP, Lo S, et al. Late incomplete apposition with excessive remodeling of the stented coronary artery following intravascular brachytherapy. Am J Cardiol 2003; 92: 587–90

153. Koster R, Vieluf D, Kiehn M, et al. Nickel and molybdenum contact allergies in patients with coronary in-stent restenosis. Lancet 2000; 356: 1895–7

154. Sousa JE, Costa MA, Abizaid AC, et al. Sustained suppression of neointimal proliferation by sirolimus-eluting stents: one-year angiographic and intravascular ultrasound follow-up. Circulation 2001; 104: 2007–11

155. Sousa JE, Costa MA, Sousa AG, et al. Two-year angiographic and intravascular ultrasound follow-up after implantation of sirolimus-eluting stents in human coronary arteries. Circulation 2003; 107: 381–3

156. Sousa JE, Abizaid A, Costa MA, et al. Late four-year follow-up from the First-in-Man experience after implantation of sirolimus-eluting stents. J Am Coll Cardiol 2004; 43: 98A

157. Takebayashi H, Kobayashi Y, Mintz GS, et al. Intravascular ultrasound assessment of lesions with sirolimus-eluting stent failure. J Am Coll Cardiol 2004; 43: 65A

158. Sianos G, Hofma S, Ligthart JM, et al. Stent fracture and restenosis in the drug-eluting stent era. Catheter Cardiovasc Interv 2004; 61: 111–16

159. Lemos PA, Saia F, Ligthart JM, et al. Coronary restenosis after sirolimus-eluting stent implantation: morphological description and mechanistic analysis from a consecutive series of cases. Circulation 2003; 108: 257–60

160. Colombo A, Moses JW, Morice MC, et al. Randomized study to evaluate sirolimus-eluting stents implanted at coronary bifurcation lesions. Circulation 2004; 109: 1244–9

161. Degertekin M, Serruys PW, Tanabe K, et al. Long-term follow-up of incomplete stent apposition in patients who received sirolimus-eluting stent for de novo coronary lesions: an intravascular ultrasound analysis. Circulation 2003; 108: 2747–50

162. Park SJ, Shim WH, Ho DS, et al. A paclitaxel-eluting stent for the prevention of coronary restenosis. N Engl J Med 2003; 348: 1537–45

163. Mintz GS, Tinana A, Hong MK, et al. Impact of preinterventional arterial remodeling on neointimal hyperplasia after implantation of (non-polymer-encapsulated) paclitaxel-coated stents: a serial volumetric intravascular ultrasound analysis from the ASian Paclitaxel-Eluting Stent Clinical Trial (ASPECT). Circulation 2003; 108: 1295–8

164. Escobar E, Mintz GS, Hong M-K, et al. Intimal hyperplasia thickness is independent of stent size in paclitaxel-coated stents. Am J Cardiol 2004 (in press)

165. Colombo A, Drzewiecki J, Banning A, et al. Randomized study to assess the effectiveness of slow- and moderate-release polymer-based paclitaxel-eluting stents for coronary artery lesions. Circulation 2003; 108: 788–94

166. Tanabe K, Serruys PW, Degertekin M, et al. Chronic arterial responses to polymer-controlled paclitaxel-eluting stents: comparison with bare metal stents by serial intravascular ultrasound analyses: data from the randomized TAXUS-II trial. Circulation 2004; 109: 196–200

167. Serruys PW, Degertekin M, Tanabe K, et al. Vascular responses at proximal and distal edges of paclitaxel-eluting stents: serial intravascular ultrasound analysis from the TAXUS II trial. Circulation 2004; 109: 627–33

168. Nishioka H, Shimada K, Fukuda S, et al. Long-term follow-up of intermediate in-stent restenosis lesions following deferral of re-intervention on the basis of intravascular utlrasound findings. Circulation 2003; 106: II-587

169. Mehran R, Mintz GS, Popma JJ, et al. Mechanisms and results of balloon angioplasty for the treatment of in-stent restenosis. Am J Cardiol 1996; 78: 618–22

170. Schiele F, Vuillemenot A, Meneveau N, et al. Effects of increasing balloon pressure on mechanism and results of balloon angioplasty for treatment of restenosis after Palmaz–Schatz stent implan-

tation: an angiographic and intravascular ultrasound study. Catheter Cardiovasc Interv 1999; 46: 314–21

171. Sakamoto T, Kawarabayashi T, Taguchi H, et al. Intravascular ultrasound-guided balloon angioplasty for treatment of in-stent restenosis. Catheter Cardiovasc Interv 1999; 47: 298–303

172. Ishikawa S, Asakura Y, Okabe T, et al. Repeat intervention for in-stent restenosis: re-expansion of the initial stent is a predictor of recurrence of restenosis. Coron Artery Dis 2000; 11: 451–7

173. Montorsi P, Galli S, Fabbiocchi F, et al. Mechanism of cutting balloon angioplasty for in-stent restenosis: an intravascular ultrasound study. Catheter Cardiovasc Interv 2002; 56: 166–73

174. Schiele TM, Konig A, Rieber J, et al. Comparison of volumetric intravascular ultrasound analysis of acute results and underlying mechanisms from cutting balloon and conventional balloon angioplasty for the treatment of coronary in-stent restenotic lesions. Am J Cardiol 2002; 90: 539–42

175. Ahmed JM, Mintz GS, Castagna M, et al. Intravascular ultrasound assessment of the mechanism of lumen enlargement during cutting balloon angioplasty treatment of in-stent restenosis. Am J Cardiol 2001; 88: 1032–4

176. Muramatsu T, Tsukahara R, Ho M, et al. Efficacy of cutting balloon angioplasty for in-stent restenosis: an intravascular ultrasound evaluation. J Invasive Cardiol 2001; 13: 439–44

177. Mehran R, Mintz GS, Satler LF, et al. Treatment of in-stent restenosis with excimer laser coronary angioplasty: mechanisms and results compared with PTCA alone. Circulation 1997; 96: 2183–9

178. Mehran R, Dangas G, Mintz GS, et al. Treatment of in-stent restenosis with excimer laser coronary angioplasty versus rotational atherectomy: comparative mechanisms and results. Circulation 2000; 101: 2484–9

179. Radke PW, Klues HG, Haager PK, et al. Mechanisms of acute lumen gain and recurrent restenosis after rotational atherectomy of diffuse in-stent restenosis: a quantitative angiographic and intravascular ultrasound study. J Am Coll Cardiol 1999; 34: 33–9

180. Sharma SK, Kini A, Mehran R, et al. Randomized trial of Rotational Atherectomy Versus Balloon Angioplasty for Diffuse In-stent Restenosis (ROSTER). Am Heart J 2004; 147: 16–22

181. vom Dahl J, Dietz U, Haager PK, et al. Rotational atherectomy does not reduce recurrent in-stent restenosis: results of the angioplasty versus rotational atherectomy for treatment of diffuse in-stent restenosis trial (ARTIST). Circulation 2002; 105: 583–8

182. Haager PK, Schiele F, Buettner HJ, et al. Insufficient tissue ablation by rotational atherectomy leads to worse long-term results in comparison with balloon angioplasty alone for the treatment of diffuse in-stent restenosis: insights from the intravascular ultrasound substudy of the ARTIST randomized multicenter trial. Catheter Cardiovasc Interv 2003; 60: 25–31

183. Kobayashi Y, Teirstein P, Linnemeier T, et al. Rotational atherectomy (stentablation) in a lesion with stent underexpansion due to heavily calcified plaque. Catheter Cardiovasc Interv 2001; 52: 208–11

184. Mahdi NA, Pathan AZ, Harrell L, et al. Directional coronary atherectomy for the treatment of Palmaz–Schatz in-stent restenosis. Am J Cardiol 1998; 82: 1345–51

185. Nakamura M, Fitzgerald PJ, Ikeno F, et al. Efficacy and feasibility of helixcision for debulking neointimal hyperplasia for in-stent restenosis. Catheter Cardiovasc Interv 2002; 57: 460–6

186. Mehran R, Dangas G, Abizaid A, et al. Treatment of focal in-stent restenosis with balloon angioplasty alone versus stenting: short- and long-term results. Am Heart J 2001; 141: 610–4

187. Shiran A, Mintz GS, Waksman R, et al. Early lumen loss after treatment of in-stent restenosis: an intravascular ultrasound study. Circulation 1998; 98: 200–3

188. Morino Y, Limpijankit T, Honda Y, et al. Relationship between neointimal regrowth and mechanism of acute lumen gain during the treatment of in-stent restenosis with or without supplementary intravascular radiation. Catheter Cardiovasc Interv 2003; 58: 162–7

189. Morino Y, Limpijankit T, Honda Y, et al. Late vascular response to repeat stenting for in-stent restenosis with and without radiation: an intravascular ultrasound volumetric analysis. Circulation 2002; 105: 2465–8

190. Schiele F, Meneveau N, Seronde MF, et al. Predictors of event-free survival after repeat intracoronary procedure for in-stent restenosis; study with angiographic and intravascular ultrasound imaging. Eur Heart J 2000; 21: 754–62

191. Wu Z, McMillan TL, Mintz GS, et al. Impact of the acute results on the long-term outcome after the treatment of in-stent restenosis: a serial intravascular ultrasound study. Catheter Cardiovasc Interv 2003; 60: 483–8

192. Mehran R, Dangas G, Abizaid AS, et al. Angiographic patterns of in-stent restenosis: classification and implications for long-term outcome. Circulation 1999; 100: 1872–8

193. Teirstein P, Massullo V, Jani S, et al. A double-blinded randomized trial of catheter-based radiotherapy to inhibit restenosis following coronary stenting. N Engl J Med 1997; 336: 1697–703

194. Mintz GS, Weissman NJ, Teirstein PS, et al. Effect of intracoronary gamma-radiation therapy on in-stent restenosis: an intravascular ultrasound analysis from the Gamma-1 study. Circulation 2000; 102: 2915–8

195. Ahmed JM, Mintz GS, Waksman R, et al. Serial intravascular ultrasound assessment of the efficacy of intracoronary gamma-radiation therapy for preventing recurrence in very long, diffuse, in-stent restenosis lesions. Circulation 2001; 104: 856–9

196. Ahmed JM, Mintz GS, Waksman R, et al. Serial volumetric intravascular ultrasound assessment of native coronary artery versus saphenous vein grafts in-stent restenosis lesions after conventional catheter-based treatment. Am J Cardiol 2003; 91: 739–41

197. Ahmed JM, Waksman R, Weissman NJ, et al. Effect of intracoronary gamma irradiation on uninjured reference segment during the treatment of in-stent restenosis: a serial intravascular ultrasound study. Cardiovasic Radiat Med 2001; 2: 58

198. Waksman R, White RL, Chan RC, et al. Intracoronary gamma-radiation therapy after angioplasty inhibits recurrence in patients with in-stent restenosis. Circulation 2000; 101: 2165–71

199. Ahmed JM, Mintz GS, Waksman R, et al. Serial intravascular ultrasound analysis of edge recurrence after intracoronary gamma radiation treatment of native artery in-stent restenosis lesions. Am J Cardiol 2001; 87: 1145–9

200. Ahmed JM, Mintz GS, Waksman R, et al. Safety of intracoronary gamma-radiation on uninjured reference segments during the first 6 months after treatment of in-stent restenosis: a serial intravascular ultrasound study. Circulation 2000; 101: 2227–30

201. Ahmed JM, Mintz GS, Waksman R, et al. Serial intravascular ultrasound analysis of the impact of lesion length on the efficacy of intracoronary gamma-irradiation for preventing recurrent in-stent restenosis. Circulation 2001; 103: 188–91

202. Castagna MT, Mintz GS, Waksman R, et al. Comparative efficacy of gamma-irradiation for treatment of in-stent restenosis in saphenous vein graft versus native coronary artery in-stent restenosis: an intravascular ultrasound study. Circulation 2001; 104: 3020–2

203. Cheneau E, Wu Z, Leborgne L, et al. Additional stenting promotes intimal proliferation and compromises the results of intravascular radiation therapy: an intravascular ultrasound study. Am Heart J 2003; 146: 142–5

204. Bhargava B, Mintz GS, Mehran R, et al. Serial volumetric intravascular ultrasound analysis of the efficacy of beta irradiation in preventing recurrent in-stent restenosis. Am J Cardiol 2000; 85: 651–3, A10

205. Takagi A, Morino Y, Fox T, et al. Efficacy of intracoronary beta-irradiation for the treatment on in-stent restenosis: volumetric analysis by intravascular ultrasound. Circulation 2000; 102: II-422

206. Hong MK, Park SW, Moon DH, et al. Intravascular ultrasound analysis of beta radiation therapy for diffuse in-stent restenosis to inhibit intimal hyperplasia. Catheter Cardiovasc Interv 2001; 54: 169–73

207. Munoz JS, Feres F, Abizaid A, et al. Long-term efficacy of intracoronary beta-irradiation for the treatment of in-stent restenosis: an angiographic and intravascular ultrasound analysis of the late catch-up phenomenon. J Am Coll Cardiol 2004; 43: 69A

208. Catalano G, Tamburini V, Colombo A, et al. Intravascular ultrasound based dose assessment in endovascular brachytherapy. Radiother Oncol 2003; 68: 199–206

209. Carlier SG, Marijnissen JP, Coen VL, et al. Comparison of brachytherapy strategies based on dose-volume histograms derived from quantitative intravascular ultrasound. Cardiovasc Radiat Med 1999; 1: 115–24

210. Kaluza GL, Jenkins TP, Mourtada FA, et al. Targeting the adventitia with intracoronary beta-radiation: comparison of two dose prescriptions and the role of centering coronary arteries. Int J Radiat Oncol Biol Phys 2002; 52: 184–91

211. Weichert F, Muller H, Quast U, et al. Virtual 3D IVUS vessel model for intravascular brachytherapy planning. I. 3D segmentation, reconstruction, and visualization of coronary artery architecture and orientation. Med Phys 2003; 30: 2530–6

212. Wahle A, Lopez JJ, Pennington EC, et al. Effects of vessel geometry and catheter position on dose delivery in intracoronary brachytherapy. IEEE Trans Biomed Eng 2003; 50: 1286–95

213. Carlier SG, Marijnissen JP, Coen VL, et al. Guidance of intracoronary radiation therapy based on dose-volume histograms derived from quantitative intravascular ultrasound. IEEE Trans Med Imaging 1998; 17: 772–8

214. Arbab-Zadeh A, Bhargava V, Russo RJ, et al. Centered versus noncentered source for intracoronary artery radiation therapy: a model based on the SCRIPPS trial. Am Heart J 2002; 143: 342–8

215. Maehara A, Patel NS, Harrison LB, et al. Dose heterogeneity may not affect the neointimal proliferation after gamma radiation for in-stent restenosis: a volumetric intravascular ultrasound dosimetric study. J Am Coll Cardiol 2002; 39: 1937–42

216. Morino Y, Kaneda H, Fox T, et al. Delivered dose and vascular response after beta-radiation for in-stent restenosis: retrospective dosimetry and volumetric intravascular ultrasound analysis. Circulation 2002; 106: 2334–9

217. Hong MK, Park SW, Moon DH, et al. Impact of geographic miss on adjacent coronary artery segments in diffuse in-stent restenosis with beta-radiation therapy: angiographic and intravascular ultrasound analysis. Am Heart J 2002; 143: 327–33

218. Dilcher CE, Chan RC, Pregowski J, et al. Dose volume histogram assessment of late stent malapposition after intravascular brachytherapy. Cardiovasc Radiat Med 2002; 3: 190–2

219. Tanabe K, Serruys PW, Grube E, et al. TAXUS III trial: in-stent restenosis treated with stent-based delivery of paclitaxel incorporated in a slow-release polymer formulation. Circulation 2003; 107: 559–64

220. Degertekin M, Lemos PA, Lee CH, et al. Intravascular ultrasound evaluation after sirolimus eluting stent implantation for de novo and in-stent restenosis lesions. Eur Heart J 2004; 25: 32–8

221. Degertekin M, Regar E, Tanabe K, et al. Sirolimus-eluting stent for treatment of complex in-stent restenosis: the first clinical experience. J Am Coll Cardiol 2003; 41: 184–9

222. Fujii K, Mintz GS, Kobayashi Y, et al. Contribution of stent underexpansion to recurrence after sirolimus-eluting stent implantation for in-stent restenosis. Circulation 2004; 109: 1085–8

223. Feres F, Munoz JS, Abizaid A, et al. Is sirolimus-eluting stent better than brachytherapy to treat in-stent restenosis at longer (12-month) follow-up? Angiographic and intravascular ultrasound analysis. J Am Coll Cardiol 2004; 43: 70A

224. Talwar K, Costa M, Teirstein P, et al. Intravascular ultrasound follow-up of the SECURE Trial: The compassionate use of sirolimus-eluting stents study. J Am Coll Cardiol 2004; 43: 70A

225. Costa M, Talwar K, Panse N, et al. Characterization of neointimal hyperplasia after sirolimus-eluting stent implantation in patients with previous brachytherapy failure: insights from the SECURE study. J Am Coll Cardiol 2004; 43: 80A

Index